Community Health Care Nursing

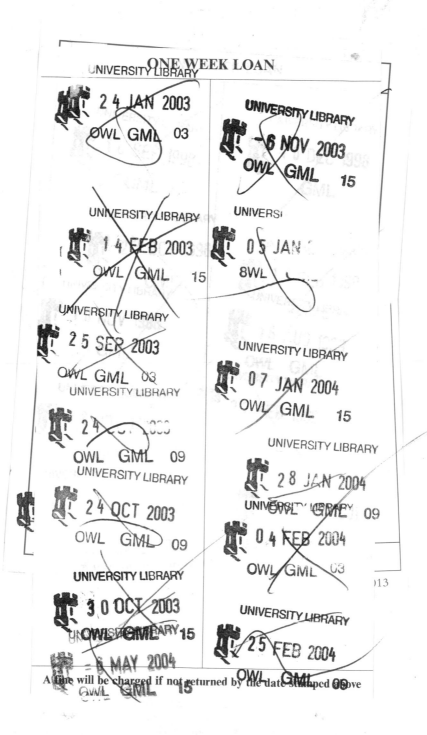

Illustrator: David Gardner

For Churchill Livingstone:

Commissioning Editor: Ellen Green
Project Manager: Valerie Burgess
Project Development Editor: Mairi McCubbin
Designer: Judith Wright
Copy-editor: Stephen Black
Indexer: Tarrant Ranger Indexing Agency
Sales promotion executive: Hilary Brown

Community Health Care Nursing

Edited by

Carmel Blackie BEd(Hons) RNT HVL RN SCM HV

Director, Primary Educare, Practice Development Consultancy Services;
Formerly Lecturer in Primary and Community Health Care,
City University, Seconded to Inner City Lecturer Team,
Department of General Practice, St Bartholomew's and the
Royal London School of Medicine and Dentistry, London

Associate Editor

Frances M. Appleby MA BEd(Hons) RGN RHV CPT CHNT

Course Director, BScHons/Postgraduate Diploma in Community
Health Care (Public Health Nursing – Health Visiting),
School of Health and Social Care, South Bank University, London

Foreword by

Jean A. Orr MSc BA RN RHV

Professor and Director of School of Nursing and Midwifery,
Queen's University of Belfast, Belfast

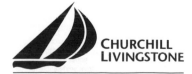

CHURCHILL
LIVINGSTONE

EDINBURGH LONDON NEW YORK PHILADELPHIA SAN FRANCISCO SYDNEY TORONTO 1998

CHURCHILL LIVINGSTONE
Medical Division of Harcourt Brace and Company Limited

First published 1998

ISBN 0 443 05291 3

British Library of Cataloguing in Publication Data
A catalogue record for this book is available from the British Library.

Library of Congress Cataloging in Publication Data
A catalogue record for this book is available from the Library of Congress

The publisher's policy is to use **paper manufactured from sustainable forests**

Produced through Longman Malaysia, P.P

Contents

Contributors

Carmel Blackie BEd(Hons) RNT HVL RN SCM HV
Director, Primary Educare, Practice Development
Consultancy Services;
Formerly Lecturer in Primary and Community
Health Care, City University, Seconded to Inner
City Lecturer Team, Department of General
Practice, St Bartholomew's and the Royal
London School of Medicine and Dentistry,
London

1 *Primary health care*
5 *Core attributes*
9 *Community health needs*
11 *Quality practice*

Dominic Blackie MB CNB MRGP LNCC
General Practioner
Formerly Senior Lecturer in General Practice,
University of Liverpool; Primary Care
Development Facilitator, Liverpool Health
Authority, Liverpool

2 *The NHS: reforms and influences upon practice*
4 *Organisation of models for service delivery*

Ros Carnwell BA MA RGN RHV CPT CertEd(FE)
Senior Lecturer, School of Health Sciences,
University of Wolverhampton, Wolverhampton

6 *Conceptual models for practice*

Marilyn Edwards BSc(Hons) SRN FETC DipPHS
Specialist Practitioner in General Practice,
Bilbrook Medical Centre, Bilbrook, Staffordshire

10 *Health promotion and health education*

Susan M. McKnight MA RGN RM RCNT RNT DN(Lond)
ENB900 ENB934 PGCEA
Lecturer, European Institute of Health and
Medical Sciences, University of Surrey, Surrey

10 *Health promotion and health education*

Yvonne T. Morris BA(Hons) MSc RNT RGN DipNurs PGCEA
Senior Lecturer, Nursing and Ethics, Thames
Valley University, London

13 *Ethics*

Penny Reid BSc(Hons) RGN RHV RNT
Pathway Leader BSc(Hons), Community
Practice, Thames Valley University, London

3 *The organisation of community care*
8 *Clients and carers: the needs of individuals and
  families*

Anne Robotham BA MEd SRN ONC DipN(Lond) RHV HVT
CertEd(FE)
Principal Lecturer in Community Health, School
of Health Sciences, University of
Wolverhampton, Wolverhampton

7 *Managing change in the contract culture*

Pam Smith BNurs MSc PhD RGN RNT DNCert HVCert
Professor of Nursing, Redwood College of
Health Studies, South Bank University, London

12 *Research*

Foreword

The publication of this book is very timely. The emphasis on the community as a location for health care is acknowledged not only in the UK but also internationally. The contribution that nurses, midwives and health visitors make to the health of the nation is well articulated in the book. The concept of community health care nursing is a relatively new one and the challenge it poses to practitioners is considerable. The main challenge is to maintain the specific focus of each speciality while at the same time ensuring there is an appreciation of each nurse's role. There is considerable opportunity for partnership and collaboration and it will be a measure of the success of community health care and nursing if we can demonstrate teamwork for the benefit of client care.

For many years the literature on community health has lagged behind the move of care into the community and there have been few critical and informative books available. The literature has also tended to be profession-specific, with little opportunity for practitioners to learn from each other and to have cross-fertilisation from discipline to discipline. The importance of multi-disciplinary and interprofessional working is a theme which runs through the book and is reflected in the authorship of the chapters. The emphasis and exploration of primary health care as a concept and reality is particularly useful and this sets the context for the rest of the book. The acknowledgement of the various professionals who work in the community is reflected in the diversity of the material covered and the authors have drawn on a wide range of evidence-based and relevant literature.

The book is timely also as community health care operates in the 'contract culture', with an increasing emphasis on managing change. This is addressed in some depth and will provide very useful material for all professionals in the community. Health care is not only about professionals; indeed some would argue that the problem with effecting health gain has been exacerbated by not concentrating more on the recipients of health care and the communities in which they live, and understanding how environmental and social factors affect health. All too often we have concentrated on what we think clients and communities need without taking into account their experiences of living in the area. That is why it is so important that community health needs are assessed in a rigorous and yet sensitive manner. Following on from this, it makes sense to explore the importance of community development and its relevance for increasing health gain. For many professionals, the political focus of community development can be challenging but is a key element in the new public health and the forming of healthy alliances with a range of statutory and voluntary agencies within a multisectorial framework.

Within any health care system we must be mindful of quality issues and how best to ensure care is relevant and responsive. All of these issues have to be set in an ethical framework and the authors also cover this important area.

This book demonstrates the complexity of care in and by the community and the challenges facing policy makers and practitioners in designing and implementing policies which will meet client, community and individual need.

Jean A. Orr

Preface

At both international and national levels, there have been significant changes in patterns of health care delivery, in particular, a steady shift in emphasis from acute care in the hospital setting to a major focus on primary care in the community setting.

This book discusses the impetus for those global changes, considers the legislative and subsequent policy changes that have directed new approaches to the delivery of care in the community, and examines the implications of these developments for community nursing practitioners.

In keeping with these changes, the UKCC for Nursing, Midwifery and Health Visiting has outlined a new framework for the education of nurses preparing to practice in the community as specialist community practitioners. The new courses seek to equip practitioners across the broad spectrum of community nursing to respond pro-actively to changing health needs and approaches.

The new preparation for specialist community practitioners acknowledges the need for specific preparation for discrete areas of practice and also the fact that the essential core approaches, knowledge and skills are required by all community practitioners in order to practice effectively in the new primary care-led NHS.

These common elements for practice, many of which are pertinent to all members of the primary health care team and not just community nurses, are explored in detail in this book.

A public health approach, including an analysis of health needs in the community, is fundamental to primary care, so a chapter is devoted to this subject to assist practitioners in this important task.

Other chapters include approaches to health promotion, ethical issues in practice, models for practice, teamwork, the needs of informal carers, individual needs assessment and care planning, quality assurance and, very importantly, research and the need for evidence-based practice.

The contributors to the book, like the editors, come from teaching, nursing or medical backgrounds and are all experienced practice educators. They share a belief in the importance of multidisciplinary cooperation and collaboration in health care, based on partnership approaches, which also include clients in the planning, delivery and evaluation of care.

We would hope that this book will encourage intending, as well as experienced, community practitioners to feel positive about, and suitably equipped for, responding to the opportunities for innovative approaches to practice provided by the current primary care legislation.

London, 1997   Carmel Blackie
                                          Frances M. Appleby

1

Setting the context of practice

SECTION CONTENTS

1

Primary health care

Carmel Blackie

The context and organisation of community health care nursing is now significantly different from that experienced by nurses in the years following the inception of the NHS in 1948. The creation of an internal market in health care and the investment of power in medical practitioners in the primary care sector mean that community health care nurses must work from a sound knowledge base in a wide range of subjects to strive to contribute equally to the care of clients in the community and the development of the profession of nursing. Equally, world-wide organisations have, through the development of strategies and targets, influenced the aims of the NHS and those who work in it. To carry out their role successfully community health care nurses must be aware of:

- **Definitions of primary health care**
- **The politicisation of health and the health service**
- **The policies and statutes which shape and drive the work of health professionals caring for clients in the community**
- **The approaches employed by health professionals in the community to organise the services demanded of them by clients**
- **The need to work with clients to deliver the care that they perceive they require.**

This chapter considers Primary Health Care (PHC), the context within which community health care nursing is practised. After reading the chapter the reader should be familiar with the following:

- Primary health care within the NHS
- The concept and philosophy of primary health care
- Definitions of primary health care
- The development of primary health care
- Factors required to achieve a service led by primary health care
- Models of primary health care organisation
- Community health care nursing and primary health care

PRIMARY HEALTH CARE IN THE NHS

What is a primary care-led NHS? The term is much used, but little understood. It means a health service led by priorities set by local service providers and service users. It integrates individual and family primary health care with the public health element required for planning and to serve the needs of communities. General practitioners and primary health care (PHC) teams are at the heart of this process and assessment of community needs is critical to its success.

Perry (1995) defined the primary care-led NHS in the following terms:

... it is about shifting decision making in primary care closer to the patient on the grounds that this is where to get the balance right between cost, quality, effectiveness and access within a framework of public health priorities. ... it is about delivering care with the GP as the co-ordinator of the primary health care team, with the patient, not the service, as focus. ... it is about new relationships with primary care in the main role and secondary services in a supporting role.

This can be summed up as a health service that is led and shaped by local commissioning, through GP fundholding or other forms of devolved budgeting. In April 1996 GP fundholding was spread to over 53% of the population served by general practice and there were 70 total fundholder/purchaser pilot sites testing the initiative for total purchasing. The prevous Government identified a significant extension of the GP fundholding scheme as a major part of its plans to achieve a primary health care-led NHS

through GP commissioning. In reality, however, many practices, for example single-handed practices in inner city areas, are ill equipped to take on the responsibilities of locally based commissioning. The inequity which this causes to the consumer must be addressed through targeting development money into smaller underdeveloped practices to enable them to develop the primary health care team infrastructure which will enable local commissioning to be effective. For some practices this is many years away and some thought should be given to the question of whether GPs actually want to, or should, lead the primary care-led NHS. Many GPs feel railroaded into taking responsibility for the service in a way for which they are neither contracted or adequately trained (Edwards 1996, Coulson 1996).

The development of primary care was central to the previous Government's intention to develop the health service. A White Paper, 'The NHS: a service with ambitions' (DoH 1996c) stated the intent to develop:

an integrated and high quality health service organised and run around the needs of individuals ... an NHS which, where appropriate, brings services to people, balancing, for each individual, the desire to provide care at home or in the local community with the need to provide care which is safe, high quality and cost effective.

The White Paper 'Choice and Opportunity' (DoH 1996b) seeks to strengthen the primary care-led NHS and recognises the valuable contribution made to health care by community health care nurses and other non-medical care providers. It seeks to give choice, opportunity and flexibility to service providers in designing local services based on need, and states the following objectives:

- To promote consistently high-quality services across the country. The organisation of these services, the mix of primary care professionals and the use of financial resources should be sufficiently flexible to meet local needs effectively.
- To provide opportunities and incentives for primary care professionals to use their skills to the full. The current legislative and contractual framework can hinder this.

Box 1.1   The principles of good primary care (DoH 1996d)

Quality

- Professionals should be knowledgeable about the conditions that present in primary care, be skilled in their treatment, and in contributing to their prevention.
- Professionals should be knowledgeable about the people to whom they are offering services.
- Services should be coordinated with professionals aware of each others' contributions [including interprofessional working] and no service gaps.
- Premises and facilities should be of good standard and fit for their purposes, and equipment should be up to date, well maintained and safe to use.

Fairness

- Services should not vary widely in range or quality, in different parts of the country.
- Primary care should receive an appropriate share of overall NHS resources.

Accessibility

- Services should be reasonably accessible when clinically needed.
- Necessary services should be accessible to people, regardless of age, sex, ethnicity, disability or health status.

Responsiveness

- Services should reflect the needs and preferences of the individuals using them.
- Services should reflect the health, demographic and social needs of the area they serve.

Efficiency

- Primary care services should be based on evidence of clinical effectiveness
- Primary care resources should be used efficiently.

- To provide more flexible employment opportunities in primary care. The primary care workforce is changing, particularly in general practice, and employment arrangements have not always kept pace with the changing needs and aspirations of GPs and other health professionals and managers who work in primary care.

The White Paper (DoH 1996b) proposes removing the present contractual restraints on general practitioners in relation to extending medical services, and encourages family practitioners to set up new models of care delivery. If adopted, this will have a great impact upon the role of community health care nurses. The White Paper also proposes that changes in practice will be voluntary. Warden (1996) outlines the key points of the White Paper as:

- participation in new general practice contracts to be voluntary
- single budgets for general medical services, other hospital and community health services, and prescribing
- contracts could reflect the full range of services
- a salaried service option
- practice-based contracts, which will include non-medical professionals
- patients' right to choose their general practitioners and the doctor's right to refuse to be retained.

The White Paper 'Primary care: delivering the future (DoH 1996d) sets out a series of practical proposals, with increases in resources, for actions to complement the opportunities for people using primary care services, providers of services and the range of services offered by the previous Paper (DoH 1996b). The principles of good primary care it sets out are listed in Box 1.1.

Achieving good primary care services depends upon team working, developing partnerships in care, appropriate research and development, extending clinical roles where appropriate, developing professional knowledge through continuing education, auditing services and performance, involving users of the service in decision making, distributing resources appropriately and developing premises. The White Paper (DoH 1996d) sets out detailed proposals for each of these areas.

WHAT IS PRIMARY HEALTH CARE?

Primary health care is now a familiar term to most people through media exposure of the NHS reforms. Familiar ideas can seem simple, but, on analysis, primary health care has many meanings and applications from the very basic to the highly complex.

Primary health care is an approach to the planning and delivery of health services. It is a concept and philosophy of how health care provision should be offered and it is also a set of activities in the provision of health care.

Primary health care: an approach

As an approach, primary health care emphasises comprehensive health care systems that encompass curative, preventative, promotive and rehabilitative activities which are developed and implemented with the participation and equal partnership of the people receiving care and services. This can mean an individual, a family or a community (Ebrahim & Rankin 1993).

Primary health care: a concept

As a concept, primary health care places reliance on several health-related activities, such as nutrition, sanitation, education and housing, finance, each of which is outside the direct sphere of control of agencies responsible for health (Ebrahim & Rankin 1993).

Primary health care: a philosophy

As a philosophy, primary health care underpins the way in which health care is offered and places the active participation of people using primary health care services, clients or patients, at the heart of any activity. This is at the level of the individual, family or community and demands proactive strategies for partnership between health care workers and services, to work towards client empowerment. Fundamental to primary health care philosophy is the notion that health is a basic human right in which the individual and wider community have a central part to play. There is a notion of personal, as well as collective, community responsibility, which embraces social justice and equity (Holzemer 1992). Primary health care philosophy, therefore, must encompass notions of equity, empowerment, self-determination, culturally appropriate services and access to services. These elements underpin the approach to community health care nursing practice.

Primary health care: a set of activities

As a set of activities, primary health care describes the first-line approach to service delivery as in the terms 'primary', 'secondary' and 'tertiary' care.

Primary health care promotes change to achieve equity in health care by:

- changing people through strategies for empowerment
- changing professional roles to enable health care professionals to work in partnership with the client
- changing health care systems' orientation from an acute medically driven base to a client-centred approach for the planning and delivery of health care.

The aim is to work with the client and not for the client, and to shift the traditional professional role of health care provider to that of enabler (Colliere 1980). It is about redistributing resources and putting the individual, family and community at the heart of health care, encouraging them to take responsibility for their own health and welfare through a process of empowerment.

In its widest sense, primary health care is concerned with bringing about social change as well as delivering health care. As Paulo Frere asserts in relation to primary health care in South America, if you encourage people to take charge of their health they can take charge of their whole lives. The role of the health professional is to enable and assist the individual, family and community to take up the mantle of personal responsibility for their health and lives, whilst not losing sight of the fact that people have different needs for support at different phases of their life and development: at times clients will be independent of the health professional, at other times they will be interdependent and at other times they will have total dependency.

Primary health care encourages a bottom-up approach to setting priorities and goals for health care that takes account of the wishes of people using services and then allows this to be translated into health service policy. In most countries of the world, including the UK, the health service is dominated by a health care system which has a top-down strategy; for example, at the top of the UK system is the Department of Health. The NHS reforms have brought about a partial re-orientation of the emphasis to primary health care in the UK health care system, mainly through devolved budgeting and locally based commissioning.

The future

Primary health care attempts to tackle inequity in the health of populations and inequity in the health care provision available. It has long been recognised in the inverse care law that the most underserved of the population are those who have the greatest health needs and the least personal resources for health (Tudor-Hart 1971). It attempts to make health care more widely available and accessible, encouraging the users of the service, whether they are individuals, families or communities, to take part in health care decisions for themselves and the wider good. It attempts to coordinate activities across sectors and to foster political support for change and development.

DEFINITIONS OF PRIMARY HEALTH CARE

Primary health care has been defined (WHO & UNICEF 1978) as:

Essential care based upon practical scientifically sound and acceptable methods and technology, made universally available to individuals and families in the community through their full participation and at a cost the community and country can afford and maintain at every stage of their development, in the spirit of self-reliance and self-determination ... it is an integral part of a country's health system of which it is the central focus and main function ... it is integral to economic and social development.

The Alma Ata conference and declaration were born from a convergence of thinking regarding new ways of planning health care and a radical approach to thinking in relation to human development. The World Health Organization (WHO) hosted the conference at Alma Ata in Russia. As a result, the experience of several nations in rela-

tion to planning and delivering health care evolved into the PHC approach as set out by the Alma Ata declaration and its goal to achieve 'Health For All By The Year 2000' (WHO 1981). From this conference, eight activities or elements of PHC were identified to tackle basic health needs through the provision of essential services (Box 1.2).

Box 1.2 Elements of PHC identified at Alma Ata

1. The promotion of adequate nutrition
2. The promotion of an adequate supply of safe water
3. The provision of basic sanitation
4. Maternal and child care and family planning services
5. Immunisation against major infectious disease
6. The prevention and control of locally endemic diseases
7. Education with regard to health problems including methods of prevention and control
8. Appropriate treatment for common disease and injury

To achieve the basic services set out in these eight elements, activity is centred in three distinct but interlocking areas. This is true whether the care offered is in a system in a developing country or whether it is offered in more sophisticated healthcare systems such as in the UK. The three areas are:

Co-ordination and collaboration. This must occur between all the sectors and agencies concerned directly with health and social care, as well as those agencies which have influence on the health of populations, such as education services, housing, environmental agencies and employers; everything has a bearing on health.

Developing a firm basis within a community. This means that the active involvement of the community can be encouraged and the views and wishes of its members brought to bear in the provision and planning of local services. This activity aims to encourage self-reliance and self-determination and promote empowerment.

Gaining support from policy makers at national and local level. In this way ideas and initiatives can be funded, encouraged and incorporated within the mainstream of the health service.

It follows then that the principles of PHC are:

- Integrated services linking PHC with communities and service users, hospitals, social services, the voluntary sector and environmental agencies promoting 'healthy alliances' through which strategy and services are planned and delivered. Primary health care services must work together and with other agencies.
- Safe, effective clinical practice in which clients can be confident and which is monitored for quality on a regular basis by the profession and is open to public scrutiny.
- Accessible and appropriate local services which are designed around local needs and are acceptable to the population using them.
- Access to named practitioners so that clients can build a relationship with the healthcare professionals caring for them and so that a clear line of responsibility for care is made between client and professional. This should also promote continuity with a minimum number of people involved.
- Services that can overcome language barriers, discrimination and deprivation, and so promote equity and equal access.
- 24-hour cover.
- Confidentiality to all users, so that people are not debarred from seeking health care because of fear of their problems becoming public.
- A range of multidisciplinary treatment choices which encompass the traditional and developing alternative views, if this is what the client wishes in the light of informed choice.
- Clarity of provision without confusion of roles.
- Services should give value for money and be effective and efficient yielding a demonstrable health gain.
- Clients should be fully involved in decision making in partnership with professionals and thereby should make informed choices (NHSME 1993a).

The UK was a signatory to the Alma Ata declaration and from this commitment stems policy such as the Health of the Nation strategy (Department of Health 1992). The declaration of Alma Ata is based on the belief that the health of the population is the most important feature of any nation and it is upon this foundation that other forms of wealth are built and created. Achieving the target of health for all involves constant action and planning and the stages of development and achievement of targets are different for each country in the world, reflecting individual national development. Critics state that the goals are largely unattainable and it is true to state that achievement of associated targets has been very slow. There are, however, three common elements to any programme trying to achieve health for all. The three elements are:

- The promotion and facilitation of healthy lifestyles
- A reduction in the burden of preventable ill health
- Reorientation of healthcare systems to a primary health care orientation so as to ensure that they respond to the social and psychological needs of individuals as well as meeting their needs for medical care.

In an attempt to achieve health for all, the European office of WHO (1985, 1986b) set out 38 targets and dates for achieving these for the 33 participating member countries within the European region. The targets can be grouped into categories which cover health for all, lifestyles, environmental factors, appropriate care provision and healthcare infrastructure (Box 1.3).

The European goals accepted by the UK government encompass other dimensions as well as health and cannot be achieved by the NHS in isolation. However, they underpin much of the NHS reforms and can be summarised as:

- Ensuring the prerequisites for health, which are peace, social justice, adequate food and safe water, decent housing, universal education and secure employment
- Equity in health
- The prevention of premature death
- The addition of health to life
- The addition of years to life
- The promotion of healthy behaviour
- The introduction of policies in all sectors of life to make it easier to adopt healthy lifestyles

Box 1.3 European targets for Health for All by the year 2000 (WHO 1985)

Health for All
Target date 2000

1. The differences in health status between countries and between groups within countries should be reduced by at least 25%. This is to be achieved by improving the levels of health of disadvantaged nations and groups.

2. People should have the basic opportunity to develop and use their health potential to live socially and economically fulfilling lives.

3. Disabled persons should have the physical, social and economic opportunities that allow at least for a socially and economically fulfilling and mentally creative life.

4. The average number of years that people live free from major disease and disability should be increased by at least 10%.

5. There should be no indigenous measles, poliomyelitis, neonatal tetanus, congenital rubella, diphtheria, congenital syphilis or indigenous malaria.

6. Life expectancy at birth in the region should be at least 75 years.

7. Infant mortality should be less than 20 per 1000 live births.

8. Maternal mortality should be less than 15 per 100 000 live births.

9. Mortality from diseases of the circulatory system in people under 65 should be reduced by at least 15%.

10. Mortality from cancer in people under 65 should be reduced by at least 15%.

11. Deaths from accidents should be reduced by at least 25% through an intensified effort to reduce traffic, home and occupational accidents.

12. Rising trends in suicides should be reversed.

Lifestyles to support Health for All
Target date 1990

13. There should be national policies to ensure that legislative, administrative and economic mechanisms provide broad intersectoral support and resources for the promotion of healthy lifestyles and ensure effective participation of the people at all levels in such policy making.

14. There should be specific programmes which enhance the major roles of the family and other social groups in developing and supporting healthy lifestyles.

15. Educational programmes should enhance the knowledge, motivation and skills of people to acquire and maintain health.

Target date 1995

16. There should be significant increases in positive health behaviour such as balanced nutrition, non smoking, appropriate physical activity and good stress management.

17. There should be significant decreases in health damaging behaviour, such as overuse of alcohol and pharmaceutical products, use of illicit drugs, dangerous chemical substances, dangerous driving and violent social behaviour.

The environment to support Health for All
Target date 1990

18. There should be multisectoral policies that effectively protect the human environment from health hazards, ensure community awareness and involvement and effectively support international efforts to curb such hazards affecting more than one country.

19. There should be adequate machinery for the monitoring, assessment and control of environmental hazards which pose a threat to human health, including potentially toxic chemicals, radiation, harmful consumer goods and biological agents.

20. All people should have adequate supplies of safe drinking water, and by 1995 pollution of rivers, lakes and seas should no longer pose a threat to human health.

Target date 1995

21. People should be effectively protected against recognised health risks from air pollution.

Target date 1990

22. There should be a significant reduction in the health risks from food contamination and measures should be implemented to protect consumers from harmful additives.

Target date 1995

23. Major known health risks associated with the disposal of hazardous wastes should be eliminated.

Target date 2000

24. All people should have a better opportunity of living in houses and settlements which provide a healthy and safe environment.

Target date 1995

25. People should be effectively protected against work related health risks.

Appropriate care provision
Target date 1990

26. Through effective community representation states should have developed healthcare systems that are based upon primary health care and supported by secondary and tertiary care as outlined in the Alma Ata WHO conference declaration.

27. The infrastructure of health care delivery systems should be organised so that resources are distributed according to need, and that services ensure physical and economic accessibility and cultural acceptability to the population.

28. The primary health care system of all member states should provide a wide range of health promotive, curative, rehabilitative, and supportive services to meet the basic health needs of the population and give special attention to high risk vulnerable and under-served individuals and groups.

29. Primary health care systems should be based upon co-operation and teamwork between health care personnel, individuals, families and community groups.

Box 1.3 (cont'd)

30. Mechanisms should exist through which the services provided by all sectors relating to health are co-ordinated at the community level in the primary health care system.

31. There should be effective mechanisms for ensuring the quality of patient care within their health systems.

Health care development infrastructure
Target date prior to 1990

32. Research strategy should be designed to stimulate investigations which improve the application and expansion of knowledge needed to support their national Health for All developments.

33. Health policies and strategies should be in line with Health for All principles and national legislation and regulations should make their implementation effective in all sectors of society.

34. There should be managerial processes for health development geared to the attainment of health for all actively involving communities and all sectors relevant to health and ensuring preferential allocation of resources to health development priorities.

35. Health information systems should be capable of supporting national strategies for Health for All.

36. Planning, training and use of health personnel should be in accordance with Health for All policies with emphasis on the primary health care approach.

37. Education should provide personnel in sectors related to health with adequate information on national Health for All policies and programmes and their practical application to their own sectors.

38. There should be a formal mechanism for the systematic assessment of the appropriate use of health technologies and of their effectiveness, efficiency, safety and acceptability, as well as reflecting national health policy and economic restraints.

- The creation and preservation of a healthy environment
- The development of health services appropriate to people's needs and wishes
- Acceptance of goals by those responsible for research, service management and training of health professionals.

THE FOCUS OF PRIMARY HEALTH CARE SERVICES

Since the NHS reforms and the NHS and Community Care Act (1990), most PHC has been centred on a general practice population.

Services should be planned and offered based on need and, in keeping with PHC philosophy, should be client-based and health-focused. Care and services should be planned and offered through teamwork within the primary health care team.

The rationale for focusing PHC services around a general practice population (NHSME 1993a) is:

- 99% of the UK population are on the registered list of a GP
- General practice is understood and accepted by clients
- Teamwork is strengthened
- Co-ordination of care is smoother
- Sharing records is easier
- There is scope for improved communication between professionals
- It allows a multidisciplinary approach to the identification of local health needs
- It allows the range of skills and abilities within the PHC team to be used effectively without duplication of effort.

Tomlinson (1992) identified that there are potential gaps in PHC services which are solely organised around a general practice population. In some inner city areas, one in seven people is not registered with a GP. Often these people include the most vulnerable in society such as the homeless, travellers, 'roofless' people, the mentally ill and substance misusers. Other groups comprise people who for reasons of culture, gender, or the nature of the services offered, for example alternative therapy or surgery hours, prefer to register at a distance from where they live. Other people prefer drop-in services such as accident and emergency or community clinics. Discrepancies also exist between provision of general practice services depending on where in the country you live. Hacking (1996) identified major discrepancies in England between the provision of general practice services which were heavily resourced in the south of the country as opposed to the north of England. This finding has implications for primary care provision and community nursing. If services in PHC are only developed through general practice based commissioning, then people who are not on the practice list will be left out of planning and will be denied access. In the past, community health care nurses (CHCNs), such as health visitors (HVs), were able to offer services to homeless families or travellers by creating time in their working patterns. In future, if GP commissioning purchases an HV to look after only under-5-year-old children on the practice list then the HV will have no time in which to explore and meet the health needs of other groups. This is a severe disadvantage to the population and restricts the autonomy of the CHCN.

The report 'Child Health in The Community' (DoH 1996a) indicated that there is a need for health visitors occasionally to work with clients in a 'patch-based' pattern rather than wholly with a GP practice list and the Audit Commission report 'Seen And Not Heard' highlights the potential limiting effect on practice of health visitor attachment to general practice.

Community health care nursing and PHC

Primary health care and community health care nursing practice are inextricably linked and complementary activities. CHCNs practise within the context and overall philosophy of PHC. Both incorporate client-focused, health-based practice which centres on clients in three domains: the individual, the family and the community. Both attempt to incorporate the client in decision making and planning. There is a focus on health promotion and disease prevention, and both enterprises require a multidisciplinary approach to the planning and delivery of health care.

In 1974 WHO defined community nursing as being concerned with the needs of the individual client and family, but also with identifying and meeting the needs of the wider population through a developmental approach in which communities and the individual members of communities are encouraged to engage in development projects related to health and welfare in the widest sense. Recent trends throughout the world have seen the reorientation of health services to PHC based on population need through local budgeting and commissioning. For reorien-

tation of health care to work effectively in the UK, it must be remembered that PHC requires more than GP services alone, and the emphasis on commissioning must be through a team-based approach which involves all the community nursing disciplines as well as other groups within the team such physiotherapy and occupational health. This view is supported by the Royal College of Nursing (1995) in a parliamentary briefing paper and in its document 'Powerhouse for Change' (1992).

In 1986 WHO published a nursing discussion paper related to targets for health for all. In this document they state that health for all implies equity and equal access to health services and that the aim of health for all is to enable people to build and maintain health, so there must be emphasis upon the promotion of health and the prevention of disease. The client population should be well informed regarding health issues which affect them and actively encouraged by health professionals to take responsibility for determining the direction, with support, of their own health and health service.

WHO envisage CHCNs as central to achieving health for all. Nurses act as the client's advocate and can integrate nursing, PHC and public health elements.

MODELS OF PRIMARY HEALTH CARE

The model of primary care which is adopted by the healthcare system has direct impact upon the development of nursing practice, the range of services which the CHCN offers and the level of autonomy which the nurse can attain. This in turn affects client access to services, choice and the development of individual nurses and the profession of nursing.

Within general practice and PHC in the UK, there is long-standing tension and debate around the relative merits of an individual focus or medical model approach to planning and delivering PHC and the community-based approach (Macdonald 1993). Nursing development, and so the contribution which could be made by nurses in an overstretched health service, is potentially curtailed because general practice, or more correctly primary medical care, has erroneously come to mean global 'primary health care' in mainstream consciousness. This includes the Department of Health, service planners and managers, and to an extent the general public (Fry 1983, Bryar 1991). This perspective has been strengthened in legislation by the NHS reforms which place the GP at the centre of a healthcare system which has as its focus a general practice based population for which the general practitioner is encouraged to act as custodian of the budget and commissioner and provider of care.

The evidence put forward by Gregson, Cartlidge & Bond (1991) and Lawrence (1988) suggests that PHC is most effectively delivered by a multidisciplinary team of equals. This is severely limited by government decisions to place medicine at the pinnacle of primary care and to make other disciplines subordinate to medicine through direct employment or indirectly through the contracting and commissioning process. Nursing development is additionally curtailed by potential conflict between the business interests of the practice and the community health needs of the population.

In order for nursing to flourish within the community, PHC should be accurately viewed as a range of activities which are community-based and to which GPs contribute primary medical services as an equal constituent of the whole enterprise, alongside nurses, social workers, the voluntary sector, education and the client population.

The identification of PHC as general practice and the location of budgetary power and so overall control of purchasing, service development and care provision with doctors alone, has implications for service choice and delivery of services to clients. It gives medicine potentially enormous influence over the professional development and practice autonomy of other groups providing PHC.

It also perpetuates a medical approach to care in the community, as opposed to medical care in a hospital setting, and so the shift in emphasis from secondary to primary care as a result of the NHS reforms is denied a true primary care focus with community needs as central to planning and delivering services. Viewing general medical practice as PHC not only controls and limits the effectiveness and development of nursing but also lessens the importance of community or population needs and limits the voice and influence of clients (North 1993). As such, it appears at odds with the move in society towards personal responsibility and choice. It weakens the express intent of the NHS and Community Care Act (DoH 1990) and initiatives to give rights to consumers of health care, such as the Patients' Charter (DoH 1993).

In order to develop the role of nurses in PHC appropriately, it is important to consider the two main approaches to primary care delivery: the community-based approach, which includes community-oriented primary health care and primary health care; and the medical approach or primary care which is currently widespread and dominant.

The community-based approach

In the UK, community-based primary health care has never had wide application but it is through this approach that the potential of nurses can be realised and consumers of health care can have a voice. Community-based PHC is located in the community, usually in health centres, increasingly in GP-based centres, as opposed to a hospital setting, and works with the population. Within a community-based approach it is the role of the CHCN to proactively contact the client population at the level of individual, family and community, to identify needs in partnership with them and develop care strategies accordingly and not merely to respond to disease.

Community-oriented primary care (COPC)

Community-based PHC in the form of community-oriented primary care (COPC), attempts to develop a community-based focus to the identification of health care needs and to the subsequent planning and delivery of services to meet those needs. It applies ideas which derive from public health and was first developed as an applied concept in Israel. COPC seeks to advance a collaborative relationship between epidemiology, medicine and community health care. Kark (1974) outlined five central characteristics of COPC which are:

- A defined population for which healthcare professionals are responsible and within which care effectiveness is audited
- Health care is tailored to meet identified needs
- The defined population, whether that be an individual, a family or a wider community, take part in assessing need and determining care
- There is a community-based, family- and person-centred approach to health care which involves treatment of disease as well as health promotion and preventive measures
- Services offered are accessible to all. This concept includes ease of physical and geographical access as well as wider issues such as financial restrictions, social class, gender and education.

In addition to Israel, COPC has been adopted to an extent in South Africa, the US, and the UK where the main proponents of the approach are the King's Fund who have backed two pilot sites at Enfield and Haringay and New River District Health Authority (Williams 1994). The concept is particularly relevant in relation to the interface between PHC and social services departments in the planning, provision and implementation of services as a result of the NHS and Community Care Act 1990.

Primary health care developed parallel to COPC and included an emphasis on health promotion deriving from the Ottawa Charter (WHO 1986b) in a way which COPC did not initially embrace. The Ottawa Charter emphasised the need for partnership between professionals and clients at all levels of interaction – power sharing, problem solving, culturally sensitive care and health promotion – as the key to enabling people and communities to maximise their potential regardless of their health status through adapting lifestyles and behaviours and encouraging community development. Today,

COPC and PHC are not distinct models, but rather should be seen as having merged; the differences between them are not enough to merit a distinction.

Why choose the COPC model?

The COPC approach:

- allows a team approach to be taken to assessing and meeting the needs of the client population
- allows understanding of the needs of the population from a multidisciplinary perspective
- provides a means by which workload planning and skill mix can be matched
- extends audit activity and brings clinical audit into healthcare planning and delivery
- addresses the prevention paradox (Rose 1992) which is 'a large number of people at a small risk may give rise to more cases than a small number of people who are at a high risk'.

Community-oriented primary care is closely linked to the WHO view of PHC set out in the Alma Ata declaration. The five principles of PHC set out and reiterated by WHO (1988) are that health services should be: equitable; affordable; effectively managed; integrated involving primary, secondary and tertiary care and other agencies and interests; and have active community participation in the planning and delivery of services.

Wearne (1993) indicates that there is some evidence to suggest strong support for community-based PHC as a result of a community-based research project to develop and test the role of the public health nurse in planning and delivering services. Wearne states:

Whilst it is important to recognise the value of the traditional medical model of primary care, it is also important to recognise its limitations. The transition from an individualistic approach to health, to a community-centred one with maximum involvement from other agencies and the community has to be the future model for PHC if we are to be prepared to meet the public health challenges of the next decades.

Community-based primary health care providing the context and philosophy of and for practice, an alteration in the employer/employee relationship between medicine and nursing and a creative approach to integration and overlap of nursing roles in primary care, could be the catalyst to primary care achieving its potential and the potential of the population.

Primary care: the medical model

Currently, PHC services in the UK have a medical need orientation rather than a community-based focus. Primary care or the medical model is located within the community, in general practice, but it does not work with the community or the individual. It is concerned with identifying disease processes and treating them, primarily to cure disease. There is an emphasis on the individual patient rather than on the family or community. The role of nursing within this model is to provide nursing care targeted at specific diseases. It is task-oriented and not able to be proactive. Because of the lack of proactive case finding in a medical model approach, underserved populations can be missed out, and staff rely on patients coming to the surgery to seek care. It is the first line of medical management offered by the health system and acts as a conduit into the secondary sector.

An example of the medical model emphasis may be found in the work of the practice nurse (PN). Practice nurses employed by the GP spend the majority of their time carrying out tasks (Davies 1993, Jeffreys, Clark & Koperski 1994) which are demanded by the GP contract (DoH 1990) and devolved to the nurse by the GP employer, for instance, screening of newly registered clients and elderly screening. There is little evidence to suggest that any of this activity yields a high level of health gain in comparison to the level of activity. Recent studies (Field 1995, Lindholm 1995, OXCHECK 1995) suggest that practice nurse activity should be more focused and that blanket screening of the practice population is expensive and more importantly is of limited use. Working in this climate and being employed by the GP restrains PNs' autonomy and the creative use of the nurse's time. It denies people direct access to a nurse who could improve the health status of many (Edwards 1987). WHO (1985) stated that 'Ideally everyone should have the same opportunity to attain the highest level of health and more pragmatically none should be duly disadvantaged'.

In the report Nursing in the Community, Edwards (1987) stated that 'there is evidence that the lack of direct access to most nurses working in the community prevents some people from seeking appropriate help'.

Given the dominance in the UK of the medical model and the intent of the Department of Health that further decision making on health care and health gain will be handed to GPs (Davies 1993), there is enormous, unprecedented and unique influence and control given to one professional group within primary care (doctors) over other professional groups (such as CHCNs) with whom the stated intent is to be equal partners. It is likely in the future that more CHCNs will find their employment linked directly or indirectly to a GP.

This control not only inhibits nursing and is unpopular (Bowling 1988), but is one factor amongst others (NHSME 1993b) that makes the development of PHC teams almost unattainable except superficially, severely limiting the potential of primary health care itself.

Community health care nursing can, if allowed to develop autonomously as an independent discipline within PHC, make significant contributions to client health. In a statement which encapsulates the potential benefits of nursing to client health, Jones (1994) states:

The emergence of professional nursing as a discrete and significant discipline in its own right rests on the competence of practising nurses to accurately define, with a high degree of specification, those areas of concern in health care for clients for which they, as nurses, are uniquely qualified to offer solutions. In making such definitions, a nurse will display a perspective towards the client's problems which is distinct from those of other care team members with whom she shares a collaborative role in providing for the needs of society at large.

Developing PHC around general practice populations

Since PHC development has gathered momentum, there has been recognition that many general practices are underdeveloped and so cannot cope with the enormity of the task placed upon them by the NHS reforms. In addition, the medical profession is trying to deal with the difficult issue of how to recognise and manage poor performers. If the reforms are to work centred around general practice, then underdeveloped practices must be enabled to develop. In March 1993, the NHSME (1993a) published a document outlining nursing in PHC, entitled 'New World New Opportunities'. Target areas for development around general practice were set. These are:

- Movement towards practice-based services
- Development of practice premises
- Programmes to enable GPs and staff to develop their management skills
- Training in PHC for general managers
- Information technology development, including shared records, the development of strategies for nurse employment, training and education
- Regionally recognised research and development programmes.

There have been several models developed to try to achieve practice development. These include a multidisciplinary team approach, involving nurses, managers and doctors, to developing practice, and a unidisciplinary approach which usually involves attaching a medical practitioner to an underdeveloped practice to act as a catalyst for change. Both models have merits and limitations, and are not contrasted here. An outline of a multidisciplinary approach to practice development within the context of the inner city and its attendant problems is outlined below.

Many of the problems of underdeveloped general practice services centre around inner city areas. There is a medical manpower crisis developing in relation to GP recruitment in some inner city areas; why practise in a deprived area where the problems are immense when you could go to the Cotswolds and have an easy life? Some critics state that the problem will not diminish until incentives are paid to doctors within inner city general practice to make the extra work and pressure more attractive.

Inner city areas of the UK such as East London, Liverpool and the Welsh Valleys exhibit and must deal with many of the stresses associated with the phenomenon of the 'inner city' in relation to factors affecting health, health status and the provision of related health and social services. The challenge to providers of health care is how to deliver appropriate and effective care, efficiently and equitably within available resources.

It is estimated that three-quarters of the UK population live in cities. By the millennium this figure will have increased (RCGP 1994). City health is therefore a major concern for providers of PHC. In the past, cities were thought of as homogeneous communities and could be divided into distinct zones: an outer zone or suburb tending to relative prosperity and health and an inner zone, the inner city, tending to relative and sometimes absolute poverty and deprivation which brings with it attendant health problems (Jarman 1981). This has been captured as the intractable phenomenon of the 'inner city'.

The view of an inner city as a geographical area requiring particular assistance due to a prevalence of major problems is, however, fast disappearing and it should be considered a way of life rather than a location. In this way the health and social-related issues which affect people in, for example, East London, may be found in areas once considered suburban, such as Epsom. It has been recognised for some time in the inverse care law (Tudor-Hart 1971) that those in greatest need receive the worst health provision. Obstacles, such as an emphasis on secondary care and a lack of development funding, have blocked the development potential of primary care and denied clients access to services which has exacerbated the situation for the most needy populations (Bolden 1981). Unfortunately this remains largely true in the mid-1990s (RCGP 1994).

Strain is placed on primary care providers and services through social factors such as the prevalence of vulnerable clients from groups such as the elderly, children, ethnic minorities, single parents, cohabiting families, the homeless/roofless, unemployed people and high numbers of social groups 4 and 5. Organisational factors such as poor access to secondary care provision and lack of social care exacerbate strain and this in turn influences the care which primary care providers are able to offer to clients (Jarman 1991, Jarman & Bosanquet 1992). The situation has been made worse by the NHS reforms (Department of Health 1990) and the introduction of an internal market for health care. This initiative has irrevocably altered the character of the NHS (Holliday 1992). Changes to the way in which community care is organised and funded have led to under provision of social care which exacerbates hardship for some vulnerable groups. In 1990 in recognition of the enormity of the problem, the Royal College of General Practitioners held a multidisciplinary conference out of which was born the Inner City Task Force in 1991, committed to developing inner city primary health care.

A multidisciplinary approach to developing PHC with a general practice population focus

The Inner City Lecturer Team was established in 1994 as a multidisciplinary initiative to develop primary health care in East London (Southgate 1993) (Box 1.4). The team was funded for a 4-year period and is a partnership between City University St Bartholomew School of Nursing and Midwifery, Department of General Practice of St Bartholomews and The Royal London Hospital School of Medicine and Dentistry and East London managers and clinicians. All of the

Box 1.4 **The Inner City Lecturer Team: aims and objectives (ICLT 1994)**

- To raise the standard of multidisciplinary primary health care and general practice within East London
- To identify issues in relation to the development of multidisciplinary primary health care
- To discover and try practical solutions to problems
- To disseminate findings
- To develop good practice
- To generate new knowledge

team members – a community health care nurse lecturer/practitioner, practice manager, general practitioner lecturers – have a clinical practice, research and lecturer function and maintain a high profile in clinical practice. The activity of the team has relevance and application to local health care and in a wider national arena.

There are three strategic layers of activity within the project (Blackie 1994).

The first layer relates to activity in the clinical area and is concerned with facilitating development within the attached practice infrastructure in clinical and managerial terms through the process of action research. This is the most visible and public face of the project activity. Issues are identified in partnership and practical solutions to identified problems are implemented.

The second layer of activity relates to the dissemination of information from the action research sites and information generated at the second level itself with other primary care providers through bodies such as the practice nurse trainer groups, the Health Authority nurse advisors and the GP forums. This level of activity is concerned with cascading information through influential bodies into all of the practices within the area. The team strives to encourage relevant groups to take a lead in the development of practice initiatives locally.

The third layer of activity relates to the attempt to generate new knowledge and theory of relevance to multidisciplinary PHC. In the past, medicine and nursing developed expertise in distinct and largely separate compartments. As the NHS reforms shift the emphasis from secondary care to PHC, the respective roles of the nurse and doctor are set to alter. There must be more sharing of roles and responsibility and it is likely that appropriately qualified nurses will assume some of the traditional roles of the doctor over time. In order to achieve this transition in a way which benefits clients, it is important to concentrate on developing a shared body of knowledge and theory which both disciplines may draw upon. The project is funded by the London Implementation Group as a result of the Tomlinson initiatives and is due to complete its remit in 1997.

Summary

Primary health care is a complex activity which is at the cutting edge of the healthcare system of the future. Community health care nurses are central to the development of primary health care in partnership with GPs and others of the primary health care team. An understanding and appreciation of the philosophy and models of primary health care and factors which enhance or limit the effectiveness of nursing within primary health care are critical to success.

REFERENCES

Blackie C 1994 Inner City Lecturer Team. Nursing first year report. St Bartholomew & The Royal London Hospital Medical College, Dept of GP and PHC and City University, St Bartholomew School of Nursing and Midwifery. Internal Document

Bolden K J 1981 Inner cities. Occasional Paper 19. Royal College of General Practitioners, London

Bowling A 1988 Team work in primary health care. Nursing Times 79(48):56–59

Bryar R 1991 What do we mean by primary health care? Discussion paper No 3. HMSO, Team Care Valleys and The Welsh Office, Cardiff

Colliere M F 1980 Development of PHC. International Nursing Review 27(6):169–172

Coulson J 1996 Are you being dumped on? BMA News Review 32–34

Davies G 1993 Report on the role and training needs of practice nurses. Team Care Valleys, Cardiff

Department of Health 1989 Working for patients. HMSO, London

Department of Health 1990 The NHS and Community Care Act. HMSO, London

Department of Health 1992 The health of the nation. HMSO, London

Department of Health 1993 The Patient's Charter. HMSO, London

Department of Health 1996a Child health in the community. HMSO, London

Department of Health 1996b Choice and opportunity-primary care: the future. White Paper. HMSO, London

Department of Health 1996c The National Health Service: a service with ambitions. White Paper. HMSO, London

Department of Health 1996d Primary care: delivering the future. White Paper. HMSO, London

Ebrahim G J, Rankin J P 1993 Primary health care: reorienting organisational support. Macmillan, London

Edwards N 1987 Nursing in the community: a team approach for Wales. Report of the review of community nursing in Wales. Welsh Office, Cardiff

Edwards S 1996 The Glaxo Wellcome debate. In: Waters J (ed) Is this simply a phase we are all going through? Health Service Journal 8–9

Field P A 1983 An ethnography: four public health nurses' perspectives of nursing. Journal of Advanced Nursing 8:3–12

Fry J 1983 Present state and future needs in general practice, 6th edn. MTP Press, Lancaster

Gregson B A, Cartlidge A, Bond J 1991 Interprofessional collaboration in primary health care organisations. Occasional Paper 52. Royal College of General Practitioners, London

Hacking J 1996 Weight watchers. Health Service Journal 2 May 1996 28–30

Holliday I 1992 The NHS transformed. Baseline Books, Manchester

Holzemer W 1992 Linking primary health care and self care through case management. International Nursing Review 39(3):83–89

Inner City Lecturer Team 1994 Internal document. St Bartholomew and Royal London Hospital Medical College, London University, London

Jarman B 1981 A survey of primary care in London. Occasional Paper 16. Royal College of General Practitioners, London

Jarman B 1991 General practice, the NHS and social deprivation. James Mackenzie lecture 1990. British Journal of General Practice 41(76):79

Jarman B, Bosanquet N 1992 Primary health care in London – changes since the Acheson report. British Medical Journal 305:1130–1136

Jeffreys L A, Clark A L, Koperski M 1994 Patterns of nurse consultation. Camden and Islington FHSA, James Wigg Practice, London

Jones I R 1994 Health care need and contracts for health services. Health Care Analysis 32:91–98

Kark S L 1974 Epidemiology and community medicine. Appleton Century Crofts, New York

Lawrence M 1988 All together now. Journal of Royal College of General Practitioners 38:296–302

Lindholm L H 1995 The impact of health care advice given in primary care on cardiovascular risk. British Medical Journal 310:1105–1109

Macdonald J J 1993 Primary health care: medicine in its place. Earthscan Publications, London

NHS and community care act. 1990 HMSO, London

NHS Management Executive 1993a New world new opportunities: nursing in primary health care. HMSO, London

NHS Management Executive 1993b Skill mix in district nursing. Value for Money Unit, York University, York

North N 1993 Empowerment in welfare markets. Journal of Health and Social Care in the Community 1(3):129–137

OXCHECK 1995 Effectiveness of health checks conducted by nurses in primary care: final results of the OXCHECK study. British Medical Journal 310:1099–1104

Perry C 1995 The IHSM Network. August 2:17

Rose G 1992 The strategy of preventive medicine. Oxford University Press, Oxford

Royal College of General Practitioners (editorial) 1994 Report of the Royal College of General Practitioners. Occasional Paper 66. Lorentzon M, Jarman B, Bajekal M, 1994 Royal College Of General Practitioners, London

Royal College of Nursing 1992 Powerhouse for change. RCN, London

Royal College of Nursing 1995 Parliamentary briefing, November. RCN, London

Southgate L 1993 The Inner City Lecturer Team. Unpublished. Joint Academic Department of General Practice and Primary Health Care, St Bartholomews and the Royal London Hospital Medical College, London

Taylor S 1954 Good general practice. Oxford University Press, London

Tomlinson B 1992 Report of the enquiry into London's health service, medical education and research. HMSO, London

Tudor-Hart J 1971 The inverse care law. Lancet 1:405–412

United Kingdom Central Council for Nursing, Midwifery and Health Visiting 1986 Project 2000: a new preparation for practice. UKCC, London

Warden J 1996 British Medical Journal 19 October 313:959.

Wearne M 1993 A report on a two year pilot project to explore the role of a public health nurse in a general practice. Mersey Regional Health Authority, Liverpool

Williams S 1994 Community oriented primary care: from concept to reality. Primary Care Management 4(8):

World Health Organization 1974 Community health nursing. Report of a WHO expert committee, technical report series 556. WHO, Geneva

World Health Organization, United Nations International Children's Emergency Fund 1978 Primary health care. Report of the international conference on primary health care. WHO, Alma Ata

World Health Organization 1981 Global strategy for health for all by the year 2000. WHO, Geneva

World Health Organization 1985 Targets for health for all. WHO, Copenhagen

World Health Organization 1986 a Nursing and the 38 targets of health for all – a discussion paper. Nursing Unit, WHO, Geneva

World Health Organization 1986b Ottawa charter for health promotion. WHO, Copenhagen

World Health Organization 1988 From Alma Ata to the year 2000: reflections at the mid point. WHO, Geneva

2 The NHS: organisational history, reforms and influence on practice

Dominic Blackie

By the late 1970s the British NHS faced organisational difficulties and required overhaul. From 1979 to 1997 the service was extensively remodelled by a radical Conservative government, in line with a particular socio-political agenda. The stated aim of incessant reform was to create a service at the same time more cost-efficient and more responsive to the needs of patients. Whether the reforms had intellectual foundations or have delivered any tangible benefits is hotly debated. However, many of the changes will not easily be reversed and community health care nurses must understand how the reforms came about and how they have influenced practice to flourish in the revised system. In particular they should be aware of:

- **The relationship between NHS inquiries and reforms**
- **The original NHS organisational structure**
- **The position of medical practitioners in relation to other professionals in the service**
- **The roots of successive reforms in a series of inquiries into the NHS**
- **The current structure of the system including the purchaser–provider concept and the internal market**
- **The nature of GP fundholding and its implications**
- **The problems that these reforms pose for community health care nurses.**

Healthcare systems are, at their core, the systematised expression of the basic human instinct to care for each other. The complexity of current systems simply reflects the sophistication of modern life in general. As they are large, expensive and socially important, they are inevitably important politically. Therefore to understand the often puzzling NHS organisational culture within which community health care nurses (CHCNs) work, it is important to know something of the history and politics of health care in the UK.

BACKGROUND TO THE NHS 1948–1984

The cultural roots of the NHS

Despite the enormous affluence enjoyed by the elite at the beginning of the twentieth century, life for the average UK citizen was characterised by insecurity, wage slavery and early death from preventable disease or involvement in colonial wars. Just as the imperial economy boomed so too did the work houses. Welfare dispensed in cases of extreme hardship was rudimentary and often arbitrarily distributed by municipal officials according to sectarian, ethnic and other prejudices. Not surprisingly, the early years of the century saw increasing dissatisfaction among 'the lower orders' and an increasingly successful struggle for civil rights.

In the health sphere too the various social pressures for reform continued unabated during the first half of the century. In response successive governments enacted disjointed legislation which, by the start of the Second World War, amounted to a patchy network of healthcare services. The lack of any overall co-ordination meant that many people fell through the gaps or were excluded by very modest incomes.

In the early years of the Second World War it became obvious to politicians of all persuasions that a people united in the sufferings of war would expect to share equally in the benefits of peace. Returning troops would expect the 'land fit for heroes' which they had been promised.

The general population, having defeated fascist dictatorship, expected a new social order. In particular, the spirit of the times called for social welfare programmes which were comprehensive, universal and egalitarian.

In 1942 The Beveridge report was published. A central tenet was that living standards could not improve without a comprehensive approach to health care. The wartime coalition government supported the recommendations and by 1943 negotiations with the various professional bodies were underway, aimed at developing a nationwide system of health care. Despite fierce opposition from the medical profession through the British Medical Association (BMA), the post-war Labour government succeeded in passing the National Health Service Act 1946.

On 5 July 1948 the National Health Service was born, based on five founding principles:

- Equity
- Universality
- Comprehensiveness
- Free to all (State funded)
- Professionally-led consensus management.

POLITICS AND THE ORIGINAL NHS FRAMEWORK

The Labour politician Nye Bevan could legitimately be called the 'father' of the NHS. In the 1940s he fought for a transformation in the delivery of health care, largely overcoming the resistance of the health care professions. Pivotal to Bevan's success was the mood of national unity engendered by war. However, in the face of strong opposition from the BMA and a parliamentary Conservative party which voted against the NHS Act, the Labour government of the day had to fight hard to deliver any sort of NHS before the decisive moment had passed.

Consequently, even from its inception the NHS was never truly unified. The strength of the professions was sufficient to ensure that the fledgling NHS was hamstrung by complex arrangements made separately with hospital doctors, GPs and various community sectors. The nursing hierarchy at the time was not sufficiently powerful to be involved in efforts to derail 'radical' new government policy – seen by some as creeping socialism, and by others simply as a threat to personal income.

Hospital doctors were eventually forced to accept direct employment and salaried service, leading to Bevan's assertion 'We have stuffed their mouths with gold'. The doctors gained the security of a good salary with a generous pension plan. Near total clinical freedom was retained, however, as was the right to practise privately – for many years even having private patients within NHS hospitals. In return, government expenditure plans were respected.

Independent contractor status

GPs undermined NHS integration by avoiding salaried service completely. They fought for and won 'independent contractor' status. The government, bankrupt after the war and in enormous debt to the US, could not afford to buy their co-operation. Dentists, pharmacists and opticians were able to negotiate similar terms.

Independent contractor status for clinical professionals within the NHS has had a negative effect on the development of the NHS. Perhaps most detrimental to standards of patient care has been the effect of dividing responsibility for general medical services among 30 000 individual contractors, self selected into some 9000 practices, making the GP sector hard to manage strategically. Variations in the standards of service made available to patients have been extremely difficult to remedy. Most noticeable for the CHCN is the day-to-day effect it has on the functioning of the primary health care (PHC) team. The problems associated with independent contractor status are discussed further in Chapter 4.

Dentists, pharmacists and opticians negotiated even more 'arms length' terms than GPs. This meant that pharmacists and opticians remained first and foremost shopkeepers running small businesses, rather than clinical service providers. The comparative looseness of their initial NHS affiliation allowed all three groups to drift away from the NHS over the years into the commercial sector. Routine optical services are no longer covered by the NHS for the majority of the popula-

tion. In the mid to late 1990s, the number of dentists leaving the NHS for private practice places the future of the public sector in question, with the poorest communities often being worst served.

ORGANISATIONAL CULTURE OF THE NHS (1948–1984)

The NHS matured into a vast institution with two main wings – general practice and the hospital service. GPs contracted with local family practice committees (FPCs) to provide 24-hour general medical services to patients registered with them. FPCs held GP contracts, paid for the services provided and loosely co-ordinated the distribution of practices. FPCs had limited influence over GPs by virtue of controlling certain payments, but did not have direct managerial powers – GPs were only accountable in the broadest sense. Except for the most serious breaches of contract, FPCs did not have authority to monitor standards in general practice.

Independent contractor status ensured that, despite major change in the balance of power elsewhere in the NHS, standards of practice for GPs are almost entirely determined by the individual GP, or small groups of colleagues. Despite recent radical changes in the role of Health Authorities, the introduction of a new GP contract and GP Fundholding in 1900, the essential nature of the relationship has remained unchanged from 1948.

The hospital service

During the initial organisational phase, from 1948 to 1973, administrative authority remained largely at hospital level. Decisions were taken by hospital boards dominated by the medical profession. The assumption underlying this organisational model was that resources would be used wisely in a system led by clinicians. In the absence of reliable data, funding of the entire system was based on the aggregate of historic spending patterns and financial accountability was vague.

In the short to medium term the new NHS

prospered. In many ways the problems it began to experience sprang from its' successes. One basic assumption had been that rapid improvements in the health of the nation would mean that with each passing year the cost of the service would go down. This was naïve in the extreme. It became apparent almost immediately that the NHS, in common with all other health systems, had a potentially insatiable appetite for resources. Consequently the history of the NHS became a saga of cash crises.

The first health charges – for spectacles and dentures – were levied in 1951 by the same Labour government which had pushed through the NHS. The subsequent Conservative administration (1951) introduced prescription charges, one shilling (5p) per script. Although abolished by a Labour government for 3 years in the 1960s and frozen throughout most of the 1970s, charges are now routinely increased on an annual basis.

NHS inquiries

The first commission of inquiry into NHS costs was established by the Churchill government in 1953. The report of the Guillebaud committee took 3 years to establish that the NHS was not wasteful or inefficient, simply underfunded. It warned however that close monitoring would be vital if costs were not to spiral.

These two themes – underfunding and the need for tight control of expenditure – have characterised every inquiry into NHS organisation since.

During the 1950s the NHS drifted administratively. It was not until 1962 when Enoch Powell, Health Minister under Harold Macmillan, produced a hospital plan that any serious thought was given to strategic management. However, lacking a unified organisational structure at its inception, the NHS simply did not have mechanisms capable of developing or implementing strategic priorities.

The 1960s was spent trying to address the need for strategic capacity through better integration of the service. Various approaches were floated by the main political parties with only minor differences. Both favoured the introduction of a strong tier of regional management which would generate strategic priorities.

The first major NHS reforms, 1974

In 1974 the Labour government enacted a reorganisation which had in fact been designed by the Conservative, Keith Joseph. In order to increase accountability and control overall costs, there was a centralisation of administrative power away from individual district hospitals. A three tier management structure was introduced across the country (Box 2.1).

For the first time a level of NHS integration had been achieved which made possible a properly planned NHS. Although subsequently associated with controlling costs, central planning in the NHS has the capacity to more effectively meet the health needs of the population.

In 1976 with the new structure firmly in place, tighter annual cash limits were imposed on the hospital service. For political and contractual reasons general practice budgets were not cash limited at this time. This led to the common practice of hospitals 'cost dumping' into the primary care sector, for example by shifting discharge medication expenses to GPs.

The changes caused unrest throughout the service. The main issues from the staff side were remoteness of decision making, the cost of the new managers, unsatisfactory pay scales and poor career structures. Despite the reorganisa-

---

Box 2.1   NHS structural reorganisation in 1974

- 14 regional health authorities (RHAs) directed 90 area health authorities (AHAs)
- AHAs supervised district health authorities (DHAs) and family practitioner committees (FPCs)
- DHAs were responsible for hospitals and community services, which became part of the NHS for the first time, formerly being under local government control. At district level 'functional budgets' were introduced in a formal way for the first time
- FPCs worked with GP contractors
- Community health councils (CHCs) with a purely advisory role were intended to provide some local accountability to patients

tion, the government remained concerned about growth of NHS expenditure.

In operation, NHS planning using the 1974 three tier structure was never very successful as each level was reluctant to defer to the priorities devised further up. AHAs had a particularly difficult time, squeezed from both directions. Even when strategic imperatives could be agreed on by managers plans often foundered on issues of professional autonomy.

The response of the Labour government of the day was to set up a Royal Commission to examine the issues, report on the situation and make recommendations on the future direction of the service.

The 'Royal Commission on the NHS' sat from 1977 to 1978. Its report recognised the considerable achievements of the system in spite of administrative inadequacies and emphasised the need for increased public spending on preventive health. Distinct from underfunding, it found deficiencies in the NHS infrastructure and made suggestions for change, backed up by specially conducted research.

Specifically, the commission recommended reorganisation to improve financial, planning and management procedures as well as information systems. In order to make decision making less remote it advised removing the awkward AHA tier from the management hierarchy and raising the status of DHAs and individual units. Consensus management was reaffirmed.

By the time the report was published the Labour government which commissioned it was beset by problems, dramatically lost public confidence during the 'Winter of Discontent' and was swept from power in 1979 by the redoubtable Conservative, Margaret Thatcher.

Until the Thatcher administration, Conservative governments had maintained the post-war consensus on the NHS, but the new government of the re-styled Conservative Party took a more aggressive approach to social policy and the extensive welfare system – or 'Nanny State' as Thatcher preferred to called it. Her new government claimed a mandate to attempt to renew British fortunes by reforming the socio-political landscape, and ultimately, the NHS was not to be immune from review.

However, the Conservatives' election manifesto for 1979 had not declared a position on health which was clearly different from its predecessors. Its first health policy document, Patients First, sought only to make the existing system work better, explicitly rejecting fundamental reform and the application of general management. In fact, it represented an updated version of the thinking of the 1960s and 1970s.

The first wave of reform under the new Conservatives occurred in 1982. Much of the reorganisation advocated by the Royal Commission went ahead but recommendations to increase public expenditure were ignored. 'Efficiency savings' and 'cost improvement programmes' were to make improvements in services self-financing. Efficiency savings were decreed by the Secretary of State at 0.2% of total budgets in 1981–1982, 0.3% the next year and 0.5% in 1983–1984. Aggravated by the economy drive in what was generally felt to be an underfunded service and despite the modifications, including abolition of AHAs in 1982, criticism from the professions remained fierce about the management system's inefficiency and unresponsiveness.

Although unclear at the time, the changes made in 1982 were to mark the terminal evolution of the original NHS organisational model forged in the deal between Bevan and the professions in 1948. This 'old' NHS had two main operating principles:

- *Consensus management:* professional teams of administrators, finance officers, nursing officers and medical officers coming together to plan resource allocation at local level
- *Strategic planning:* this was always part of Bevan's socialist vision but was only actually possible after the reforms of 1974.

The tension inherent between these two principles was never properly addressed by the original NHS, the central problem being the lack of a mechanism to make doctors accountable to nondoctors.

Despite this, the collegiate system worked well in the initially stable environment. Regardless of outdated bureaucracy and chronic underfunding, by the early 1980s the NHS was undeniably successful in many ways. Almost universally popular with the British people, the NHS was capable of delivering care to a world-class standard that was remarkably cheap compared with the systems of other developed countries. Although by the early 1980s it was the largest single employer in western Europe, it cost only 5.8% of gross domestic product (GDP). The international mean for comparable economies in 1980 was 7%. Among western style European states only Greece and Turkey committed a lower proportion of GDP to health. After 35 years the NHS in the UK, even with its many imperfections, had become arguably the most cost effective health service in the developed world. The obvious question, then, is why change the NHS fundamentally even if it does have some problems?

Even its staunchest defenders could not deny that the old collegiate style of management sometimes impeded rather than promoted better care or that by the 1980s there were real problems, for example queues for hospital procedures and the lack of productivity in some areas of physician practice (Scheffler 1989, Light 1990, 1991). Most importantly, it did not equip the service to deal with rapid change.

The rate of social change this century has been much more rapid than at any other time and has continued to increase during the growth of the NHS. An ageing population, recurrent economic problems, increasingly expensive medical technology, AIDS, consumerisation and medicalisation of society, moral relativism, political apathy, multiculturalism, family instability, information technology: all have demanded increasingly nimble health services management if system failure was to be avoided. Clearly, so huge and important a national institution as the NHS could not be allowed to simply drift into the twenty-first century. Regardless of political persuasion any government in power from the mid-1980s would have been obliged to reform the NHS once more.

By a quirk of history, the task fell to a radical 'free market' Conservative administration to determine the nature and extent of the restructuring. This is central to understanding why the reforms from 1984 on led to a 'new' NHS and not simply a more highly evolved, better funded version of the quintessentially socialist original. The key point is that NHS reforms of the 1980s and 1990s were as much to do with restructuring the UK socio-economically as they were about seeking the best health policy, inevitably reflecting the thinking prevalent in the Conservative government at the time, that is, the rebuttal of post-war socialist ideas.

ORGANISATION OF THE NHS FROM 1984

The Griffiths Inquiry: introduction of general management

Against this background, in February 1982 the Conservative administration commissioned yet another NHS management review. In keeping with the spirit of the age the brief was given to four businessmen led by Roy Griffiths, manager of a successful nationwide chain of grocers. They were required to produce a short, incisive critique of NHS management as viewed against the yardstick of 'best practice' organisation and management in the private sector. The report – a 24-page typed letter – reached the desk of the Health Secretary in October 1983. The opinions which the businessmen held and the suggestions they made resonated precisely with the overall approach being taken by the government on socio-economic issues. The report was accepted in full and so the NHS was committed to 'general management'.

The report (Griffiths 1983) made clear what its authors felt was the major organisational problem in the NHS:

One of our most immediate observations from a business background is the lack of a clearly defined general management function ... By [which] we mean the responsibility drawn together in one person ... for planning, implementation, and control of performance. [Its] absence ... means that there is no driving force.

To the outsider, it appears that when change of any kind is required, the NHS is so structured as to resemble a 'mobile' designed to move with any breath of air, but which in fact never changes its position and gives no clear indication of direction.

In short if Florence Nightingale were carrying her lamp through the corridors of the NHS today she would almost certainly be searching for the people in charge.

General management, commonplace in the commercial sector, is at its most basic a clear cut organisational hierarchy with named individuals responsible for key decisions at each level. The presumption is that by giving individual managers personal responsibility for direction and strategic decision making, greater accountability and thus efficiency can be achieved.

General management did not in itself alter the central concept of a unified NHS. In fact the establishment of general management principles was *necessary* to the strategic direction of the service, which had always been intended. It is important to recognise that although the radical 1991 market reforms required the adoption of general management suggested by Griffiths, it did not arise inevitably from it.

Following the Griffiths report, all administrative units of the NHS were ordered to introduce line management and to appoint a general manager by 1985. The new management hierarchy had twin peaks, the political and the operational. Politicians exercised overall control via the supervisory board (now the NHS policy board) chaired by the health secretary. The other peak was the NHS management board (now the NHS Executive) headed by the new NHS chief executive.

The new management philosophy did not affect all parts of the system uniformly. Ancillary staff were rapidly subject to the new approach. Nursing staff managed to gain substantial representation within the new structures, but conceded in large measure the principle of professional self government.

Consultants and GPs, as in the 1940s, were more difficult to convert. In many cases medical staff simply continued to operate as in the days before general management, aware that there was little that managers could do. Information systems inherited from the 'old' NHS were crude, especially relating to prices, costings and outcomes. This meant that weight of evidence could not be used to 'persuade' clinicians to change established practices. Terms of NHS entry negotiated in the 1940s protected clinical autonomy, so under the existing system there was no real sanction which could be brought to bear on consultants' work pattern or behaviour. GPs, as independent contractors, were even more difficult to convert to an appreciation of and acquiescence to the new managerialism.

So, even after implementation of a general management structure throughout the 'old' NHS, no hospital or general practice could be compelled to improve its performance. Poor performance relative to other similar units did not carry the risk of losing money or closure. In fact the reverse was often the case, with money being thrown at problem units. Moreover, outstanding units often attracted not more resources but more work.

This is the central paradox of all government-operated public service monopolies. In theory, an optimally administered institution is capable of tremendous efficiency, through economies of scale and so on. In practice, this is at times not the case, probably due to human nature. The new Conservative administration was in no mood to tolerate 'inefficiency' in any public sector enterprise. The preferred solution for the public utilities was to expose supposed inefficiency to the disciplinary effects of market forces. Privatisation or the sale of state owned assets was the mechanism. In most cases the effect was to create private monopolies in, for example, gas or electricity. For practical and political reasons this approach, at least in one step, was entirely untenable in relation to the NHS.

THE INTERNAL MARKET REFORMS (1991): THE 'NEW' NHS

The government had decided that only by overcoming the inertial effects of professional autonomy could 'genuine', commercial sector-style efficiency be achieved within the NHS, although it was repeatedly stated that increased efficiency, quality and accountability were the motivation behind the change. Throughout the continuing period of reform, assurances have been made at prime ministerial level that there is no wish to move the system away from founding principles. Whether these claims bear scrutiny in the light of experience is discussed below, following an overview of the new structure.

'Working for Patients' (Department of Health 1989) laid out the framework for the first radical reorganisation. The ideas were formalised and brought into effect by the NHS and Community Care Act 1990. At the heart of the reforms is the purchaser–provider distinction.

The purchaser–provider concept

In the mid 1980s in the US, health systems expert Alain Enthoven developed the concept of an internal market for healthcare services in which health maintenance organisations (HMOs) with not less than 50 000 patients each would act as purchasers of health services from hospitals, physicians and other providers.

Enthoven developed the concept of the purchaser–provider distinction in relation to the NHS during a research visit to the UK. He proposed that the purchasing role of the HMO could be carried out by modified health authorities in the UK. As in the US, hospitals and other secondary care services would be provider units, the central dynamic being the establishment of a more equal power balance between producer and consumer in order to control costs. Although philosophically the health sectors in the UK and the US were at the time poles apart (Box 2.2) the same model was touted as being capable of transforming both.

In the UK Enthoven concluded that, although a state-run monopoly, the NHS was also tightly controlled by providers. For the Conservative government the attraction of Enthoven's purchaser-provider concept was not principally reduction of costs, already good by international comparison. Rather, here was a mechanism for setting up a 'market' framework. A whole new set of operating principles were created, leaving the professions struggling to reposition themselves. Almost as a side issue, introducing market forces held the promise of at last being able to deal with the long-standing issue of professional underperformance, as well as making

> ### Box 2.2 Purchasers v. Providers in the USA 'free market' health system
>
> The US health sector, in theory, clearly distinguishes purchasers from providers. In reality the strength of the medical institutions and profession, and the fundamental differences between health care and other 'commodities', allows the supposed 'free market' to operate as a series of producer cartels which offer US consumers of health services (patients and insurance companies) little choice. For example open heart surgery can only be purchased from a cardiac surgeon and can only be carried out in an operating theatre. Therefore, providers have no need to compete seriously on price for individual or corporate consumers as long as they stick together.
>
> Individuals cannot challenge doctors or hospitals, and many US 'for profit' health insurance companies, by virtue of operating nationally in a crowded market sector, do not represent sufficient patients in any one locality to have much bargaining power either. Doctors and hospitals set the price, often to the limit which the market will stand.
>
> In principle, a locally-based HMO representing 50 000 individuals in a particular provider's catchment area becomes the most important single customer for that provider. This changes the situation considerably in the purchaser–provider relationship. Unless any one HMO represents too large a proportion of the population in one particular area, a consumers' cartel is avoided.
>
> The US reality of unregulated market forces in the health sector demonstrates how providers inevitably dominate in such a situation. This encourages costs to escalate, principally through high wages, profit-driven over-investigation of minor complaints and the unrestricted use of technically exotic, highly expensive and/or unproven procedures. The outcome of this is that, despite spending a much larger proportion of a bigger GDP on health, the richest country in the world is unable to afford basic comprehensive health care for the 20% of its people who cannot pay private health insurance premiums.

it easier to support and expand successful units.

In the US context Enthoven's suggestions work to control costs for the benefit of patients by creating a large new consumer unit, powerful enough to begin to regulate the market. A 'bulk' purchaser can destabilise the cartel and induce real competition between providers. Regulation of the market by this mechanism could be said to limit choice. In fact, by lowering costs it enhances access and increases options for the majority of the population, for whom the so-called 'choices' were always beyond financial reach.

Implementation in the UK

An important change was made to Enthoven's concept prior to its introduction in the UK in 1991 – the size of the purchaser unit was reduced from 50 000 patients to 11 000. This was suggested by Alan Maynard, a Conservative health policy adviser. It was accepted largely on the basis of political expediency – units of 11 000 patients are much easier to assemble, particularly if they need to be attached to a group of GPs. Even with blocks of 11 000 the scheme could not be 'rolled out' fast enough to keep pace with similarly radical changes in other public services. Consequently, the size of the minimum purchasing block fell with most public spending rounds, for example in 1992 to 9000, in 1993 to 7000. 'Community fundholding' reduced the minimum purchasing unit to 3000 patients. However, Enthoven's first principles seem to suggest that too small a purchasing unit completely emasculates the purchaser–provider concept. A large number of small, competing units cannot influence the behaviour of providers effectively.

The NHS internal market

On the basis of the scheme first discussed in Working for Patients (Department of Health 1989) and enacted in 1990 as the Health and Community Care Act, the structure of the 'new' NHS is in principle very simple (Box 2.3).

The regional tier of NHS management, although key to the initial implementation of the reforms, ceased to exist in April 1996. NHS Executive regional offices are expected to undertake the strategic role, but with much less power than former regions, less direct control over resources and faced with a greater number of much more autonomous units. It remains unclear as to whether and how national and regional priorities can be driven. Interestingly, GPs *as providers* of primary care services have not yet been subjected to the market forces applied to secondary and community services.

In theory and without formally dissolving the NHS or, technically, moving away from the founding principles, a market for health services has been created. Purchasers are able to 'shop' around for a better deal and providers, faced for the first time with the real prospect of losing income, are encouraged to compete for business. The forces of competition thus created are said to promote efficiency, quality and more rapid innovation. More correctly an 'internal market' was set up since there are strict rules governing the nature of the trading allowed and the extent to which publicly funded providers can enter the commercial world.

Key players: Purchasers

District health authorities, originally created by the 1974 reforms and bolstered by the changes following the 1982 Royal Commission, merged with family health service authorities to become joint commissioning authorities in April 1996. Now called Health Authorities, they make all purchasing decisions for patients not registered with a fundholding GP (see Table 2.1) as well as being responsible for most of the expensive or important areas of spending not controlled by GP fundholders. JCAs combined the functions of both previous roles.

1. Previous functions of district health authorities:
   - Purchasing services for their residents
   - Managing units which remain under their control
   - Assessing the population's need for health care
   - Public health

Box 2.3   **Structure of NHS internal market**

- Purchasers – district health authorities, fundholding GPs and private patients, who buy secondary care and community health services
- Providers – NHS trusts, directly managed units (DMUs) and the private sector, who make this care available
- A series of contracts links the two sides
- The market is regulated – to a greater or lesser extent depending on prevailing political circumstances – by the NHS Policy Board and NHS Executive and by the purchasing decisions of DHAs because of their scale

2. Functions of FHSAs:
   - Managing the contracts of family practitioners, plus dentists, pharmacists and opticians
   - Assessing the population's need for primary health care
   - Planning services to meet those needs
   - Managing GP development funds.

GP fundholders. GPs, the so-called 'gate keepers' for the secondary and community services, traditionally could only refer patients to hospitals and other secondary units directly managed by the local DHA within whose catchment area the patients happened to live. There was choice between individual clinicians, but consultants with a good reputation tended to be over-subscribed. Additionally, in theory, it was always possible to refer to any part of the 'old' NHS. In practice, with the exception of acute trauma and unusual life-threatening disease, referral outside DHA boundaries was likely to mean an even longer delay for patients as local referrals received higher priority. The catchment area concept was, and still is more strictly observed by high demand, under-resourced units, for example psychiatry and gerontology. GPs had no direct say over which units cared for their patients, nor could they direct patients away from units perceived to be substandard, unless fortunate enough to live in a major urban centre with a choice of hospitals.

GP fundholders do have a choice. Instead of relying on purchasing decisions made by a DHA, GP fundholders receive a set amount of money each financial year to buy a defined range of services for their patients. The amount is fixed on the basis of historical spending and the practice's business plan, which is simply a projection of the services the GPs expect to have to buy in the next financial year together with associated costs (primarily pharmaceuticals and practice staff). As data systems become more sophisticated, the amount of money will come to be fixed strictly by list size, weighted to allow for various factors such as age, gender and so forth.

The basic range of services purchased (in standard fundholding) is:

- Out-patient care
- Diagnostic tests
- In-patient and day-care treatments where there is some choice over time and place of treatment.

The cost of these services, plus the cost of prescribed drugs and staff expenses, sometimes as much as £1 million per annum, is deducted from the financial allocation of the health authority which would otherwise be responsible.

To protect 'expensive patients', practice liability for any one patient in a particular year is limited to £6000 – the excess is covered by the DHA. Treatments not specified in relation to fundholding status continue to be purchased by the DHAs.

If the practice is able to achieve 'savings' in a particular year, that is it has provided all necessary care with money left in the budget, it is able to spend the 'excess' on practice improvements of a general nature, not including paying GPs more.

The three key freedoms therefore available to GP fundholders are:

1. The ability to alter the mix of spending between the three main budget areas – secondary services, drugs, staff/practice
2. The freedom to 'shop around' in the internal market
3. Licence to spend 'savings' on practice-related projects.

Several factors guaranteed that the GP fundholding scheme mushroomed in the first 5 years of operation:

- The new 'freedom' was intrinsically attractive to some GPs
- Hefty financial inducement to those first to come forward; for example, £16 000 start-up grant, £33 000 p.a. management allowance, 100% reimbursement of computer expenses
- Rapidly falling threshold (size of purchasing blocks) for entry to the scheme
- Increasingly 'innovative' approaches after the limited number of larger practices joined:
  - 'fundholding consortia' – groups of small practices assembled to reach the threshold for standard fundholding by FHSAs driven to meet targets

Table 2.1 UK population covered by fundholding (April 1996)	
Region/county	Percentage
Anglia & Oxford	54.5
Northern & Yorkshire	54
North Thames	55.8
South Thames	52
North West	55
Trent	54.5
West Midlands	60
South & West	54.3
Wales	53
Scotland	40
Northern Ireland	45

Based on government figures released Sept. 95, including 3100 'sixth wave' practices live from 1.4.96.

- 'community fundholding' for very small groups indeed, unable to face the full rigour of standard fundholding
- A ratcheting system of annual targets for fundholding imposed on RHAs and FHSAs.

As a result of these measures, in 5 years (1991–1996) the GP fundholding scheme spread to cover just under half the UK population in some form (Table 2.1). With such extensive coverage, any future government would find it difficult to reverse the process. However, the recently elected Labour government has decreed that hospital treatment must be based on need, and not on whether the patient belongs to a GP fundholding practice.

Possible future developments: fundholding

Direct employment of CHCNs by GPs. All GP fundholders indirectly employ community nurses through contracts with community trusts. Some already choose to purchase their community nursing service from a geographically distant provider. In principle there is no reason why a fundholding practice cannot directly employ and manage a team of community nurses. There are many implications for nurses if this occurs.

Total fundholding. Pilot projects are underway in which GP fundholders buy all services for their patients, bypassing the DHA completely.

Another scenario currently being considered is that purchasing of services is devolved to consortia of GPs holding funds in common for their patients in one locality.

Health authorities. Significant changes were also made to the allocation of resources to HAs and to the way in which money was to be spent. Funds are now allocated to *purchase services for residents*, but not necessarily to fund existing hospitals and service providers. For this reason the resources received by HAs from central government are no longer adjusted for flow of patients across boundaries. Instead, authorities receive a fixed per capita annual budget from which they pay directly for patients to be treated outside their districts through contracts negotiated with providers. The establishment of a funding system for secondary services in which money follows patients is intended to create a stronger incentive for hospitals to be sensitive to the 'wants' as well as the needs of patients as consumers of health care.

The potential impact of this radical change of emphasis is enormous, although the long planning cycle means that it is still only beginning to feed through. Despite GP fundholding, DHAs will remain the biggest single customer for every provider unit. Formally accountable only directly to the Secretary of State, with legal rights to allocate resources wherever they see fit and not *bound* to observe the strategic policy suggestions of NHS Executive regional offices, DHAs are likely to emerge as the dominant force in the new NHS.

THE NHS MARKET REFORMS: A CRITIQUE

The NHS reforms have permanently altered the structure of the NHS. The central questions remain:

- In principle, can marketisation of the NHS solve both its long-standing problems and any new ones?
- In practice, what have been the costs and benefits of the new NHS?

The special nature of the healthcare marketplace

It is recognised that there are a number of highly unusual factors at play in any so-called healthcare market. Several examples of these factors will be highlighted and discussed here.

1. The consumer seldom pays directly at the time of use

In member countries of the Organisation of Economic Co-operation and Development (OECD), 75% of healthcare expenses are paid from the public purse. Only the US and Turkey now have public proportions of less than 50%. Much of the 'private' expense is covered by insurance so that the link between demand and payment remains indirect. In such circumstances demand for services is much higher than if the individual must pay directly per use. One study (Newhouse et al 1981) suggested that spending was 60% higher when patients were covered than when they were responsible for payment. In other words, most of us tend to be much less careful about spending what appears to be 'other people's money' than we are about spending our own.

2. A relatively small number of users account for a high proportion of expenditure

This is entirely consistent with basic biology which demands that in any large, flourishing population the vast majority of individuals must enjoy good health most of the time. If this were not true, the group could not prosper in its environment and would withdraw or become extinct. It can also be reasoned from first principles that those individuals in need of most support will be pregnant females, the very young, the old, the acutely ill or injured, and the chronically ill.

Clearly, the group needing care can never be anything other than a minority at any one time, although each individual will pass through most of the subgroups at various stages of life and for varying periods.

Costs remain concentrated around birth and death, with only sporadic need during the mature adult stage and then usually in relation to trauma. Although on a life-time basis healthcare needs differ dramatically, ultimately everyone becomes ill and/or old and dies. The fact that most people are healthy most of the time has allowed politicians to make health policy into a party political football.

3. What people generally want is not health care, but health, which they cannot always have

A market obviously depends upon something being available for purchase. While health care is always available to buy, health is not for sale. It may or may not be achieved through the application of health care. Although the relationship between intervention and result may be direct, provable and dramatic, it is complicated by several factors:

- If a patient recovers he or she may have done so anyway
- If a condition worsens it may be through no deficiency in currently available care
- The 'care' may actually damage the patient
- Disease and death are, ultimately, not optional.

4. Health care is personnel intensive

Inevitably, caring for people is largely a 'hands on' activity. It is difficult – intellectually, physically, emotionally and spiritually – and demands much of those who undertake it. Educating and supporting the very large work forces involved is necessarily expensive – salaries and wages account for 80% of spending on hospital and community health services.

5. When important health care is needed timing is usually not optional

In the usual course of events the absence of a commodity for a period is not life-threatening to the consumer, so it is possible to 'shop around' for the best deal. However, as stated earlier, people cannot choose in relation to illness, and so providers are always in the stronger position.

6. Demand is heavily influenced by supply

In a real free market for basic goods and services – that is one where there are many suppliers of commonly available commodities – demand and supply are independent. Two main differences from this situation are inevitable in health care:

- The medical establishment is the only provider of care
- The choice of services available for 'purchase' is limited, or inflated, by available technologies.

Just as the indirect method of paying for health services distorts the market, so too does the role of the physician as both principal supplier and the patient's advisor and agent. For example, variations in the use of surgical procedures within and between countries cannot be explained on the basis of epidemiology (Ham 1988). They mainly reflect 'the clinical fingerprint' of the particular medical culture and the level of availability. One explanation for the increase in surgery is that there are now more surgeons.

During the life of the NHS, medical technology has developed explosively. In the early years of this century, all the average doctor or nurse could offer a dying patient was sympathy and comfort – tremendously valuable, but cheap. Today they can offer invasive, often uncomfortable, sometimes useful technology, at a price. Another problem with medical advances is that they do not actually save money even if they are cheap and effective. They simply release resources to be used in treating other conditions.

7. It is morally unacceptable to deny access to 'basic' health care

Distribution of services invariably becomes more uneven. However, the right to basic health care is accepted by members of civilised societies at the same level as the right to food, water and shelter. A 2-year-old victim of severe burns undeniably has the right to the best treatment. On the other hand, no one could describe immediate access to cosmetic mammoplasty as a human right, even in Beverley Hills. The difficulty is in agreeing what constitutes 'basic'. (These issues are discussed in greater detail in Chapter 13).

The 'new' NHS: market or command hierarchy?

It is clear from consideration of basic economic principles that in civilised societies so-called health markets can never really operate as free markets; the socio-political consequences are unacceptable. If not a 'market' what then is the new NHS?

There is still an enormous and unresolved tension about whether the NHS is best thought of as a market or a command hierarchy (Best et al 1994). There are clearly market-like forces at play in the 'competition' between providers. However, this 'market' has overall social aims and a global spending limit.

The tension is felt most by purchasers and providers who are, it seems, expected to face both ways at the same time – behaving as entirely independent 'competitors', while observing a stream of hierarchical strategic directives from the NHS Executive and the government. In practice, this amounts to much more than basic regulation of the market. Detailed commands on how particular players must behave are issued regularly – regardless of the impact on competitive positioning. Precisely how a notional 'internal market' can deliver any of the putative advantages of competition between providers while simultaneously responding strategically to health needs and meeting national socio-political aims, is not clear.

In his classic work on markets and hierarchies, Williamson (1975) proposed that hierarchies were generally better than markets when:

1. The transactions between players have a high degree of uncertainty
2. Decision makers must act in the light of insufficient information
3. There are relatively few competitors in any particular market.

Hierarchies are better in these cases because the central value system and level of trust that pervade a hierarchy improve the organisation's ability to cope flexibly with uncertain transactions. If markets operate in these conditions high transaction costs can be expected as players in the market clarify in contracts the precise nature of the agreements reached. The costs of this formalisation are both financial – an army of contract managers replace implicit agreements between professionals – and cultural in terms of lost trust and spontaneous collaboration. Imposing 'market forces' on public services runs the very real risk of destroying 'professionalism' in its truest sense.

Markets, however, are better where real competition exists and there is easy access to information about product specifications, quality and costs. For various reasons, even after several years, this is not yet the case in the 'new' NHS. Although there is some evidence from within the NHS, and elsewhere in the public sector, that market forces and contracting out can improve local efficiency and service quality, such improvements may be at the expense of service provision to the wider community as individual players feel no reponsibility for the performance of the market as a whole. As discussed earlier, this is one of the central problems of 'markets' which have to deliver services with social value.

The NHS is currently, therefore, *both* a market and a hierarchy with at least two distinct features:

1. The overall performance of the 'market' is more important than the performance of any individual players
2. Ministers are accountable to parliament for the performance of the 'market'.

Unless a theory and practice of market management appropriate to the NHS is urgently developed it may suffer the worst of both worlds: bureaucracy at the top combined with purchaser-provider confrontation locally.

The purchaser–provider split

Distinguishing between the theory and practice of the internal market has been obscured by the considerable controversy generated by the reform process. In such a highly charged and ideologically partisan environment, both the advocates and the opponents of market-based solutions have tended to promote their respective claims by reference to political philosophies and economic theories rather than practical experience.

The 'new' NHS is not popular with most of its workers. Exhaustion and confusion in the face of seemingly endless, unfocused upheaval whose rationale is widely questioned, is common throughout the NHS. The reforms in general have been received with great scepticism by the professions and the mass media. The credibility of the reforms is being strained by murders committed by mentally ill patients 'under care' in the community, and by the deaths of patients whilst being shuttled between hospitals in search of the appropriate care. So, have any benefits been recognised as a result of this radical reformation of the NHS?

Benefits of the NHS reforms

Temporary extra resources, or 'start up costs', were allocated to the NHS in the first 2 years. Predictably, this small amount of extra cash in the chronically underfunded NHS allowed increased productivity and a fall in waiting times.

Separating the roles of purchaser and provider also facilitated a new clarity of outlook for NHS managers. Both health authorities and trusts have shown that their new powers can be used to tackle long-standing weaknesses in the delivery of services and to bring about improvements for patients.

Health authorities have negotiated contracts with providers which make more explicit how resources should be used. The introduction of these contracts has helped to enhance the accountability of providers to purchasers, and has opened up a debate about the standards of care that should be delivered and service priorities.

Some NHS trusts have used the new freedoms to improve the position of low paid staff and to introduce greater flexibility in the provision of services to patients. Local pay bargaining has two major problems however:

- Encouraging wage inflation – staff are the single biggest expense for the NHS. Anything which causes wages to rise out of control is bad news for service provision
- It has the potential, if abused, to lower terms and conditions of employment and remove job security, particularly for groups of workers who are easy to replace.

General practice fundholders have demonstrated their ability to innovate and use resources differently. This includes:

- Providing additional services through primary care teams
- Negotiating for the provision of some out-patient services in practices
- Changing prescribing patterns to achieve better value for money, the savings being available to the practice
- Using those hospitals prepared to deliver the standard of care specified by fundholders.

One of the most valuable, though perhaps unanticipated, gains has been the shift in emphasis to primary care. In part this has been promoted by GP fundholding, but more fundamentally by health authorities having to listen more closely to primary health care terms (PHCTs) to inform purchasing decisions.

This gain has been complemented by the most important potential benefit of the reforms, which has been the change in the traditional power balance in the NHS. The alliance between health authorities and GPs and the stimulus provided by GP fundholding have brought hospitals under pressure and have started to move resources towards primary care. However developments around the country have been uneven. Given the party political significance of the reforms news stories are often polished prior to release.

Whether 'progress' has been a result of increased funding made available to smooth transition or represents an advantage of the new system itself is a matter of debate (Maynard 1993). It can be argued persuasively that the same effects could have been achieved by simply using the extra funds spent on reorganisation to target areas of concern, and without the enormous damage to professional culture and staff morale.

Perhaps in another 50 years the 'new' NHS will have been as successful as the original in meeting the healthcare needs of the people in the UK – although the early signs have not been encouraging. Whether the internal market reforms have caused current NHS problems – differences between providers in costs, quality, outcomes, competence levels and so on – or simply highlighted pre-existing inadequacies, remains a fiercely contested issue. Similarly, the debate regarding whether the dynamism of a managed market or the strategic capability of a command hierarchy can best serve the UK population, is certain to continue. The nagging concern about the 'new' NHS is quite simple: there is no guarantee that the sum of multiple purchasing decisions will add up to an appropriate pattern of service provision.

PROBLEMS WITH HEALTHCARE SYSTEMS

No healthcare system is free of problems. In the US, where per capita health spending is more than double that in the UK and rising more rapidly, one in seven of the population is without even basic health cover (see Table 2.3). In 1993 some 87% of US citizens wanted major change in their 'non-system' which at the time was being used as a model for the 'new' NHS (Mott 1993). At the same time in Alberta, Canada, the government announced a 20% cut in health spending to be phased over 4 years, mirroring a similar plan introduced by the Australians in 1991. In Europe, the Germans have introduced severe controls on prescribing costs, while the Danes have restricted referrals. All healthcare systems must wrestle with the same 3 problems (Macara 1994).

1. The need to secure resources for health

Since the oil crisis of the 1970s and with the emergence of 'high-tech' pacific rim economies, there

Table 2.2 A summary of the history of the NHS

	Health service event	Background	Major socio-political events
1911	**National Insurance Act**	Free care guaranteed by Lloyd George's Liberal Government to particular income groups e.g. manual workers	
1914	NI extended	Free drugs and other benefits	WORLD WAR 1
1918			
1919	*A period of prosperity follows the war but the Wall Street Crash of 1929 (the catastrophic failure of the New York Stock Market, mainspring of US capitalism) heralds world wide economic collapse – the 'Great Depression' Poverty and mass unemployment permit political extremists to seize power in much of Central and Eastern Europe. Germany – particularly battered by the depression – embraces National Socialism.*	
1938	*The Nazi Third Reich unleash an orgy of violence and destruction unparalleled in human history*		
1939			
1942	**The Beveridge Report**	Wartime coalition government agrees the necessity of a post war "Welfare State" including a comprehensive approach to universal health care	WORLD WAR 2 *For the first time in history machines of mass destruction kill more people than disease & famine*
1943– 1945	*Negotiations with 'producer' groups. Opposition from the professions. Doctors resist vigorously via the BMA*		
1946	**National Health Service Act**	"We have stuffed their mouths with gold!" Nye Bevan	
1948	**NHS Day One**. July 5, 1948	The NHS commences operation. Founding Principles: Equity, Universality, Comprehensive, State funding, Management Style: Professionally-led Consensus	
1949	*During this organisational phase administrative authority remains largely at Hospital level. Clinicians dominate. Financial accountability is vague. In the absence of reliable data funding is essentially demand led i.e. based on historic spending patterns. It assumes that resources are used wisely because the system is led by the professions. There are sporadic eruptions of concern but no wholesale attempt at reform i.e. the system is modified but no attempt is made to move away from the Founding Principles.*		
1973	*GPs become increasingly discontented with their position in relation to hospital doctors. 'GPs Charter' in 1966 seeks to redress the balance and revive GP as a career option.*		
1974	**Major NHS Reform** Region, Area & District Authorities Established	Centralisation of Administrative power away from hospitals and clinicians. Purpose: Increased accountability and control of costs. Main changes: Three Tier NHS Structure – Region, Area & District / District Level 'Functional Budgets' / Community health services are transferred from local government to NHS 'Consensus Management' remains	
1976	Tighter annual cash limits imposed	This adds to existing unrest about the remoteness of decision making following the 1974 reforms, the cost of managers, and concern about growth of NHS expenditure in general. *Not applied to GP services.*	
1977 –1978	**Royal Commission on the NHS**	Recommends re-organisation to improve financial, planning and management procedures as well as information systems. Emphasises need for increased public spending.	

Table 2.2   *(cont'd)*

	Health service event	Background	Major socio-political events
1979		Incoming government proceed with much of re-organisation but less keen on increasing expenditure, insisting on 'efficiency savings' and 'cost improvement programmes'	THATCHER GOVERNMENT ELECTED *'There is no society, only individuals'* MARGARET THATCHER
1982	Area HAs abolished	Districts and Units strengthened – an attempt to reduce bureaucracy Despite this criticism from the professions remains fierce about the inefficiency and unresponsiveness of the system. This led to:	*A new generation of conservative politicians promote radically different social values. Out goes 'One Nation' Tory-ism In comes 'Greed is Good' Thatcherism*
1982 1983	**The Griffiths Inquiry**	A short incisive critique of NHS Management as viewed against the yardstick of 'best practice' organisation and management in the private sector	
1984	General management introduced	The Griffiths Report is critical of NHS management at all levels. In particular dismisses consensus management as incapable of delivering the drive and imagination needed by a modern service.	
1986	The Cumberlege Report	A Community Nursing Review recommends far reaching organisational changes.	
1987	Promoting better health	A government 'discussion' paper touting the virtues of disease prevention leads to the new GP Contract 1990. Preventive programs attract payments for GPs if targets are reached.	
1989	**Working for Patients**	Prime Minister's Review Paper published in Jan 89. Proposes RADICAL reformation of all NHS organisational structures in line with 'New Right' political opinion	*UK society moves sharply away from the centrist social consensus politics which had persisted since the end of the War, towards an uncompromising free-market approach. All public services are remodelled or privatised. Public concern grows about standards of service from the new private monopolies and in NHS and schools. The government is repeatedly shaken by scandals involving 'sleaze'.*
1990	**NHS & Community Care Act**	'Market Forces' are unleashed within the NHS: The INTERNAL MARKET, NHS Trusts, GP Fundholding and GP New Contract imposed.	
1991	The health care 'market'	For the first time an organisational review begins to move the NHS away from its traditional values.	
1992	**The Health of the Nation**	A strategy for health in England is published.	
1995	**Patient's Charter Towards a Primary Care led NHS**	Basic standards to be expected by the public are published and distributed widely. NHSME document acknowledging the central role of PC in the new NHS is circulated.	
1996		Regional Health Authorities abolished, FHSAs combine with District HAs to form joint commissioning authorities. Regional Offices of the NHSME – a direct civil service branch of the Department of Health – strategically regulate the new market driven NHS	*Feb. 96 THE SCOTT REPORT – an inquiry into the conduct of government and standards in public life during the 15+ years of Conservative rule is heavily critical.*

has been a redistribution of wealth from developed western economies to oil producers and the Far East. This has meant that expansion each year of the economies of the west, with consequent ever-increasing tax revenue to finance generous social welfare programmes, can no longer be relied upon. Growth at a rate of 1% or 2% is now seen as a considerable achievement. There are increasingly frequent times of recession when the economy stagnates. During the 1980s the US, unable to break the habit of perpetual boom, spent huge sums of tax dollars to boost the

Table 2.3   NHS spending and international comparisons.

	Percent of GDP	Per capita spending (US $)	As % of UK spending	% public spending
Turkey	3.9	175	20	37
Greece	5.1	371	44	89
Portugal	6.3	464	56	62
Spain	6.3	644	77	78
Ireland	7.3	658	79	84
New Zealand	7.1	820	98	85
United Kingdom	5.8	836	100	87
Denmark	6.3	912	109	84
Belgium	7.2	980	117	89
Japan	6.7	1035	124	73
Italy	7.6	1050	126	79
Finland	7.1	1067	128	79
Austria	8.2	1093	131	67
Australia	7.6	1125	135	70
Netherlands	8.3	1135	136	73
Luxembourg	7.4	1193	143	92
Germany	8.2	1232	147	72
Norway	7.6	1234	148	95
France	8.7	1274	152	75
Iceland	8.6	1353	162	88
Sweden	8.8	1361	163	90
Switzerland	7.8	1376	165	68
Canada	8.7	1683	201	75
United States	11.8	2354	282	42
Average	**7.4**	**1059**	**127**	**76**

Source: Data from Health Care Systems in 24 countries, Schieber et al, Health Affairs 10, 3 (Fall 1993), 22–38
GDP spent gives an idea of the relative priority the society gives to health
Per capita spending reveals the huge gulf in spending in absolute terms
Average spending is 27% higher than in the UK.
Public spending relects the society's desire for equity.

domestic economy. Unfortunately, most of it was spent on imports, so America moved from being the world's largest creditor nation to being the biggest debtor in less than a decade.

Fortunately for the NHS, the UK continues to value it highly in the struggle for funds (see Table 2.4) with other public works such as education, defence and transport. Ultimately, the decision about exactly how much money is spent on health is not taken directly by the public or health professions, and can, in theory, be affected by other political agendas at any time.

2. The issue of priorities

No society can possibly afford to make available to all its citizens every technology which medical scientists invent (Macara 1994). Unfortunately, public tolerance of individual suffering is lower than at any time, and most of us expect that eventually medicine will answer all the problems of the human condition. Unrealistic expectations have been encouraged by politicians, in the Patients' Charter for example (Department of Health 1992a), doctors (assisted conception, cosmetic surgery) and the media ('Race against time for leukaemia girl', a headline from the Sunday Times on 18 February 1996).

In every choice there is a sacrifice (Kierkegaard). If sacrifices are not to be borne by those least able to demand attention there must be rational debate about priorities. This is true regardless of level and source of funding. 'Rationing' is an emo-

Table 2.4 UK health spending 1978–95		
	Health Spending £billions	Spending in 1991 values £billions	% of total public spending
1978–79	7.8	19.9	12.0
1979–80	9.3	20.3	12.1
1980–81	12.0	22.0	13.0
1981–82	13.5	22.6	13.0
1982–83	14.7	22.9	12.6
1983–84	15.5	23.2	12.7
1984–85	16.7	23.7	12.7
1985–86	17.6	23.8	12.7
1986–87	18.9	24.7	12.9
1987–88	20.7	25.6	13.4
1988–89	22.8	26.4	14.1
1989–90	24.7	26.8	13.8
1990–91	27.7	27.7	14.2
1991–92 est	31.4	29.4	14.4
1992–93 est	34.4	30.8	n/a
1993–94 est	36.6	31.5	n/a
1994–95 est	38.5	32.2	n/a

Source: H M Treasury 1992 Public Expenditure Analysis to 1994–95. HMSO, London

tionally loaded synonym for 'prioritisation'. It can imply that there is some sort of conspiracy to deny patients what they have an absolute right to expect. In fact, making choices at some level about who gets what is inevitable. Whether this should occur near to patients – for example, a fundholder delaying a hip replacement until the next financial year to pay for an infertility treatment – or further away from the patient is a subject of heated debate. However it seems invidious to impose this burden on individual practitioners. A universally acceptable explicit system of prioritisation has yet to be produced. In fact, it is far from clear that explicit rationing is more effective than implicit rationing in securing a sensitive and equitable use of resources. It also has the undeniable potential to politicise health care even further and restrict clinicans' individual and collective freedom to make choices.

The reality is that the problem of the equitable distribution of healthcare resources is simply too complex to rely on mechanical indices in decision making. No formula can ever be devised to cover all aspects of healthcare priori-

tisation. Inevitably, someone has to make the choice.

Public debate about priorities in health care can be usefully harnessed through the development of health targets which focus on health outcome rather than health care as in the Health of the Nation document (Department of Health 1992b). Once the general direction is agreed the public empower the professions to determine the means by which the targets are best attained. This solution involves the public, but is sensitive to the role of the professions. The purchaser–provider split is actually useful in this regard in that it frees public health professionals from close involvement with the details of provision and allows them to take a more appropriate strategic approach.

3. The quality of outcomes of health care

The third challenge faced by health systems is quality control.

Simply trusting the stewardship of implicit standards to individuals (the matron) or professional groups is no longer viable. This is true for a number of reasons:

• Sophisticated populations expect their health services to provide uniformly high clinical standards, to be sensitive to individual needs and to use public money wisely. Educated, affluent, empowered citizens expect all aspects of society to function with due public accountability. Politicians, professions, judiciary, police – all must now earn the respect and trust which in former times was expected, usually granted and sometimes, deserved. Increasing scepticism, suspicion or cynicism clouds the public–professional relationship. This should not be overstated, particularly with regard to the nurse–patient relationship, but is a factor nonetheless.

• The process of medical care is increasingly complex, both in terms of the medical technologies applied and the organisational context within which it occurs. However, without effective organisation whatever promise medical knowledge and technology offers cannot benefit patients. The importance of management skills is not often appreciated by practising clinicians.

• Some of what clinicians do – collectively and individually – has no rational basis. The premise that *every* medical advance is necessarily beneficial to patients can no longer be accepted because it is wasteful and unscientific; for example, the use of expensive new drugs with no clearly proven advantages over older treatments.

• The cost of many medical technologies is now so high as to be beyond the financial means of any society to apply them carelessly, if at all; for example, transplantation, reproductive technologies, and growth hormone treatment to delay ageing.

• The commercial health industry globally is enormous and will drive the health agenda if allowed to.

Applied research and clinical audit are potentially the most important tools in the quest for quality. They can lead to evidence-based practice, effective organisation of service and rational setting of priorities. Clinical guidelines or protocols can be useful in establishing and maintaining standards, but are not without drawbacks.

The most problematic aspect of the search for quality in health care is the measurement of outcomes. This is notoriously difficult; generally agreed measures of outcome are few and far between. Professionals focus on the technical while patients view subjective indicators as of equal or greater importance. These issues are discussed in greater detail in Chapter 12.

Summary

The NHS exists as the result of historic acts of social democratic political will stretching back to the turn of the century but rooted even further back in human social behaviour. Even though, to the medical establishment of the 1940s, it was an intensely controversial project it rapidly became an unquestioned part of British social life. Pre-1984 it enjoyed remarkable unanimity of approach from alternating governments and evolved through successive Inquiries into a world-class system of care that cost less as a proportion of GDP than any comparable OECD country. As such it was seen by people of all political persuasions as the best example this century of the enduring capacity of British society to make appropriate, pragmatic responses to evolving social issues.

The NHS reforms of the 1990s were also, undeniably, an ideological experiment introduced without information on the impact of markets or their likely costs. Secretary of State for Health, Kenneth Clarke, freely admitted to Parliament in 1989 that he had 'no idea' how much the reforms would cost (HMSO 1989). Once again the medical establishment resisted fiercely, although less effectively.

It is an unfortunate, but inevitable, characteristic of health care reforms that the political debate generated by the ideology – in the 1940s socialism, in the 1990s Thatcherite neo-conservatism – diverts attention away from an objective assessment of how well the suggested mechanisms meet the needs of the population.

Health is not a commodity. Attempts to deliver cost-effective, universally available and comprehensive health care services through unregulated market mechanisms will prove unacceptable morally, politically and economically; for example, the USA spends the highest proportion of the worlds largest GDP on health, to achieve the worst coverage of any developed country.

No health care system is free of problems. The three central issues of finance, rationing and quality will permanently dog health care delivery regardless of the organisational model determined by local socio-political realities. Clinicians and managers working together with mutual respect can optimise the outcome for patients with, or despite, politicians.

The effect on patterns of working of the latest wave of reforms imposed on the NHS in the early 1990s will take time to develop fully. Predicting the future development of the service is difficult in view of recent political changes in the UK. However it is clear that CHCNs must maintain an assertive, politically aware presence in the working environment in order to overcome practical obstacles raised by both reforms and long-standing organisational inadequacies. CHCNs must also maintain and develop the profession's due status as a primary deliverer of care. Client advocacy is an increasingly important role for CHCNs, facilitating effective lay contribution to the planning and delivery of services at all levels, in the face of sometimes daunting professionals.

To cope with the challenges of the extended role now emerging, and to exert due influence at all levels, CHCNs must be as politically aware as they are clinically skilful.

REFERENCES

Best G, Knowles D, Matthew D 1994 Managing the new NHS: breathing new life into the NHS reforms. British Medical Journal 308(6932):842–845

Department of Health 1989 Working for patients. HMSO, London

Department of Health 1992a The patients' charter. HMSO, London

Department of Health 1992b The health of the nation. HMSO, London

Ham C 1988 Health care variations: assessing the evidence. Research report 2. King's Fund Institute, London

HMSO 1989 House of Commons Paper No. 214, Resourcing the NHS. HMSO, London

Light D W 1990 Bending the rules. Health Service Journal 100:1513–1515

Light D W 1991 Embedded inefficiencies in health care. Lancet 338:102–104

Macara A W 1994 Reforming the NHS reforms. British Medical Journal 308(6932):848–849

Maynard A 1993 Competition in the UK NHS: mission impossible. Health Policy 23:193–204

Mott P 1993 American view of the NHS reforms. British Medical Journal 306

Newhouse J P, Manning W G, Morris C N et al 1981 Some interim results from a controlled trial of cost sharing in health insurance. New England Journal of Medicine 305:1501–1507

Scheffler R M 1989 Adverse selection: the Achilles heel of the NHS reforms. Lancet 950–952

Williamson O E 1975 Market and hierarchies. Free Press, New York

FURTHER READING

Bloor K, Maynard A 1994 An outsider's view of the NHS reforms. British Medical Journal 309(6951):352–353

Davan C M 1993 Provider power: an important lesson from the US health care market. Journal of the Royal College of Physicians 27(3):238–241

Dwyer O 1995 NHS trust loses £3.5m on business venture. British Medical Journal 301

Gore R 1996 Neanderthals – the dawn of humans. National Geographic 189(1):2–35

Ham C 1994 Where now for the NHS reforms? British Medical Journal 309(6951):351–352

Ham C, Maynard A 1994 Managing the NHS market. British Medical Journal 308(6932):845–847

Holliday T 1992 The NHS transformed. Baseline Books, Manchester

Moorbath P 1994 A guide to documents on the NHS reforms. Nursing Standard 9(3):30–34

Robinson R, LeGrand J 1994 Evaluating the NHS reforms. King's Fund Institute, London

Royce R G 1995 Observations on the NHS internal market: will the dodo get the last laugh? British Medical Journal 1311

Scheffler R M 1992 Culture versus competition: the reforms of the British NHS. Journal of Public Health Policy 180–185

3

The organisation of community care

Penny Reid

In primary health care, staff from a variety of professional groups must work together to provide services for clients. The difficulties faced by staff in trying to work together in an environment where services have been split into social care and health care must be analysed by community health care nurses to allow them to make suggestions that will develop effective collaboration. In this context, it is important for the community health care nurse to:

- Understand why care in the community is emphasised so heavily in primary health care
- Understand what social policy measures have been necessary to create an organisational structure for care in the community
- Understand the roles of the voluntary and private sectors
- Comprehend the issues involved in working with other disciplines.

ORGANISATION OF CARE IN THE COMMUNITY

POLICY BACKGROUND

Following the post-war period there was consensus that local authority social services departments had a central role to play in the provision of formal services such as acute hospital care. However, due to the rising cost of this since the

41

1970s, attempts have been made by successive governments to minimise the role of the state in caring for those unable through illness or infirmity to care for themselves. The experience of clients receiving formal care in the community has, therefore, changed so that many services are now means tested. This has led to a growing proportion of care being delivered by the informal care sector, particularly the family, as discussed in Chapter 8.

Bornat et al (1993) identify three main dimensions to the policy that emerged during the 1980s. The first is the promotion of the private sector. The government encouraged a switch in the provision of residential care in the early 1980s from the public sector to the private sector. Resources available to local authorities were cut by 4.9% in 1979/80 and 6.7% in 1980/81 (Walker 1986).

Second, the Department of Health and Social Security (DHSS) not only agreed to meet the full cost of care in private residential and nursing homes for those on income support, but also allowed local DHSS offices to set limits on board and lodging payments as deemed appropriate. As a result the number of places in private residential homes for older people and people with physical and mental disabilities nearly doubled (97%) between 1979 and 1984, and by 1990 had risen by 130%.

From 1979 the government tried unsuccessfully to cut public expenditure. So, third, the DHSS acted in 1984 by freezing limits and then, in 1985, imposing material limits for board and lodging payments, although these still represent a major form of income to the private sector. Many proponents of these policies emphasised the increasing choice a mixed economy of welfare offered to clients. The range of choice, however, seems to have been restricted because the number of private sector homes and day homes has increased at a greater rate than those in the public sector.

Factors affecting choice

The choice of residential care is usually arrived at under the pressure of a crisis in informal care leaving little time to explore all the options.

A study of the private sector by the Centre for Policy on Ageing (1984) found that only one-quarter of residents exercised any choice about the home they were admitted to, and around one-quarter said that their admission resulted from unsolicited arrangements by a third party. Choice of private homes is also restricted by geographical location and by the admission criteria applied, which often exclude confused or demented people or those who are difficult to control. Thus there is a tendency for private residential homes to select less severely dependent people, leaving those with greater needs to be cared for in the small number of specialist nursing homes.

Residential homes can be under private ownership or administered by the local health authority. Generally, they do not expect their clients to need any nursing care, although the level of client dependency has increased over time as the population of older people has grown. Nursing homes, which again can be privately owned or local authority run, provide a 24-hour nursing service in an attempt to ensure that standards of care are maintained.

Under the Registered Homes Act 1984, local authorities were given powers to register and inspect residential care homes. The monitoring of standards in nursing homes, however, is a health authority responsibility. Small homes with less than four residents were excluded from the 1984 Act, although concern was expressed about the standards of care in these homes (Social Service Inspectorate 1991). Similarly, the Act did not apply to residential care in the public sector, despite evidence of poor standards here as well (Day 1985). More recently, the government has responded to demands for the independent registration and inspection of local authority homes (National Institute for Social Work 1988), and local authorities are now required to establish inspection units to examine standards in both private and local authority homes.

At the same time as cutting resources and encouraging the growth of private sector nursing homes, the government also embarked on the large scale closure of mental institutions, resulting from the belief that it is better for people with mental health problems to be cared for in their communities. The care being given to people with mental health problems and learning difficulties at the time was deemed not to be of a satisfactory standard. Three main forms of action were taken: money was set aside, a hospital advisory service (now health advisory service) was established to visit suspect hospitals, and a major policy review was announced. In the White Papers, Better Services for the Mentally Handicapped (DHSS 1971) and Better Services for the Mentally Ill (DHSS 1975) it had been argued strongly that hospitals should be abandoned as the mainstay of provision for these two groups. Both papers contained targets for running down long-stay hospital provision and an increase in community based services to replace them.

The next major policy development was the production of the consultative document Care in the Community (DHSS 1981a) which contained a wide-ranging analysis of available options for speeding up the transfer of patients into the community. During the 10 years to 1986 the average number of daily occupied beds in mental illness hospitals fell from 109 000 to 82 000, and in mental handicap hospitals fell from 59 000 to 42 500, but the decline accelerated during the late 1980s as the government's discharge programme took effect. The Conservative government received heavy criticism for instigating these changes without proper planning, preparation or consultation, and without any agreed understanding of what community care would entail.

It seems that the rapid decanting of people with mental disabilities and of those with mental health problems into an unprepared community led to them simply being placed in smaller institutions. For example, between 1976 and 1985 there was an increase of 70% of people with learning disabilities in local authority staffed homes and 154% in private homes. Most of the increase (133%) in the numbers of these groups in private homes occurred between 1981 and 1985, and the majority of the rise (47%) in public sector homes took place between 1976 and 1981. Many of these people end up in residential homes, that is, private nursing homes, inappropriately because there is no realistic alternative

and private sector places are subsidised by Department of Social Security (DSS) board and lodging payments.

Following criticism from the Social Services Committee about the speed at which care in the community was being implemented, the government ordered a deceleration in the discharge programme and, in a White Paper (Department of Health 1989) it was stated that ministers would not approve the closure of any mental health facilities unless it could be demonstrated that adequate alternatives had been developed.

The NHS and Community Care Act

Since 1982 a series of seemingly unrelated policies can be seen as part of an evolving strategy to remove local authority social services from the central role of care provision to one of residual care – providing care for those who have no other option – a 'safety net' rather than a 'catch-all'. For those in need of more general care in the community, the aim of placing greater responsibility on quasi-formal voluntary help and informal support was reflected in Community Care (DHSS 1981b).

The Audit Commission's report on community care (1992a) came to the same conclusion as many other previous independent studies – that joint planning and community care were confused and offering poor value for money. In response to the debate following the Audit Commission report, Sir Roy Griffiths was appointed in March 1986 to try to find a way of improving the organisation of community care and to explore the idea of putting the whole service for older people under the control of a manager who would purchase from whichever public or private agency was appropriate (discussed in greater detail in Ch. 2).

The National Health Service and Community Care Act 1990 was the culmination of the Griffiths report and provided a new framework for the operation of the NHS. The objectives behind the new Act included seven key measures:

1. To ensure more delegation of responsibility to local level thus enabling the health and

community care services for the mentally ill, those with learning disabilities, the physically disabled and the increasing numbers of elderly persons to become more relevant and responsive to local needs.

2. To improve the flexibility of hospital services and give a number of hospitals more freedom to make decisions to benefit patients. The new self-governing status, called NHS hospital trust, was introduced with the aim of allowing certain hospitals more control over their budgets. Trusts also have the right to determine rates of pay for their staff. NHS trust hospitals remain within the NHS and must continue to provide essential services.

3. To update community care funding.

4. To alter primary health care funding – changing GP contracts – and to computerise records.

5. To reduce hospital waiting lists for patients needing consultant advice and for operations. Over 3 years 100 new consultant posts were created to meet this aim.

6. The RHAs and DHAs have had the numbers of their members reduced and the selection process changed. The Family Practitioner Committee was renamed the Family Health Service Authority (FHSA) and their membership reduced and changed periodically, and they became answerable to the RHA rather than the Department of Health as had hitherto been the case. This is discussed in greater detail in Chapter 2.

7. A new medical audit service was introduced throughout the NHS. The Audit Commission now carries out the audit of the financial accounts of health authorities and other NHS bodies. These changes were implemented with the purpose of ensuring that wide ranging studies would be constantly carried out.

All family doctors now produce a practice leaflet providing details of the services offered to their patients and the sorts of staff they employ in the practice. They are also now encouraged to carry out child health surveillance for children under the age of 5 years, and each FHSA keeps a list of

GPs who offer this service. The Act also encouraged GPs to train in and to offer minor surgical procedures on their premises. Again, the FHSA keeps a list of doctors offering this service.

Patients registering with a new GP are offered a medical examination and the opportunity is taken to offer individual health advice at this initial interview. Initially, those aged 16–74 were offered a similar service every 3 years, if they had not been seen by the GP in the meantime.

Patients aged 75 years and over are also invited to visit the surgery if they are able or are offered a domiciliary visit annually by the doctor, or increasingly by the practice nurse, in order to observe matters which may affect the patient's general health including, where appropriate, the patient's:

- Sensory functions
- Mobility
- Physical condition, including continence
- Social environment
- Use of medicines
- Reliance on carers.

From this information the health needs of the client and her likely involvement with the healthcare services can then be established.

Under the Act the emphasis on community care is much more on prevention than on cure. This has had implications for nurses who find themselves taking on a wider range of skills designed to prevent ill-health occurring rather than focusing on physical care, for instance health promotion activities.

The role of social services

The Griffiths report recommended that social services authorities should be given the lead agency role for community care. A primary objective of the community care reforms was to make proper assessment of need and good case management the cornerstone of high quality care (Department of Health 1989) while the subsequent policy guidance devoted a whole chapter to this issue (Department of Health 1990). The policy guidance outlined the three stages of a proper care management system; namely:

- Assessment of the circumstances of the client, including any support needed by carers
- Negotiation of a care package in agreement with clients, carers and relevant agencies, designed to meet identified need within available resources
- Implementation and monitoring of the agreed package, together with a review of outcomes and any necessary revision of services provided.

Practice under previous systems involved slotting people into a limited number of inflexible and traditional services which often did not meet their needs or were organised to meet the requirements of service providers rather than service users and their carers. The policy guidance argued that the new system of needs-driven assessment and care management could overcome these major weaknesses in existing practice by being much more flexible about its approach to paying relatives and friends to care, and reimbursing them for travel and so on, achieving six major objectives, which are:

- Ensuring that resources available are used in the most effective way to meet individual care needs
- Restoring and maintaining independence by enabling people to live in the community wherever possible
- Working to prevent or minimise the effects of disability and illness in people of all ages.
- Treating those who need services with respect and providing equal opportunities for all
- Promoting individual choice and self-determination and building on existing strengths and care resources
- Promoting partnership between users, carers and service providers in all sectors, together with organisations of and for each group (Department of Health 1990).

The progress in achieving these positive care management strategies has been slow and hesitant largely due to the gaps in service provision of long-term and respite care. Also, local authorities find themselves facing considerable uncertainty and disagreement about what care

management is and how it might be able to help within the new community care arrangements.

Means testing is the major stumbling block here as the care managers have to operate as gatekeepers to the services available. Until such issues are resolved it is difficult to clarify the core tasks of care management, and how this relates to existing assessment skills associated with social workers, home care organisers, community nurses, occupational therapists and others.

Central government has acknowledged that this is a very complex task and that changes will not come about overnight. The Audit Commission's report (1992a) 'Community care: managing the cascade of change', summarises very clearly how under previous arrangements the client was expected to fit in with existing service requirements, and the service received was often more dependent on which agency received the initial request for help rather than on actual needs, even for people in very similar situations (Means & Smith 1994).

Putting the client and her needs first involves a radical change of thinking and operating; key strategic decisions need to be made about whether or not to develop a mixed economy of care in order to meet those needs, or whether to develop an internal split within social services between purchasers and providers; these decisions then have to be supported by new and appropriate financial, structural and procedural arrangements. Social services authorities also need to develop new assessment systems and forms which are needs-driven, that is decided upon according to the needs of the client, and which are acceptable to a wide range of agencies. Decisions have to be made about who will be a priority for services, given that resources are likely to be limited (Lightfoot 1994). Also, how wide a range of staff within and outside social services will be capable of performing the role of care managers must be addressed. Such a structure would allow a needs-led assessment and care management system to be put into operation.

HEALTH AND SOCIAL CARE

The other major area of confusion in the new

community care arrangements is the split between health and social care. This is particularly important to the client because it affects how the service is paid for; if it is provided by the NHS it will be free at the point of delivery, but if it is provided by social services it will be means tested and clients may have to pay part or all of the cost. The government's view is that there should be no national definitions of what constitutes health and social care, but that local definitions should be agreed instead.

This is vital because lack of clarity about the respective responsibilities of health and social services undermines the idea of a seamless service in which people flow easily between health and community care.

The more effective authorities have taken individual users and analysed their care to identify where the level of nursing skill required is such that it can be offered only in a healthcare setting, for example a long-term community care bed or nursing home, and they have then drawn up agreements to meet the client's needs.

The voluntary and private sectors

The role of the voluntary and private sectors in health care waned during the expansion of the welfare state; however, under the recent policies a revival of their input is being encouraged by the government. It is, therefore, necessary to include a brief section here about these two very important deliverers of community care.

During the nineteenth century the voluntary organisations were the main agencies providing welfare. The function of the state was to fill the gaps in the network of private charity. The development of the welfare state during the early part of this century was expected to cause a reduced need for the voluntary sector. However, this did not happen, and voluntary organisations continued to provide mainly for the poor and the old, relatively powerless groups who were not in a position to press for greater priority.

The 1948 legislation which set up the National Health Service was limited in its application, and local authorities were not empowered to supply a total range of services even to the elderly, the

blind, the mentally ill and children, the main groups they existed to serve. There was no comprehensive family care, and very little was done for the disabled in general or for other persons who did not fit the legislative categories. While these services remained inadequate, the voluntary organisations continued to fill a need providing, as they always had, for the welfare of the elderly, the disabled and children. The local statutory departments were in no position to take over the responsibilities of the voluntary sector, especially in the case of the expensive residential care, where for instance voluntary homes still catered for more than half the children in residential care.

The intervention of the state extended rather than reversed the long tradition of voluntary effort. Demand for services was intensified once the local welfare departments were active beyond their capacity to meet it, making for greater dependence on the voluntary services.

It has been argued that the main focus of the White Paper on community care (Department of Health 1989) was on the need for local authorities to develop their lead agency role through enabling and co-ordinating services, rather than through actually delivering them. Their responsibility was to create a market in social care by involving the independent and voluntary sectors in service delivery, particularly in residential care. This represents a major cultural shift for both local authority and voluntary sector organisations. It is therefore important to consider what the main prerequisites are for enabling markets to work in social care. Clearly a balance is needed between the supply of voluntary and independent sector services in order that one may complement the other so that demand from clients can be met.

The Conservative government sought to promote the private provision of community care in a number of ways. Voluntary organisations involved in community care received increased funding from central government. The health authorities were urged to co-ooperate with them (DHSS 1981c). In 1985, voluntary organisations were included in the strategic planning process along with the NHS and local authorities. At the same time a statutory duty was placed on health authorities to consult the voluntary sector. Informal care by families, friends and neighbours was also encouraged (see Ch. 8). The government stressed that care of the elderly and other vulnerable groups was a community responsibility and must increasingly mean care by the community. For many, this meant a heavy burden of individual responsibility. There are more than 6 million informal carers in the UK regularly looking after sick, elderly or disabled persons. One-quarter of them spend at least 20 hours a week caring for someone. Most carers (around 58%) are women, and one-quarter of women in the 45–64 years age range are carers (Green 1988).

Working together

Professionals and organisations have been encouraged in policy documents to work more closely and effectively for many years, but the reality is still a confusion of services, fragmented by professional, cultural and organisational boundaries.

Hudson (1987) suggests three main strategies available to foster collaborative working despite these problems. These are:

- Co-operative strategies
- Incentive strategies, based on financial inducements to encourage joint working
- Authoritative strategies, where agencies or individuals are instructed to work together.

Deciding which is to be the lead agency in co-ordinating the services is a major problem. The demarcation line between health care and social care has always been traditionally disputed territory, in terms of both institutional provision and domiciliary services. Individual health and social services departments tend to find their own solutions, but this unsystematic approach does not aid workers in their efforts to work together in the long term. The problems of improving and co-ordinating services need to be tackled in many different ways and at all levels of service provision; through joint planning, major restructuring of services, development of models for primary health care, joint projects, refinement of procedures, production of guidelines and not least through the co-operative efforts of workers at ground level. Much work has been done in these areas; however, there are still innumerable examples of failure in collaboration. A few attract publicity, but many more go unnoticed except by those involved, who are aware that the help provided could have been better.

Successful collaboration

At the point of delivery, services have to be combined and individualised; and, if needs are to be met adequately, it is crucial that practitioners relate well to each other. Any structural approach to problems in collaboration must be accompanied by a relational approach, that is one which is concerned with the human element in working together.

If help can be provided from a single agency or within one department of a large agency, working relationships can develop over time, in teams or other groups, supported by agency structures. Although there may be collaborative problems between workers of various professions and training, these are compounded by the need to work across the agency or departmental boundary (Cowley 1993). Often, when help is needed from more than one agency it has to be assembled to meet a particular situation, each situation requiring a slightly different set of services, workers and skills. It is important to build a good team by selecting people who have complementary strengths to meet the health needs of a particular caseload or local population.

Hindrances to collaboration can be reduced by efficient procedures and the development of organisational structures designed to encourage interprofessional relationships, such as health centres, the siting of various agencies in close proximity and multidisciplinary projects. However, restructuring professions and agencies can never provide quite the whole answer and, where there are complex problems, there will always be a need for highly skilled collaboration between the different professional groups. It is therefore essential to deal with the collaborative difficulties that stem from human relationships in the context of helping.

Hornby (1993) identifies the common causes of collaborative failure which arise from relational rather than organisational factors. One of the first problems she discusses is the difficulty professionals sometimes have in knowing whether it is the individual or the family who is the client. In the case of children, the family unit, whatever form it takes, will invariably be involved; but with adults the 'user-unit' may include relatives, friends or neighbours with whom the client has a personal relationship. Although they may contribute positively or negatively to the situation, recognition of these people is important. Responsibility for self-care is often taken away from the client and clearly this diminishes his autonomy and self-esteem and encourages dependence. It is crucial that workers recognise and understand the roles clients and the family play in the situation if they are to help them to help themselves.

There is often also ignorance about the different roles and functions played by other agencies and professions, leading to inappropriate referrals and duplication of work. This usually results from too narrow a view of the situation and from being too restricted to a single profession or agency, thus losing a proper overview of the services available. Where different professionals do not know each other it is almost inevitable that they react initially to a stereotype. It takes time to build relationships and for each to recognise the other's qualities and the limitations of their role. In trying to overcome ill-feeling caused by stereotyping, there is a tendency to emphasise the things different professional groups have in common rather than stressing the different qualities and emphases of their role; this can lead to a sense of uncertainty and a feeling of not being valued. To establish a sense of self-image each professional must be aware of the things she alone can contribute and of the qualities that make her different from everyone else. Failure to use professionals from another agency when their help could be useful is a common problem in collaborative working. Collaboration will be enhanced by developing respect and recognition both for the differences and for the similarities between agencies. Above all, practitioners need to nurture their own self-confidence and self-esteem for their chosen professional path, if collaboration is to be encouraged. This can help to avoid defensiveness or animosity arising, since practitioners will be able to explain readily the contribution they could make to client care. They would then be able to justify their practice to colleagues, to the managers and doctors who control and contract for their services and, most importantly, to the users of their services.

Of crucial importance to collaboration is the terminology professionals use which may not be easily understood by others, thus hindering interagency communication. Practitioners will also sometimes hold different opinions about which interventions are likely to be helpful. The attempt to resolve differences or to find a compromise is only likely to succeed if motivation to do so is strong, and time is made for discussion with all interested agencies including the client. Nurses cannot assume that all the agencies involved agree on the basic aims of helping strategies. In many cases, such differences do not affect the help that is needed nor the collaborative process. Only when conflicting assumptions affect attitudes to the client or the choice of methods to help, do fundamental differences of approach form serious problems for working together.

Different agencies need to make time to reflect on their failures, otherwise relationships between workers can suffer and have a long-term detrimental effect on collaboration. If a collaborative failure can be worked through, with faults being owned, it can often lead to increased mutual understanding and improved working relationships.

In recent years professionals in all the caring agencies have had to work within organisations undergoing radical change. This often leads to role insecurity and role ambiguity, which in turn leads to a perception that seemingly intractable problems are unsolvable and may lead to professionals retreating behind professional and agency

Case study 3.1

Mr Reid, who is 85 years old, had a cerebrovascular accident 2 years ago. He now has a right-sided hemiplegia, is incontinent of urine and faeces, his speech is slurred, and he is very confused. He is cared for by his elderly wife, whose mobility is becoming increasingly limited by arthritis.

The couple's only son was killed during the Second World War. Mr Reid was the youngest of four brothers, all of whom are now dead, and apart from a nephew and niece with whom he lost contact many years ago, he has no other relatives. Mrs Reid has a younger sister, but she lives more than a hundred miles away and so they rarely see each other.

The Reids live in a terraced cottage in a small village. The house has not been modernised, so the only heating is by open fires, supplemented when necessary with a paraffin heater. There is no bathroom and only an outside toilet.

Mr Reid is cared for in a living room, which in addition to the large double bed contains a comfortable clutter of rather old-fashioned furniture. Mrs Reid rarely goes further afield than the village post office where she does most of her shopping especially since the bus service to the local town was stopped some months ago. She is finding this task increasingly difficult as her mobility becomes more limited.

The district nurse could be identified as being the most likely professional to deal with the problems faced by Mr Reid. Clearly, some reason needs to be established for his confusion. He also needs some help in dealing with his faecal and urinary incontinence. She may give advice on aids available to help him. She may also be able to help Mrs Reid to bath him.

Social services could be asked to provide a sitting service for Mr Reid while his wife takes some time out from the continuous task of caring for his needs. A home help might be arranged to do the shopping and some cleaning should it be needed. In some areas, these social services are means tested, so the Reids may be asked to pay for them, whereas health care is provided free at the point of delivery.

boundaries, thus creating a major hindrance to collaboration. Case study 3.1 describes a scenario where multi-agency care is required and offers a possible collaborative solution.

Assessing needs and setting priorities

Needs assessment is pivotal to the work of practitioners in health and social care, especially since the community care reforms. The White Paper 'Caring for People' (Department of Health 1989) highlights the role of needs assessment which, with sound case management, is intended to form the 'cornerstone of high quality care'.

The concept of need and the practice of needs assessment are both subject to a wide range of interpretations, and are discussed in greater detail in Chapter 9. Clear definition is important for individual assessment, for the development of multidisciplinary tools and in gathering planning information. Clarity in thinking and talking about need, and consequently about needs assessment, is essential to the multidisciplinary, collaborative ethos required to care for people in the community generally.

One definition from the community care literature states that 'needs are said to show a requirement for individuals to enable them to achieve, maintain or restore a respectable level of social independence and quality of life, as defined by the particular care agency or authority' (Social Services Inspectorate/Social Services Group 1991). This definition employs constructs of dependency and quality of life in an attempt to define the concept of need. The meaning of the term 'need' can be clarified by distinguishing between any identified difficulty and the help which is required to alleviate it. A person's difficulties are indicators of potential need: for example, difficulties with preparing food might indicate a need for prompting, for physical assistance or for aids and adaptations. Such difficulties can be identified independently of the inference of actual need, perhaps through the observation of behaviour. Clearly, the assessment of needs is not the same as the assessment of difficulties, because assessing needs requires some evaluation of the services that are available in order to distinguish met need from unmet need. So assessing needs is vital in determining the ability of someone to live successfully in the community and is also important because an assessment of a person's needs alone does not specify what is required to address those needs. The needs should be assessed with a view to how they might be met and what services are available to achieve this, rather than looking at the suitability of clients for particular services.

What often happens though, is that the assessment involves looking at the actual services available, while focusing on the particular difficulties of the client. McWalter et al (1994) describe how patients with dementia are assessed by means of an assessment tool in an attempt to quantify their difficulties along some dimension. Similarly, the assessment of carers' needs may involve assessment tools that examine some dimension of either the difficulties carers face or the effects of those difficulties. These have contributed to a recognition of the problems associated with stress on carers and their ability to cope.

District nursing

There are serious problems in the community care policy which are directly relevant to district nursing. First, the powerful professional interests within the hospital and residential sectors, while not being opposed to community care in principle, have resisted any reduction in resources in their own specialties. Second, the structural separation between health and social services has prevented effective planning and implementation of co-ordinated policies. Third, expenditure cuts in the 1990s seriously eroded community services, particularly for the elderly; faced with the loss of government grants, local authorities have been forced to assess ability to pay for services, such as meals on wheels, home helps and day care places.

In promoting care in the community since 1986, there has been a move to identify patient groups for priority care; one such identified group is older people, and district nurses spend 75% of their time with them. This is seen as a priority, especially for those living alone (DHSS 1982).

Informal carers

One of the main problems facing the domiciliary services and district nurses is the needs of infor-mal carers. The shift from care in the community to care by the community has wide implications for informal support. As discussed in greater detail in Chapter 8 'families are, as they have always been, the principal source of support and care' (Webb & Tossell 1991). The majority of carers are women and many are elderly, frail spouses or elderly sons or daughters. Frequently the health of carers is poor. It is not possible to estimate the size of the problem, because the relevant figures are unavailable. However, the numbers of women available to care in the 45–60 years age group was predicted to fall from 1980. In addition, the increase in marital breakdown, divorce and remarriage will mean that complicated patterns of family responsibility will occur in the future.

The burden of caring can be discussed in terms of the physical, emotional, social and financial costs. The physical demands include time spent on caring tasks, wear and tear from lifting, and sleepless nights. Second, there is much evidence to support the claim that caring is stressful (Webb & Tossell 1991); one study showed that the continuous emotional demands, and resulting heightened tension between family members, were more difficult to cope with than the physical tasks of caring. Third, carers often become socially isolated because of giving up outside employment and interests, at the same time becoming emotionally isolated from help except in times of crisis. Finally, the financial costs are considerable, such as loss of income and career opportunities; benefits are inadequate, particularly for married women who are not eligible for invalid care allowance. This is compounded by the direct costs of caring, such as financial outlay on heating, laundry and special equipment.

There are two main reasons why this should concern district nursing. Admission into hospital is often caused by stress and exhaustion in the family and breakdown of the caring relationship; sleep disturbance and faecal incontinence have been found to be poorly tolerated by relatives and causal factors precipitating admission (Sandford 1975). Furthermore, support for carers

Case study 3.2   **An example of discharge planning**

Mr James was admitted to hospital in December following a cerebrovascular accident with left hemiplegia. He was extremely dependent in all the activities of daily living and had no swallowing reflex. A gastrostomy tube and a urinary catheter were inserted.

Mrs James was determined to care for her husband at home. Although the multidisciplinary team were not optimistic about the success of this they were willing to help as it was what both Mr and Mrs James wanted.

As the statutory services were unable to provide continuous 24-hour care in the community, it was considered important for Mrs James to be able to undertake some aspects of her husband's care, particularly gastrostomy feeds and catheter management. A multidisciplinary assessment was carried out with the medical social worker as assessment co-ordinator. A meeting was arranged between Mrs James, two of the James' daughters, the medical social worker and the liaison officer. This gave Mrs James and her daughters the chance to discuss their needs, expectations and wishes for Mr James' future.

While Mrs James was determined to have Mr James home at all costs her daughters were concerned about the level of support that would be available at home for Mr James' needs. The medical social worker and the liaison officer explained the availability of the services and tried to impress upon Mrs James the enormity of the task she was taking on, although they would support her in every way possible. Most carers are unaware of the stresses involved when they take on this role.

Following this meeting the medical social worker and the occupational therapist visited the patient's home to examine the possibility of nursing Mr James there. It was decided that he should be nursed downstairs to accommodate the equipment that would be needed. Also at this time, a hoist and sling were delivered to the ward for Mrs James to learn how to get Mr James out of bed safely. A meeting was then arranged in the ward with the liaison officer and all members of the community care team to discuss Mr James' requirements following discharge.

The care package was planned taking account of Mr and Mrs James' needs and wishes. A provisional discharge date was set, the multi-agency assessment was completed and the care plan was finalised by the medical social worker in collaboration with the liaison officer and the primary nurse.

The supply of gastrostomy feeding equipment required a meeting with the dietician and the liaison officer to discuss any system suitable for use in the community. Following this the liaison officer met with the feed manufacturer representative, who explained the benefits to the patient, carer and district nursing service and also the cost that would be incurred to the primary care directorate for feed items not available on prescription (around £1000 a year). Funding was approved and several discussions ensured delivery before discharge.

A visit to the patient's home was planned the week before discharge to ensure all equipment had been delivered, was in the correct position and was working effectively, and that Mrs James was happy about using it.

The liaison officer had frequent meetings with Mrs James during this time in order to provide support and reassurance during such an emotional and stressful period. 6 weeks after discharge Mrs James was coping well with her husband's physical care, and he showed a slight improvement through being at home. She has accepted that she will need to make use of the respite care in the future.

The care package arranged for discharge included the following on a daily basis:

- During the morning visit the district nurse assists with general nursing care, catheter and pressure area care. The nurse assists Mrs James to use the hoist to transfer Mr James out of bed into a chair.
- During the lunchtime visit the community care worker (social services) helps Mrs James transfer Mr James back to bed using the hoist.
- At the teatime visit the community careworker (social services) helps Mrs James transfer Mr James out of bed using the hoist.
- During a late evening visit the district nurse (out-of-hours service) assists Mr James back to bed using the hoist and gives general nursing care as required.

Other care required at assessment included:

- Referral for respite care to the hospital to be arranged following discharge
- Domiciliary physiotherapy each week
- A telephone answering system used to obtain help in an emergency installed before discharge
- Night sitting service (by district nursing service) probably weekly to relieve the carer and enable her to have a full night's rest.
- Laundry service to supply and collect sheets on a weekly basis
- Delivery of gastrostomy feeds and equipment each month.

at home is frequently inadequate and at best patchy. Provision has been criticised as being inflexible, unimaginative and not sensitive to the individual and heterogeneous needs of carers (Allen et al 1983). The district nurse has been described as the 'linchpin and co-ordinator' of community care for the dependent elderly (Wade et al 1983). If this is so, then it is essential that she recognises the support needed by families to continue caring and help with physical tasks, provides information about other services available, and, above all, gives the 'listening kind' of help often most appreciated by carers.

Case study 3.2 demonstrates clearly the need for professionals from many disciplines to work together in order to achieve the best possible care for both the client and the carer.

Summary

This chapter has discussed the changes in community care organisation and their impact on clients and carers. The changes have had a major impact on the way in which professionals work together. The current community care policy has located the family at its hub, and the role of family, friends and neighbours has been stressed increasingly. It is important that health and social care professionals act to support the carers as well as the clients in order to meet the growing need in the community.

REFERENCES

Allen I 1983 The elderly and their informal carers. In: Department of Social Services, Elderly people and their service needs. HMSO, London

Audit Commission 1992a Community care: managing the cascade of change. HMSO, London

Audit Commission 1992b Homeward bound: a new course for community health. HMSO, London

Bornat J, Pereira C, Pilgrim D, Williams F (eds) 1993 Community care: a reader. MacMillan, Basingstoke

Centre for Policy on Ageing 1984 Home life: a code of practice for residential care. Centre for Policy on Ageing, London

Cowley S 1993 Collaboration in health care: the education link. Health Visitor 67(1):13–15

Day P 1985 Regulating the private sector of welfare. Political Quarterly 56(3):282–285

Department of Health 1989 Caring for people: community care in the next decade and beyond. HMSO, London

Department of Health 1990 Care in the community: making it happen. HMSO, London

Department of Health 1994 Regulation of residential care and nursing homes and independent hospitals. HMSO, London

Department of Health and Social Security 1971 Better services for the mentally handicapped. HMSO, London

Department of Health and Social Security 1975 Better services for the mentally ill. HMSO, London

Department of Health and Social Security 1978 Collaboration in community care: a discussion document. Central Health Services Council and Personal Social Services Council, HMSO, London

Department of Health and Social Security 1981a Care in the community. HMSO, London

Department of Health and Social Security 1981b Community care. HMSO, London

Department of Health and Social Security 1981c Care in action. HMSO, London

Department of Health and Social Security 1982 Nurses working in the community. Office of Population Censuses, London

Green H 1988 General household survey 1985: series GHS15A Informal Carers. HMSO, London

Hornby S 1993 Collaborative care: interprofessional, interagency, and interpersonal. Blackwell, Oxford

Hudson B 1987 Collaboration in social welfare: a framework for analysis. Policy and Politics 15(3):175–182

Lightfoot J 1994 Identifying needs and setting priorities: issues of theory policy and practice. Health and Social Care 3:105–114

McWalter G, Toner H, Corser A, Eastwood J 1994 Needs and needs assessment: their components and definitions with reference to dementia. Health and Social Care 2:213–219

Means R, Smith R 1994 Community care: policy and practice. MacMillan, Basingstoke

National Institute for Social Work 1988 Residential care: a positive choice. Report of the independent review of residential care (the Wagner report). HMSO, London

Registered Homes Act 1984 HMSO, London

Sandford J R A 1975 Tolerance of disability in elderly dependants by supporters at home: its significance for hospital practice. British Medical Journal 3:471–473

Social Services Inspectorate/Social Services Group 1991 Assessment systems and community care. HMSO, London

Wade B, Sawyer L, Bell J 1983 Dependency with dignity: different care provision for the elderly. Bedford Square Press, London

Walker 1986 Community care: fact and fiction. In: Wilmott P (ed) The debate about community. PSI, London, pp. 4–15

FURTHER READING

Alderson P 1990 Choosing for children. Oxford University Press, Oxford

Baggot R 1994 Health and health care in Britain. Macmillan, Basingstoke

Bornat J et al 1993 Community care: a reader. Macmillan and Open University Press, Basingstoke

Burnard P, Chapman C M 1993 Professional and ethical
    issues in nursing. The Code of Professional Conduct, 2nd
    edn. Scutari Press, London
Doxiadis S 1987 Ethical dilemmas in health promotion. John
    Wiley, Chichester
Husted G L, Husted J H 1995 Ethical decision making in
    nursing. Mosby, New York

Jensen U J, Mooney G (eds) 1995 Changing values in medical
    and health care decision making. John Wiley, Chichester
Means R, Smith R 1994 Community care: policy and practice.
    Baillière Tindall, London
Richardson J, Webber I 1995 Ethical issues in child health
    care. Mosby, London

The primary health care team

Dominic Blackie

Although the community health care nurse must be aware of the policies and overall organisation that shape primary care services, it is of even more direct relevance to appreciate how that care is actually delivered to people day to day, and why the primary health care team is now so central. To make sense of the complex working environment it is also necessary to be familiar with the operational realities of general practice. Similarly, familiarity with the normal processes involved when a group of individuals attempts to work together as a team is vital for any community practitioner to function effectively. It is necessary therefore to understand:

- The necessity for team work in the community and its potential advantages
- The basic concepts and definitions of the primary health care team
- How the current team structure developed
- The context of teamworking in the organisational environment of general practice
- The fundamental dynamics of teams
- The reasons why teams succeed or fail.

THE NEED FOR TEAM WORK IN PRIMARY CARE

Primary care has been succinctly defined by Starfield (1994) as 'First contact, continuous, comprehensive and co-ordinated care provided to populations undifferentiated by gender, disease or organ system'. This is a Herculean labour, impossible for any one professional group. Clearly an alliance between community services and general practice is required. Some form of primary health care (PHC) team to which both sectors contribute resources is the obvious basis for joint health care provision. Although the PHC team has long been recognised in theory (Ministry of Health 1920) as the optimal way to deliver community based care, NHS events in the first five years of the 1990s have made its existence and successful functioning critical; for example, the tasks of 'Caring for People' (DoH 1989) alone demand that health professionals in the community form effective teams (Dowrick 1992).

On a practical level, too, there is an urgent need for effective teamwork in primary care. All community nurses, however employed and regardless of role, have a very close professional relationship with GPs and their practices: the great majority work with, or for, GPs and increasingly under the same roof. This interdependence is likely to increase as the NHS Management Executive vision of the entire service being directed by the needs of the population as seen from Primary Care is implemented – as set out in the paper 'Towards a Primary Care led NHS' (1995). Familiarity with the general practice 'facts of life' will enable CHCNs to understand the merits and limitations of the current arrangements, and to function more effectively within those constraints.

Although teamwork is necessary, it is undeniably difficult, so it is worth considering the main potential benefits it offers:

- The care given by the team can be greater than the sum of individual episodes
- Rare skills can be made more available
- Continuity of care between professions is encouraged
- Peer influence and informal learning within the team can raise the standard of care
- Team members can have increased job satisfaction and are better supported
- Prevention and curative roles can be more effectively co-ordinated.

Ultimately patients can receive more efficient and holistic care.

THE PRIMARY HEALTH CARE TEAM

BASIC CONCEPTS AND DEFINITIONS

Fundamentally, a PHC team consists of a number of individuals from a variety of professions working together on problems in health and social care which are appropriately handled jointly or interprofessionally.

Above all the PHCT must be meaningful as a day-to-day resource for practising clinicians. It is vital to avoid defining PHC team membership so inclusively that it becomes an exercise in political correctness. On occasion the term PHC team is stretched to include virtually anyone who works in a general practice building! Basic team dynamics means that team size can be critical – too big a team spells trouble. For reasons of utility a team should be as small as possible, so it is most useful to consider the operational, or core, PHC team as health professionals delivering care to patients. Although some definitions of the PHC team include infrequent clinical visitors – for example, audiologists, chiropodists, physiotherapists – in day-to-day *clinical* practice the PHC team means the health visitor (HV), district nurse (DN), practice nurse (PN) and GP.

Other definitions of the PHC team very often include administrative staff – for example, receptionists, practice managers and accountants. Efficient administrative support and a robust managerial framework are certainly central to success and the individuals carrying out this important work are clearly part of the *wider* practice team, but they do not provide *clinical* care on a daily basis. It is therefore useful to distinguish between the *core* PHC team and the *extended* PHC team.

Core PHC team. This refers to those clinicians who work together day by day caring for the same group of patients. An essential skill for the core PHC team is the ability to act autonomously in a *clinical* role and be willing to collaborate in a team approach to relevant problems.

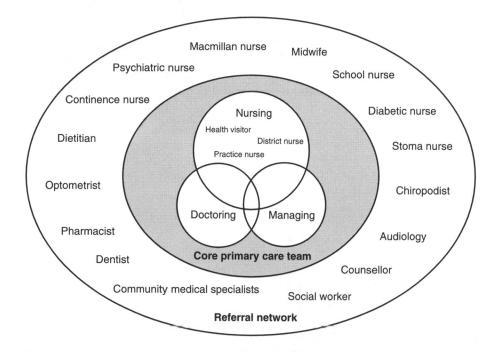

Figure 4.1 Model of PHC team (Thomas 1994)
1. Midwives sometimes fulfil the criteria for membership of the core team
2. Community specialists (nursing or medical) are defined by their skills with special needs groups and by their case mix. They are not alternative clinical generalists because most do not have training which emphasises broadly based clinical competencies
3. Many core team members can relate to the same outer ring of specialists if a clear referral relationship is maintained
4. Social workers must sign a confidentiality agreement with the core group before they can become full PHCT members
5. Public Health medicine provides support to PHCT in relation to health needs assessment
6. Health Commissions support PHCT managerially and often with training

Extended PHC team. Members of this section of the team always include the support staff whose efforts make possible the work of the core PHC team, and sometimes regular visiting practitioners.

Whatever distinctions are made regarding membership of the core or extended team, all members connect with a wider supporting referral network (Fig. 4.1); however, although clearly useful for clinicians to operate within an integrated unit, it is important to appreciate that the large majority of episodes of care will be delivered by one practitioner to one patient. For example, on a typical day in 1992 GPs alone saw 650 000 patients, practice nurses in general practice saw around 110 000 and health visitors and district nurses, combined, saw about 150 000. It follows that most episodes of primary health care in the UK do not involve clinical teamwork.

TEAMWORK MODELS

Multidisciplinary teamwork

Andrews (1987) describes the multidisciplinary team as a group of professionals who each provide their own expertise *irrespective* of the techniques used or the goals set by other team members. This approach could mean that while attending the same terminally ill patient in rotation a DN may advise one approach to symptom relief, the GP another, and the Macmillan nurse something different again. Although this might seem unlikely to happen in practice, it *is* part of the everyday experience of community practitioners. To extend the terminal care example, attitudes to narcotic analgesia vary considerably in relation to when to start it, how much to give, how to deliver it and so on. The multidisciplinary team approach can lead to pointed disagreements between professionals which do nothing to encourage confidence in the patient or her family.

This model partitions the patient into a collection of clinical and social problems (McGrath & Davies 1992) which are then allocated to different professionals, assessed and treated. Using this approach the individual disciplines work alongside each other but essentially independently (Box 4.1). Often a medical model will dominate in this situation.

Despite its limitations the multidisciplinary team model is the approach most commonly adopted by PHC teams as it respects existing role boundaries making it relatively unthreatening for professionals new to teamwork. However, to function effectively even this level of collaboration requires open communication and a decision making process which involves the whole team, not just one or two powerful members. The multidisciplinary team approach also requires of its members the capacity to examine relationships in an honest straightforward manner, and inevitably calls for some 'role blurring', that is, the ability to develop a more fluid conception of individual professional roles and the willingness to learn from others. These requirements are not always easy to ensure.

Box 4.1   Key features of multidisciplinary teamworking

Advantages:

- The disease process is reliably measured which makes evaluation of outcome simpler
- Existing role boundaries are respected so that the expectations of each therapist are clear
- Conceptually easy to grasp for team members, so no major investment in learning new behaviours is required

Limitations:

- Defines the patient in terms of disease processes, for example the diabetic asthmatic versus the lady with asthma and diabetes
- Definition of the patient's problem may be limited to the number of professions available to treat it; some problems 'slip between the cracks', for example, in a team dominated by biophysical therapists the psychological or social aspects may be overlooked

---

Interdisciplinary teamwork

Interdisciplinary teamwork (McGrath & Davies 1992) is a more sophisticated model, capable of delivering true integration between professional groups. Consequently, it has the potential to address those patient problems which are not clearly the province of any one discipline, and which might otherwise go unattended. The essential difference to the multidisciplinary team model is that goal planning involves all team members *structurally*, at formal team meetings, and is explicitly patient centred, focused on what the patient needs rather than what the individual therapist can do (Box 4.2).

To be successful an interdisciplinary team must meet regularly to review progress and make plans (Andrews 1987). It is also essential that each member of the team has an understanding of the techniques being used by others and accepts that there will be some overlapping of roles. On occasion joint consultations with the patient may be useful.

To return to the example of terminal care, an interdisciplinary team would meet regularly to plan a general approach to pain relief and devel-

Box 4.2   **Key features of interdisciplinary teamworking**

Advantages:

- No hierarchy of professions
- The patient is treated holistically
- The practical usefulness of teamwork is much clearer to the patient and may improve involvement and motivation

Limitations:

- Role blurring can be uncomfortable and cause problems
- Requires very highly developed teamworking skills

op a strategy which all involved could feel comfortable with. So if, for example, the DN was attending to carry out an unrelated procedure and it was apparent that the patient was in pain, it would be clear what to do next.

Similarly, if PN, HV, GP and midwife all take the same approach to cervical screening and work together using this model, it is likely that a higher uptake rate can be achieved and death from cancer of the cervix reduced.

True interdisciplinary teamwork which delivers co-ordinated, non-hierarchical holistic care, while actively involving patient and family, is extremely difficult to deliver in practice. Nonetheless, it is perhaps the model of PHC teamwork which should be worked towards.

PHC TEAMWORKING THEORY VERSUS PRACTICE

The concept of the PHC team has, for some health service planners, become the panacea for every problem in the organisation and delivery of care to communities (Marsh 1991). So many reports have supported the idea, and so much discussion has occurred that there has arisen the mythology of universal teamwork in primary care. There is of course usually a big difference between theory and practice, and the PHC team is no exception. Indeed, it has even been argued with some merit (Iliffe 1995) that 'Primary care does not exist, it is an abstract concept invented

by policy experts to describe a patchwork of community services through which people access health services'. If primary care doesn't exist as a functional sector of the NHS, what chance is there for the PHCT? Fortunately for patients and health professionals, the working arrangements experienced by CHCNs do not wholly support Iliffe's view. In the mid-1990s, the typical community nurse can expect to be employed by a community trust and work attached to several general practices, often based in one, as one of a range of nurses (PN, HV, DN) providing care to a group of patients defined by the practice list. Most practices are in a position, notionally at least, to use the PHC team model to deliver care.

However Iliffe's rather extreme position does correctly focus attention on the fragmented organisational arrangements which do not assist team-based delivery of primary care in practice. In order to understand the operational difficulties faced occasionally by all community practitioners, and to appreciate Iliffe's position, it is important to know how the present situation arose and to be aware of the current status of the PHC team.

Origins of the team

Historically, the key providers of health care in the community – HVs, DNs, GPs, school medical services – developed quite separately and consequently had different operating systems. Even so, the idea of teamwork in primary care is not new. It can be traced back at least as far as the Dawson report of 1920 (Ministry of Health 1920) and there were one or two notable examples in the 1930s (Ashton & Seymour 1988). However, there was no potential for teamworking to become a commonplace reality before the creation of the NHS, and even after the NHS came into being in 1948 the hoped for integration of the various basic elements of primary care could not be achieved.

The first practical steps, system-wide, to foster teamwork in primary care were not taken until 1966. Up to this point the fees paid to GPs by the NHS had not recognised the inevitable expenses associated with providing medical services – either support staff or buildings. Consequently, many doctors worked entirely on their own from rooms in their own home – or the cheapest available premises – supported by the apocryphal 'doctor's wife'. Employment of a receptionist was unusual, expensive nurses virtually unheard of. In response to concerns about standards in general practice, as well as to counter falling recruitment, a package of benefits was introduced – the GP Charter. This allowed for 70% reimbursement of ancillary staff costs. This cash incentive gave impetus to the widespread creation of the Mark I PHC team – GP plus administrative support. A few new PNs also appeared at this time, usually the doctor's wife. This first step had no real impact, however, on the relationships between the various community practitioners.

For several decades after the birth of the NHS providers of community health services continued to operate independently, communicating only when absolutely necessary. In fact, until the major NHS reforms of 1974 community units were part of local government not the health service.

After 1974, community services continued to operate in parallel with general practice, and duplication of services was common, for example, family planning, child health surveillance. All the main professions providing services to a given community generated their caseloads from geographical patches or localities.

Organising the delivery of care based on discrete geographical units can be very effective, particularly if the patches relate to an existing, real community. However, they usually appear to be arbitrarily derived from maps. The local authority roots of community nursing meant that their localities were often electoral wards, which usually represented one or more functional communities. The great strength of the system was the direct connection which CHCNs could build up with the community they served.

GPs were free to, and did, recruit patients at random from a very much wider catchment area. As the bulk of GP income has always been capitation-based, once on the list GPs are reluctant to lose patients. Although there has been a gradual tendency to move towards much tighter practice areas in recent years, a radius of several miles from the practice is still the norm. In densely populated urban areas, where there are several practices competing for the same community of patients, each practice area overlaps with many others.

Clearly, the probability of GP and CHCN patches overlapping neatly was extremely remote. Furthermore, the healthcare workers did not usually even share a building – CHCNs operated from NHS-owned purpose built clinics, most GPs from modified houses or shops, often 'privately' owned. This meant that, for example, one HV could be expected to establish a useful working relationship with every GP who had patients in the patch, which not uncommonly meant several practices and maybe 10 or more GPs spread over not less than two sites. Although, of course, individual practitioners made local arrangements to overcome some of the more ridiculous situations, only senior management level initiatives could possibly resolve the problems system-wide.

The Gillie report (1963), whose main recommendation was to promote group practice, was also the first to propose that community nurses should be attached to practices. The suggestion was not implemented with particular enthusiasm. In the mid-1980s, a wide-ranging review of the organisation of community nursing services was undertaken. The result, the Cumberlege report (DHSS 1986), was critical of the community service management structure and recommended many changes.

General practice-based service delivery

Ultimately, to rationalise the framework for the delivery of care, the community service and/or general practice had to revise the way in which catchment populations were defined. Politically the only option available was for the community service to fall into step with general practice. It did this by attaching named community nurses to particular general practices, not to particular GPs (CHCNs worked *with* GPs *for* the practice population). Although CHCNs were the largest professional group operating from the most developed network of facilities and serving real communities, as opposed to random lists of patients, they were obliged to fit in with GPs. The political expediency here was the independent contractor status of GPs; they could not be required to realign according to a centrally determined model.

Attachment did not necessarily imply being physically based in the general practice. Initially many small practices did not have sufficient space to provide a permanent base for attached staff. Although many practices have since created on-site space for attached staff, a significant number have not been prepared to make the investment, particularly in deprived inner city areas (for example, the London Implementation Zone).

The attachment of CHCNs to practices produced the Mark II edition of the PHC team – GP, CHCNs. More importantly, it reinforced the position of the general practice as the basic organisational unit of primary care. This position was further strengthened by the introduction of GP fundholding.

The growing demands placed on primary care by the NHS reforms have produced the current, Mark III version of the PHC team – GP, administrators, CHCNs and PN. In particular, the new GP contract of 1990 emphasised targeted health promotion programmes, chronic disease management clinics, regular health checks, all of which attract payments, and mandatory annual visits to patients over 75. The enormous additional workload for practices, coupled with new cash, caused an explosion in PN numbers. The rapid emergence of practice nursing is both a huge opportunity for community nursing and a threat to the established order. Although Mark III is the current model, it is unlikely to be the final version.

Current status of the PHC team

Wholesale change in the NHS has, in principle, made teamwork easier through the formal attachment of CHCNs to practices and the massive expansion of practice nursing, and more

essential through policy documents such as Caring for People (Department of Health 1989) and The Health of the Nation (Department of Health 1992). A great deal of PHC team facilitation work has been undertaken by health authorities to help the 'teamwork for all' vision to become a reality. It is undeniable that the term PHC team is now generically applied to more or less any group of clinical professionals working in the community for the same population of patients. However, despite all the encouragement from professional bodies and government, the *truly* integrated team is still rare in primary care.

Collaboration between primary care professionals has certainly increased over the years as a result of structural and functional proximity. However, *genuine* teams form under conditions of interdependence. As well as simply sharing the same patient base and facilities, effective clinical teamwork requires shared objectives and involves, according to McWhinney (1989), three behaviours:

- Recognising the strengths and limitations of personal role
- Understanding and valuing other roles
- Communicating sensitively and effectively.

Present to varying degrees in different individuals and valued and promoted during training to a greater or lesser extent by the various professional groups, these key behaviours are not always sufficiently practised to make teamwork effective. Developing teamwork is an active process demanding leadership, commitment and time. Often, the general practice-based PHC team functions only as a network, important for information exchange rather than co-ordinating care. Although harnessing the behaviour of the various individuals is invariably a challenge for any team, the key factor inhibiting genuine teamwork in many GP-based PHC teams is the nature of the structural relationship between doctors and all other team members. Drury (1988) observed that 'One thing that can be said for certain about teamwork in primary care is that there is not a lot of it about'. Despite real progress, the

---

Box 4.3   Qualities of the effective PHC team

1. Members are more generalist than specialist. Flexibility of response is achieved through an overlapping skills mix
2. Members work on a daily basis from a common centre – informal contacts enhance communication
3. A broad range of medical and nursing skills is available
4. Common healthcare objectives are shared and made explicit
5. Staff stability is the norm so that personal relationships with the community are steady
6. Core team size is 3 to 12 people
7. The team as an operational unit must be its own manager in relation to its specific work

---

widespread operation of genuine functional PHC teams remains some way off.

The future PHC team

The constitution of the PHC team in the future is uncertain because needs differ in various locations, and because the NHS itself is in flux. Its local composition should be determined by a consideration of the qualities of the effective PHC team (Box 4.3). These characteristics are likely to mean that clinical generalists (nursing and medical) will continue to be the core of the team supported by a practice manager and reception staff.

One probably desirable additional component to these qualities is 'one management structure for all members of the team'. Given the power of GPs the way this is likely to occur is through practice-employed integrated nursing teams. This could help solve the problem of so much specialisation in nursing. (Figure 4.1 on page 57 includes 10 different community nursing specialties.) Some professionals feel that under current GP contractual arrangements it would be inappropriate for community nursing to be taken over by GPs.

Hasler (1994) described one vision of the twenty-first century PHC team:

Organisations will come to resemble clover leaves. A care team, generally made up of professionals, is the essential element which drives the activities forward. Not all the work is done by care workers: some of it is contracted out to others. The third component is the part-time labour force that can expand or contract as demands change.

A list of 8000 in the next century might be cared for by a team of around four or five doctors and 10 to 11 nurses. Some doctors and nurses will be part-time: some will be partners, some self employed under contract and some employees. The average list size per doctor will be higher than in the mid-1990s but because of the large proportion of work done by nurses (many of whom will be graduates) consultations will be longer than now. A higher percentage of patients than now will consult the nurses directly, and nurses will do most of the prevention and long-term disease monitoring. Rigid divisions between the various nursing activities will have gone. Nurses will work with doctors to provide out-of-hours work, which will be largely based on central treatment areas.

The practice will have a clear strategy and each individual will have a personal development plan. Regular meetings where everyone can contribute will be held and audits demonstrating quality of care will be published regularly. Morale will be high.

This is only one version of the future of PHC teamworking, but it does represent the vision of some influential practitioners. Many elements are beginning to happen already and in the medium to long term many of the changes indicated will probably happen in some form. Hasler's suggestions will appear radical to some and tame to others, for example, the increasing overlap between medicine and nursing. Reliance on a part time workforce which can expand or contract could lead to casualisation of professional work and place healthcare professionals in the ranks of seasonal workers. This pattern is perhaps already being established: in 1992 there were 13 320 whole time equivalent bank nurses compared with only 11 050 in 1987, an increase of 20% in just 5 years (Nursing Standard 6.4.94). The career instability this can cause is likely to be profoundly damaging to morale and is advantageous only to managers and accountants. Ultimately, professionals and the public are notoriously conservative in their response to health system changes and these limiting factors are likely to delay the rate of change.

The other major factor will be cost. Hasler's

(1994) assumption must be that the new order will be cheaper, or at least no more expensive. Recent work comparing costs of nurse and GP consultations shows that nurses are actually more expensive because they take much longer. It is extremely unlikely that changes which increase per capita primary care costs will be politically acceptable whatever the proposed quality dividend.

TEAMWORK IN PRACTICE

GENERAL PRACTICE: THE CORNERSTONE OF PRIMARY CARE

Although always centrally important to the operation of an effective national health system, general practice was seen principally as the gateway to specialist services. The acceptance in the 1980s that attachment of CHCNs to general practice was inevitable despite its organisational inadequacies, confirmed it as the basic operational unit for the delivery of care to communities. Fundholding has extended the influence of GPs still further and reaffirmed the general practice as the basic organisational unit of the new primary care, and thus of the NHS.

Given the symbiotic relationship between community nursing and general practice it is important for the CHCN to be aware of the dynamics of the typical general practice. This will assist in understanding some of the more puzzling situations encountered when working with GPs, as well as the serious obstacles the current system raises to effective PHC team-based delivery of services.

The most important organisational consideration for GPs is their contractual relationship with the NHS (see Ch. 2). Technically GPs are self-employed physicians engaged by the NHS via health commissions to provide the range of services laid down in the new GP contract (1990). Likewise the organisations through which they provide services – the general practice – although entirely NHS funded (directly and indirectly), are not technically part of the NHS. The premises and contents belong to the GPs and the staff are employed directly by the doctors. Each general practice is, therefore, an 'independent', privately run business. Although this 'independence' is essentially manufactured (GPs are entirely dependent on the NHS as a market for their services), the concept has been fiercely defended by GPs as a means of minimising managerial 'interference' in organisational and financial matters.

Independent contractor status means that, whether they like it or not, on one level GPs and their practices are obliged to function as small businesses. They must concern themselves with partnership agreements, income and profit, competition with similar 'businesses', etc. (Box 4.4). Perhaps the most important point to grasp is that GPs in a practice partnership do not have a guaranteed income. A GP's pay is the share of practice income from fees and allowances left after expenses have been met. The size of the share is negotiable between partners. It is this fundamental difference from other NHS clinicians which can make GPs appear intransigent at times to other health professions.

The degree of financial unpredictability created by this system acts as both benign and perverse incentive, that is, although good at controlling costs, it can tempt some GPs to adopt a commercial rather than a public service ethos.

Box 4.4   Independent contractor status

Problems with ICS for the NHS and GPs include:

- Strategic management of the GP sector is extremely difficult, for example:
  - ensuring equity of service provision in 'difficult' areas
  - developing the role of practice nursing
- Coverall GP contract without explicit performance standards means:
  - underperformance is a matter of opinion, so dealing with problem practices is very difficult
  - unlimited personal 24-hour liability of GP for primary medical services
- Conflict of interest between 'practice profits' and service quality:
  - individual GPs are forced into an invidious position of balancing personal income with practice and service development
  - the less spent on services, facilities and staff the higher the GP's wages
  - this creates a powerful perverse incentive which can reduce quality

> **Box 4.5   Main requirements of the 1990 GP contract (Department of Health 1989)**
>
> 1. Doctors should render services to patients accepted on their lists to include:
>   - Health advice
>   - Consultations
>   - Vaccinations
>   - Referrals
> 2. Additionally they may provide:
>   - Contraceptive services
>   - Child health surveillance
>   - Minor surgery
>   - Maternity medical services
> 3. Consultations for screening should be offered:
>   - To new patients
>   - To those patients not seen within 3 years
>   - Yearly to patients aged 75 and over
> 4. GPs are required to:
>   - Keep adequate records
>   - Issue prescriptions
>   - Prepare practice leaflets
>   - Prepare annual reports

In reality there are very few full-time GPs who make less than so-called intended net remuneration (£45 000 in 1996). The more common problem thrown up by the system is underinvestment in various aspects of the practice to raise 'profits'.

The GP contract

Notwithstanding certain minimum standards (particularly with respect to hours of availability, premises and the provisions of national legislation applying to health and safety at work), as independent contractors GPs are free to organise themselves any way they choose to provide the services expected of them. Various factors restrict the range of practical options and inducement is given to encourage certain organisational traits such as employment of support staff, use of computers, and type of premises. In addition there are rules related to where a practice may be set up and maximum list size per GP. Perhaps the most important choice facing a GP is whether to work alone or in partnership with other GPs.

Partnerships

The majority of GPs in the UK work in groups of 3 or 4, a few in groups of 7 or more, and a large minority are still in single-handed practice.

A general practice partnership is a legal entity bound by a partnership agreement. Agreements cover such issues as profit shares, ownership of property, and so on. They are not policed or externally refereed and new partners must negotiate for themselves to obtain a fair deal. Partnership breakdown is not at all rare, while dysfunctional partnerships are as common as bad marriages – for many of the same reasons.

The list

General practice partnerships contract with their local health commission to provide services to a particular group of patients, universally referred to as 'the list'. Most general practice lists are simply random collections of individuals and families within a very broad geographic area who over the years have either chosen a particular doctor or practice or have been 'inherited' by remaining GPs when a colleague relinquishes a list. The most important factor in patient choice of a practice is location (Salisbury 1989). Provided the practice is close at hand, patients are known to be loyal and uncritical of their GPs.

Patients are free to move between GPs, but the uniquely valuable feature of the UK system is that their medical record follows them to their new GP. This means that for every UK citizen there is a single 'cradle to grave' medical record. This is the optimal way of keeping medical data, having many advantages for patient and health system, but is unusual world-wide and nowhere else as efficient as in the UK.

GPs are free to accept or reject applicants. More controversially, GPs are free to remove patients from their list without explanation, provided only that they are not in need of acute treatment at the time. 'Unpopular' patients are 'allocated' to a new GP by the health commission and the practice must then provide services for a minimum of 3 months.

The average list size in the UK is around 1750. This varies widely, in inner city areas sometimes being very much higher, principally because of difficulties in recruiting GPs and 'entrepreneurial' GPs. Lists as large as 4000 people are 'cared for' by one GP while 'looking for' a replacement partner. Curiously, FHSAs have been remarkably slow to act on behalf of patients in such circumstances, even though they have a duty of care and the powers to remove patients in excess of 2500. The list size per GP determines the income of the GP.

Practice area

General practices are not bound to strict geographical patches when it comes to recruiting patients. Provided patients live within a 'reasonable' distance of the practice and that the address is within the boundaries of a health commission with which the GP has a contract to provide services, they may join the list. 'Reasonable distance' simply means the distance from which the patient is prepared to travel and at which the doctor is prepared to guarantee visits. This can cause problems for attached CHCNs. In particular, HVs may be frustrated to find that a high dependency family have moved miles away to a new estate, but the GP has agreed to keep them on the list. More organised practices are moving towards high density practices, which have compact population areas, to facilitate access to the service as well as PHC teamwork.

Practice income

The large bulk of a practice income is from NHS activity. Broadly speaking, in 1997 intended gross income to the practice is about £100 000 per full-time GP per year, of which some £45 000 p.a. is intended net remuneration. The remainder covers practice running costs.

Patient related income

Capitation and deprivation payments. These fees represent about two-thirds of total NHS income. The underlying idea is that since the amount paid is fixed it is in the doctor's best interest to maintain a healthy population. Annual fees vary

Table 4.1 Payments to GP per patient registered July 1996

Capitation payments		Deprivation payments	
Basic – All GPs, All patients		Paid according to Jarman Index	
Under 65	£15.35	High	£10.75
65–74	£20.30	Medium	£8.05
75+	£39.25	Low	£6.20
New Registrations Per new patient		£6.80	
Child health surveillance Per child (0–5) registered		£11.15	
Payment made for each child whose parent signs a form agreeing to attend GP rather than trust clinic. Whether the work is done by the GP and to what standard is not monitored. The child can still attend trust clinics.			

depending on the patient's age – older people create more work (Table 4.1). In some areas deemed 'deprived' – as determined by the Jarman Index – additional payments are made. The idea of weighted capitation is to allow GPs with difficult caseloads – for example providing services to an elderly population in a deprived inner city – to maintain high standards by having a smaller than average list size while still achieving an income comparable with colleagues operating a rather bigger list in an 'easier' location. Unfortunately no explicit performance standards are linked to capitation payments, which is particularly worrying with respect to deprivation. In many inner city settings it is possible to operate a very large list of highly deprived patients, and to receive equally large deprivation payments. Some practices have such high capitation and deprivation payments that they are immune to the quality enhancing effects of the various target programmes.

Item of service payments. Some services currently offered have been added since the original agreements were made as to what was covered by basic capitation (Table 4.2). For example, contraceptive services are seen as non-core and therefore attract an extra fee. Income from health promotion activity has formed a separate catego-

Table 4.2 Item of service

Average claims per patient 1994/95	
Health promotion	1.46
Maternity services	1.47
Night visits	1.26
Contraceptive services	0.99
Minor surgery	0.53
Other	1.61
Total per patient	7.62

Table 4.3 Chronic disease management clinic fees

Payment is made simply for providing the clinic	
Asthma	£380
Diabetes	£380
The fee stated is for the average list – 1 April 1996	

ry since 1996 with an annual figure being paid by the health commission to the practice, if the plan is approved. The amount is £2200/average list of 1750 patients, which alone is enough to pay the 30% proportion of the nursing salary which the typical practice is required to find per GP per year.

Targets. Childhood vaccinations and cervical cytology programmes have long been promoted in general practice by payment of a fee for each completed test or course of vaccine. Two big changes were made in the new contract of 1990:

- The potential income available was increased (and became much more important to overall practice finances).
- To qualify for any payment a hurdle has to be jumped – one patient short of a target and either no money or only the lower fee is paid.

The idea was to use motivational methods from industry to breathe new life into important public health programmes which in some areas had stalled. Equally important was to raise the profile of preventive measures in a service which has traditionally focused on curative measures. For every 1750 patients a typical practice in 1995 could gain £2900 for higher target performance in childhood vaccinations and a further £2500 for similar achievement in cervical cytology. Lower performance offered only £1800 for both.

Chronic disease management. To promote better management of asthma and diabetes and to move the locus of care from hospital to community, a fee is available to those practices providing specific clinics for these conditions

(Table 4.3). Most such clinics are run by practice nurses.

Income not directly patient related

Basic practice allowance. A fee independent of list size is paid for each GP. In 1996 this was £7200 per full-time principal.

Staff reimbursement. Staff costs are the biggest expense for most partnerships. Prior to the 1990 contract the deal was that each full-time GP could employ up to two full-time support staff at Whitley council rates and the NHS would directly fund 70% of the salary (but not pension) costs. Practices could always employ more staff but would not attract 70% reimbursement. Even with this generous inducement, in 1994 the average GP employed just over one whole time equivalent staff member, despite the marginal expense to the practice.

The new contract changed the rules. The level of reimbursement for staff is now negotiable up to 100%. Existing arrangements have generally been frozen, but the health commissions will be able to exercise some discretion as new staff are appointed. For example, to facilitate a useful project 100% funding may be given.

Postgraduate education allowance. A fee of £2260 per year is paid to each full time GP to support continuing professional development.

Computer expenses. Prior to 1990 50% of computer expenses were met directly by the NHS. Now, discretion similar to staff costs applies. Computer expenses related to fundholding are met 100%.

Seniority. There are three levels of seniority payments to GPs which are intended to recognise the accumulation of skills but are not linked to explicit performance criteria or reaccreditation. Payments range from £445 to £5015 per year.

Fundholding. Fundholding is intended to be cost neutral to practices with various management allowances available. It is certainly not meant to increase practice profits and there is some evidence that fundholding GPs actually take home less pay than their non-fundholding colleagues.

Premises related income

If a practice rents approved accommodation, for example a trust-owned health centre, the entire cost of the rent is met by the health commission. Rent is therefore not a consideration for the practice. In all cases operational expenses (utilities, maintenance) come from practice profits.

If a practice owns (or is buying, building or modifying) premises the NHS meets the mortgage interest payments (100% for new build, 60% for conversions) under the cost rent scheme. If and when the notional rental value of the site exceeds the mortgage payments (or the mortgage is paid off), the practice can choose to receive the notional rent instead of the lower cost rent.

The detailed operation of the scheme is hugely complicated but is essentially this:

1. The NHS buys the building, but pays rent to the GP forever
2. The GP owns the building, effectively at no cost, and may sell it when leaving.

The GP can profit in two ways:

1. The excess of notional rent over actual costs is available as yearly profit
2. Increased market value (including that made possible through use of fundholding savings to improve the real estate) can be harvested at retirement.

Non-general medical service (GMS) income

Most GPs seek additional income through various sessional jobs to supplement the NHS basic intended income of £45 000. Insurance medicals (DHSS and private), teaching (nursing and med-ical students, GP registrars), forensic medical examiner, medical director of nursing home are some possible roles. One session per week is worth about £5000 p.a.

The general practitioner

Training, postgraduate education and current workforce

Doctors wishing to enter general practice (about 50% of all graduates) are required to complete a minimum 3-year period of approved training following the houseman year before being eligible to practise as an unrestricted principal. The time is composed of 2 more years of hospital-based training, followed by 1 year as a GP registrar in a training practice.

The 2 years in hospital must be spent in a mix of specialties of general relevance to family medicine. Most registrars try to include paediatrics, obstetrics and gynaecology, psychiatry and accident and emergency as a minimum. Apart from these general guidelines there is no mandatory programme of experience required by all GPs.

The year in practice ideally comes when hospital experience is complete, but can happen any time in the process; therefore not all GP registrars are equally experienced when in the practice setting.

At the end of the training period, the registrar must have obtained 'certificates of satisfactory completion' of training posts. This means that in the opinion of the supervising principal or consultant the registrar seemed to perform adequately. It is extremely uncommon for registrars to be refused certificates. Unlike nursing and all other medical specialties, compulsory final examination is yet to be implemented.

It would be reasonable to suggest that membership of the Royal College of General Practice (MRCGP) should be mandatory, in common with other medical specialties. This is the policy of the College and the National Association of Health Authorities and Trusts (NAHAT 1994). Most registrars choose to take membership in order to enhance their opportunities. However mandatory summative assessment has been fiercely resisted by a section of the profession because it points towards the eventual introduction of explicit performance standards and periodic re-accreditation for established GPs: a threatening prospect for certain sections of the profession. It is justified on the basis of defending the important principle of self-regulation.

The principle of summative assessment was conceded in 1995, provided that the exam was not the MRCGP. Implementation of the decision was delayed over a dispute about who should pay for the administration of the new exam (Hayden 1996).

Once the training period is over, and having identified a suitable vacancy, the doctor is able to apply to join the list of general medical practitioners contracted to a health authority (Box 4.6). Most GPs are fully trained at age 28–30 and are likely to spend the next 30 or 35 years practising family medicine. There are no further requirements to undergo training or ongoing education although postgraduate education is encouraged by the payment of a fee, Postgraduate education allowance (or PGEA), up to £2260 per year. This is available for those GPs able to produce certificates to prove that they have attended the equivalent of 5 days' education in the previous year. Postgraduate sub-deans vet the outlines of proposed courses but standards remain variable.

The practice administrative team

Practices are supported administratively by a group of clerical and 'managerial' staff.

The practice manager. Generally, the individual designated practice manager is in fact the practice administrator, since the GPs themselves will inevitably decide practice policy, in particular maintaining tight control of financial and personnel details. However, this is still a key role as a good practice manager is vital for an effective PHC team. Their contribution, actual and potential, is often undervalued by clinicians and truncated by GPs.

Main duties include general management of the practice staff, premises, health authority returns (sending in claims for fees for general medical services and so on), operation of practice-based complaints procedure (mandatory since 1996), overseeing smooth operation of the appointment system and patient liaison.

The receptionist. Simply listing the main duties of a receptionist fails to reveal the tremendous importance to the post of personal qualities. The receptionist is the public face of the practice and can ensure the success (or otherwise) of, for example, a vaccination programme. In this way they can be of direct importance to patients' health. Moreover, the local knowledge of most receptionists is invaluable at PHC team meetings.

Main duties include the reception of visitors,

Box 4.6 Current medical workforce in GP (BMA 1996)

The medical workforce in UK family medicine is composed of:

- 32 000 fully trained GPs, otherwise called unrestricted principals
- 1800 GP registrars
- 630 assistants (doctors employed by practices, not partners)
- 160 restricted principals (GPs with a limited responsibility, that is, providing services to a specific population)

Box 4.7 Basic employment options for CHCNs

- Trust employed
  - Community clinic based: school nurses, family planning, a few HVs/DNs
  - GP attached: health visitors, district nurses (the large majority)
- GP employed
  - Directly: practice nurses: all; HV's and DNs: very few, but likely to increase*
  - Indirectly*: health visitors, district nurses: about 50%

* As fundholders become more adept at managing resources more will choose to provide 'in-house' alternatives to trust-provided CHCN services (i.e. HVs and DNs)
** Via fundholding contracts practices pay trusts for attached CHCNs. This establishes virtually an employer–employee relationship between doctor and nurse

operation of appointment, telephone and filing systems, processing repeat prescriptions, dealing with requests for visits, processing mail, and basic secretarial work.

The fund manager. If the practice is fundholding there is an extra 'manager' who co-ordinates the paperwork involved in tracking contracts and expenditure. In smaller practices this will be a part-time position and the responsibilities of fund administration are sometimes added to the existing work of the practice manager.

Other personnel. The core staff listed above will be found in all but the smallest practices, where all of the administrative functions may be undertaken by a senior receptionist with perhaps a part-time assistant. Larger practices, particularly fundholders, may employ more specialised administrative staff, for example a data entry clerk, call/recall clerk, computer systems manager, audiotypist and so on. The ethos and scale of most practices, however, means that most people do more than one job.

Implications of NHS reforms for delivery of care

The impact of the reforms (discussed in Ch. 2) at practice level for CHCNs has mainly been produced by GP fundholding. Although so far this has not significantly affected day-to-day work patterns it has indirectly made about 50% of HVs and DNs employees of general practices. In effect, rather than working *with* GPs many now work *for* them. Some GP fundholders already directly employ all community nurses in the PHC team.

The new fluidity within the NHS means that the CHCNs have a new set of opportunities. Many PNs already routinely manage chronic diseases such as asthma and diabetes, as well as running women's health programmes, traditionally carried out exclusively by physicians. It is likely that the role, responsibilities and status of nurses in primary care will continue to grow.

For perhaps the majority of primary care clinicians the most serious implication of the reforms is the impact on equity (Box 4.8).

Box 4.8   Fundholding and equity

Equity is one of the founding principles of the NHS. Fundholding has the capacity to undermine equitable distribution of health care in several ways:

- Favouring one group of patients over another regardless of clinical need
- Redirecting funds from deprived areas to more affluent areas through open and hidden administrative costs
- Administratively 'better' practices attracting resources at the expense of 'weaker' units
- Retention of 'surplus' funds may promote:
  - further transfer of costs to patients, for example medication, causing increased non-compliance in low income groups
  - substitution of generalist for specialist care inappropriately
  - encouragement of enrolment in private health insurance schemes, so saving referral costs and reducing the critical pressure exerted on the NHS by more affluent patients
- No formal requirement to follow public health agendas when making purchasing decisions
- Creation of controlling institutions that serve the interests of a professional group (GPs) and exclude public influence – mergers between Fundholders could produce mini-Health Authorities controlled by GPs, where there is no prospect of institutionalised public influence or control

---

Current organisational structure in general practice: a critique

Many factors combine to make GPs the arbiters of organisational culture within practices. For CHCNs, especially PNs, physician domination can restrict autonomy and often limits the contribution which nursing professionals are permitted to make. These factors are important to the understanding of the roots of much day-to-day frustration and for full awareness of the potential implications for nurses and nursing of shifting contracts to practice level.

At practice level

The practice is now the basic organisational unit of primary care. Independent contractor status ensures that virtually all decision making power is invested in GPs, who directly or indirectly employ everyone else. Even in the most progressive practices managers, nurses, administrative staff and patients are unable to materially influence the service unless given authority by the GP. Despite the new GP contract of 1990, the fundamental nature of the arrangement between GPs and the NHS remains the same. In fact, fundholding has made GPs even more powerful. Non-medical health professionals employed by or attached to general practice-based PHC teams are effectively powerless.

The status of GPs system-wide

The most problematic authority conferred on GPs by independent contractor status is the power not only to decide on the day-to-day details of service provision but more importantly to determine service development priorities. Individual GPs make development decisions for their practices for their own reasons, which do not have to be made clear to the public, regardless of whether they serve any wider public health agenda or indeed are led by health needs at all. Chapter 2 raised the concern that in the 'new NHS', there is no guarantee that the sum of multiple purchasing decisions will add up to an appropriate pattern of service provision. In just the same way the likelihood that the disconnected development decisions made by over 8000 independent small businesses will produce the optimal primary care system for the British people in the next century is remote.

Co-ordination of GP services by local and national public health planners, explicit national, contractually enforceable performance goals and a clinical reaccreditation process are the three elements of quality control necessary to regulate general practice. Although not appropriately supported by the current system, health authorities and trusts have inherited the responsibility for strategic management and quality control in the primary care sector. Independent contractor status ensures that this responsibility has always been, and still is, particularly difficult.

The financial structure of general practice

Independent contractor status can either be viewed as a good example of performance-related pay or an unethical system of 'piece work' driven by conflict of interest. Although it has been notably unsuccessful at providing uniformly high standards of family medical services it has been particularly effective in one dimension – control of costs. Although for many years GP spending was not cash limited, cost per head of population was always a fraction of that delivered by the cash limited hospital sector, and rose less rapidly. Much of the difference is of course inevitable – comparing treatment costs between community and hospital sectors is like comparing apples and oranges. However, the simplistic notion that lower per capita costs in general practice must reflect greater financial efficiency has become a central tenet of 'new NHS' thinking. The deeply flawed financial and

---

Box 4.9 Power resources used at practice level

The extent to which A has influence over B is determined by the resources at A's disposal, B's dependency on those resources and B's alternatives. What are some of the resources which B might perceive A to have that would be important to B's decisions?
French & Raven's (1960) classic analysis suggests the following six categories of power resources:

1. *Rewards:*
   higher salary, better terms of employment
2. *Punishment:*
   reduce perks, impose unpleasant tasks, terminate employment
3. *Information:*
   'she knows something I don't . . .'
4. *Legitimacy:*
   B feels A has the right to make this request due to the hierarchy or precedent
5. *Expertise:*
   B feels that A is qualified to make the request
6. *Referent Power:*
   B admires A's personal qualities and is predisposed to acquiesce

There is a structural imbalance of power between professions at practice level. Although the GP can control any of the above, CNs must rely on 4, 5 and 6. The first two power resources generally trump all the others. This explains why a GP who is not respected for professional expertise or personal qualities can dominate a PHCT

contractual GP model provided conservative politicians of the 1980s with much of the conceptual basis for the 'new' NHS, that is:

- Link professional and personal income directly
- Tolerate vague implicit standards of performance while measuring 'manufactured' indices
- Allow notional independence from central control.

Unfortunately, as well as any benefits this model may offer, the problems associated with it – lack of accountability, conflict of interest, perverse incentives, maintenance of standards and loss of strategic control – which have retarded UK primary care for half a century will now come to haunt the rest of the NHS.

Ultimately, the system operates at practice level, it is here that the inherent conflict of interest occurs and is most visible to CHCNs. Two centrally important aspects of the current financial system put pressure on the GP's personal and professional roles:

- The GP's personal income is not clearly identified – the various fees, allowances, target and deprivation payments which make up practice income are paid together in one block; *whatever is not spent supporting the service can be kept as pay*
- Fees and so on are determined nationally – the sums paid reflect national average expenses, *not* actual practice specific expenditure.

Put very basically, the less a GP spends on service development and running the practice the higher the personal income.

Box 4.10 Parallels between general practice and the 'new NHS'

- 'Independent' service providers competing for business
- Money following patients
- The encouragement of 'efficiency' through establishing concrete links between performance and personal/institutional financial well-being
- Higher income
- Insecurity

This is more a criticism of the system than of individuals. Doctors are placed in an invidious situation, trying to balance the conflicting demands of personal and professional responsibilities. The impact of this potential conflict of interest cannot be overstated.

Workforce gender

Medical schools now produce equal numbers of male and female graduates. Statistics relating to appointments to GP training schemes and as principals show a small excess of females in recent years. This has taken several decades to achieve. Consequently, women doctors are still very much outnumbered by male colleagues (Fig. 4.2).

Furthermore, the majority of women are under 40 and many are part-time. Consequently, as a group women GPs are much less influential than their increasing numbers seem to suggest. Within individual practices too, young part-time female GPs are often treated as decidedly junior partners.

If the ratio of men to women in general practice is at last changing (it was around 2.5:1 in 1994) the same is certainly not true of community nursing. By far the majority of CHCNs are female.

From a gender perspective, general practice operates a profoundly retarded organisational model – high status, unaccountable, male auto-

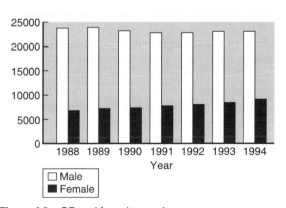

Figure 4.2 GP workforce by gender.

crats controlling large groups of disempowered women.

Critique summary

There is much to celebrate about general practice. The best UK general practices are the equal of any in the world and have always been more cost effective than most which operate at the highest level. Moreover, the UK system of universal registration of every citizen with a personal physician gives rise to the unique resource of a 'cradle to grave' medical record which is always available when the patient presents. These two principles originate in the UK and should form part of any rational primary care system. The average practice provides a broadly satisfactory level of service and an acceptable base for attached CHCNs.

However, because of the various organisational inadequacies, from the perspective of the population's health general practice is ill-equipped to become the foundation of a reconfigured health service, since the quality of medical care provided is so variable and so difficult to change. Although this may be a logical objection to the notion of a primary care-led NHS, political imperatives from both right and left combine with professional ambition to promote this policy option (Iliffe 1995).

TEAMWORK THEORY

It is important to consciously recognise that most teams are disparate groups of human beings brought together by circumstance and professional necessity. Effective teams do not just happen. The disparate group who form the typical PHC team will not spontaneously transform into a high-performing team simply because they should. Assuming that all prospective team members are competent at their particular role, there are four key determinants of success:

- Composition
- Size
- Leadership
- Time.

TEAM COMPOSITION
The Apollo team

Belbin (1981) is responsible for the best known work on the importance of team composition. Initially, he put together 'Apollo teams' composed exclusively of the brightest and the best from other teams. Surprisingly, they frequently came last in terms of performance. Too much time was spent in debate and not enough on carrying out the task. Belbin also found that poor results were produced when a team was made up of people with similar personality types. Further work enabled Belbin to produce his now classic analysis of preferred team roles.

Belbin's work indicates that in order to be successful, a PHC team not only must have all the relevant clinical skills but should be composed of individuals with a broad range of personal traits and preferred group roles. Table 4.4 summarises Belbin's (1993) categorisation of preferred roles within teams. It is not the only model but it is widely recognised as being useful. An individual may be a composite, or may have a different role preference in different teams. In a small group, individuals will have to be capable of more than one role if the team is to function.

Unless an appropriate balance is achieved the conflicts created will hamper effectiveness and may even break up the team. The other avoidable problem is the team with too many like-thinking individuals. Although it is certainly pleasant for colleagues to like each other personally, agree on fundamentals and be generally supportive, too much cohesiveness and homogeneity can be stifling.

The danger of 'groupthink'

The principal danger facing very close teams is the tendency towards oversimplified decision making – so-called 'groupthink'. Groupthink occurs when too high a priority is given to maintaining harmony and morale. Loyalty to the team's previous policies, or to the group consensus, overrides the conscience of each member. 'Concurrence-seeking' drives out the realistic appraisal of alternatives. No bickering or conflict

Table 4.4	Belbin's team roles	
Role	Definition	Characteristics
Co-ordinator (chairman)	The team controller	Calm, self-confident, controlled
Shaper	The slave driver	Highly strung, outgoing, dynamic
Plant	The source of original solutions	Individualistic, serious-minded, unorthodox
Monitor–evaluator	The analyser of problems	Sober, unemotional, prudent
Resource–investigator	The creative negotiator	Extroverted, enthusiastic, curious, communicative
Implementer (company worker)	The effective organiser	Conservative, dutiful, predictable
Team worker	The internal teamwork facilitator	Socially-oriented, rather mild, sensitive

is allowed to spoil the cosy 'we-feeling' of the group. So even the brightest, most highly motivated and well-intentioned team can get into deep water.

Team size and group interaction

Most people know from personal experience that a team can be either too small or too big. This intuition is borne out by research. In the drive towards the 'new' primary care based on the super-PHC team there is a danger that this simple truth will be overlooked or its importance underestimated. This would be particularly unfortunate because, of all the variables affecting team performance, it is the easiest to get right. The best known work on small group interaction was done by Bales & Cohen (1979) using the SYMLOG approach, a System for Multiple Level Observation of Groups. One study using the system analysed the interactions of groups ranging from two to seven people (Bales & Borgatta 1956). The findings indicated that very small groups show more tension, agreement and asking for opinion, while larger groups show more tension release, as well as giving of suggestions and information. It appears that in small groups an emphasis is placed on everyone getting on well together and people having time to develop their ideas and arguments. In larger groups, getting on is not such a priority and team member behaviour becomes more directive.

Interestingly, there is evidence that groups with an even number of members behave differently from groups with an odd number of members. The even-numbered groups have greater difficulty in obtaining a majority, and there is more tension, antagonism and disagreement.

Slater (1958) later confirmed Bales' findings but extended the research to include member satisfaction. He found an interesting relationship between group size and satisfaction. Participants in his study were most satisfied when working in a team of five. Although the actual number five was to some extent a function of the task involved in the experimental situation, the reasons subjects gave for choosing it are more generally applicable. It also happens to be the size of the suggested clinical core PHC team – DN, HV, PN, GP, and manager. Smaller teams were found to be tense and non-direct, while larger groups failed to allow time for everyone to speak. Slater summarised that very small groups provide physical freedom with psychological restrictions, while larger groups are physically restricting but psychologically less tense.

Team size and effectiveness

The relationship between team size and performance is largely dependent on the nature of the task. In the PHC team, where performance depends on the quality of the group's interaction, the addition of new members will become increasingly less beneficial. With each new member the contribution of extra skills and knowledge to the existing pool becomes less significant, while the difficulty of co-ordinating team efforts increases. At some point the co-ordination problems will begin to outweigh the gains in skill and knowledge until further increases in team size may actually worsen performance (Yetton & Bottger 1983).

One of the great strengths of teamwork is the choice it provides about how to undertake a piece of work, for example who should be involved in setting up a new clinic. However, too much choice can give rise to a situation referred to as 'option paralysis'. In this there are simply so many possibilities that the individual or organisation is unable to move beyond the basic decision making stage.

The maths of team interaction

Subgroups. Table 4.5 demonstrates that with a team of only four people there are at least 11 different ways of tackling a job. Even this number assumes that those not present in the main subgroup are not active, that is, where groups of three are listed the possible member not included is neither supporting nor opposing the activities of the main group.

If the members not included in the main subgroup are actively 'doing their own thing' or forming other subgroups, the number of possibilities is much greater. With a subgroup size of two it is clearly possible to have two independent, or even opposing, subgroups. Perhaps most significantly the basic maths begins to indicate the great number of potential relationships and shifting factions which can arise within even a small group. With so many ways to interact it is easy to see how team relationships can rapidly become dysfunctional. The possibility of subgroup formation increases very rapidly with each additional team member (Table 4.6).

Table 4.5 How many ways can a team of four work?

Group size	Possible group membership	Number of variations
4	ABCD	1
3	ABC, ABD, ACD, BCD	4
2	AB, AC, AD, BC, BD, CD	6
Minimum number of possible ways for a team of four to work on a task		11

Table 4.6 Subgroups

Group size	Possible groups and subgroups
2	1
3	4
4	11
5	24
6	48

Lines of communication. Another way of looking at the complexity of team interactions is to calculate the number of lines of communication. This can be expressed as $(n^2-n)/2$, where n is the size of the team. For example, a team of four has six lines of communication, a team of 12 has 66 and a team of 15 has 105 lines of communication. If 10 minutes per week are spent on each channel the time costs are considerable.

Solving the size problem

The army solves the problem of maintaining cohesive units despite massive size by imposing tight hierarchies and strict line management. The PHC team needs to be more flexible – more like a football team than an army platoon. Furthermore, professional sensibilities do not take kindly to imposed management structures, so solutions in general practice have to be more organic. In both cases, teams must share values and culture if they are to work effectively. This is especially important in the case of the PHC team with its general absence of explicit form or hierarchy.

There seems to be general agreement that good teamwork is best achieved with three to six people (Belbin 1981) and is unlikely with more than 12. The amount of time and energy spent on communication provides diminishing returns as team size increases.

In the case of the PHC team it is also important to remember that many individuals are not exclusive members of one team. In particular attached staff with external management have even more lines of communication to inhibit effective primary teamwork. For this reason many argue that the future PHC team should have one management structure for all members. In large urban centres, specialist multidisciplinary networks can be so extensive and have such a rapid turnover of staff that core PHC teams may spend large amounts of time simply trying to keep up with the changes. It is for these reasons that the core primary care team is recognised as quite distinct from the multidisciplinary network of community-based specialists and sub-specialists which intermittently supports it.

TEAM LEADERSHIP

Effective leadership of the type required by clinical teamwork springs from individual qualities rather than from role. Also, in principle, team leadership can be collective rather than individual. Moreover the style or individual right in one situation will be wrong on another occasion. PHC team leadership should therefore be flexible and open to any member of the team. In practice this does not happen.

Some members of existing PHC teams can use their power not to lead but to control. GPs tend to assume that they are the 'natural' team leader based on their position as 'managing director' of the practice and in line with the hospital model of physician domination. PHC team leadership in general practice usually fails for one of two reasons.

Role overload

This occurs when the expectations and demands of a role exceed the role occupant's ability to respond. This can happen to a particular individual or affect anyone who is given the position. The person can be too small or the job too big. Overload is more likely to appear in situations where the precise nature of the job is ill-defined and the limit of responsibility vague. When expectations are unclear more and more demands are made of the individual or role. The number of projects the individual must become involved in can quickly become unmanageable. Despite this, it is difficult to say 'no' because few clear regulations exist as to how time should be spent.

Research on the effects of role overload shows that in general it produces dissatisfaction, fatigue and tension. Moreover, it has been shown to be related to medical symptoms. One study of US government (Caplan 1972) found higher heart disease rates and higher levels of serum cholesterol in people subject to role overload.

Although most community practitioners are affected to some extent by role overload, the GP could reasonably claim to be most severely afflicted. Even before the full workload implications of the primary care-led NHS are realised, existing expectations of GPs are probably too great; clinician, businessman, educator, health service planner and so forth. In the circumstances what is surprising is not that sometimes GPs perform badly as team leaders, but that most are competent and some are good.

Status incongruence

This state exists either when someone in a particular position performs well on a few dimensions which are valued for the role but poorly on others, or when personal characteristics are generally inappropriate for the position held. This can work both ways, that is, a person can be overqualified for a job or not up to it. Status incongruence, particularly affecting the leader, impedes effective team dynamics. Adams (1953) found that people feel strongly that it is not fair to have an incompetent person in a high-status position. It is not equitable. This creates a type of cognitive imbalance within the team. When there are incongruent characteristics for team members to deal with, psychological tension is created. This state is both unpleasant and dissatisfying. Motivation is reduced, behaviour problems appear, and team performance deteriorates.

There are two main solutions to the problem of status incongruence:

1. Select or promote only those people whose characteristics are all congruent with the job
2. Change the team's values about what is congruent and what should lead to high status.

In practice, neither of these approaches is particularly useful because of the power imbalance in PHC teams.

TIME

Even when composition, size and leadership are right a team will not form immediately. Any group of human beings have to wear off the rough edges before they can mesh together smoothly as a workforce. If individuals can be brought to apply the same piercing insights to their own behaviour as they do to their co-workers, an effective team will result, but only after passing through a series of stages. No group, however experienced or motivated, can skip any stage. Whether stages are successfully navigated and how long it takes depends on appropriate composition, size and leadership, as well as previous experience and motivation.

Stages on the road to effective teams

Tuckman (1965) suggested that the process of team formation follows four main stages:

Forming. During this stage the individuals get to know each other and attempt to define the purpose of the team, roles, status, leadership and so on.

Storming. A stage of conflict follows when the initial, often false, consensus on purpose, roles and so on is challenged and re-established. Personal agendas are often revealed at this stage and inter-personal hostility is generated, which must be resolved. This stage is important for establishing norms of trust.

Norming. Group norms or standards are determined. These cover all group behaviours, including matters such as time keeping, hours of work, levels of output, quality and decision making. Individuals test the group to assess the appropriate level of commitment.

Performing. When the team has grown through the three previous stages it is fully mature and able to perform optimally.

Many PHC teams never resolve all of the issues of the first three stages and effectiveness is

---

Box 4.11 Hallmarks of effective teams

- Relaxed friendly atmosphere
- Everyone participates
- A clearly stated and agreed objective
- Ideas are encouraged, listened to, and discussed
- Disagreements about process or method are faced and resolved
- Team decisions are accepted by the individuals
- Criticism is open, helpful and positive
- Expression of feelings or emotions is acceptable
- Individuals know what is expected of them, the value of their work and where it fits into the overall purpose and objectives
- Leadership of the team is open and democratic
- Team performance is appraised and ways to improve results, methods or relationships are sought

---

permanently compromised. The hallmarks of a team which has successfully evolved are outlined in Box 4.11.

WHY DO TEAMS SOMETIMES FAIL?

Teams fail when any one of the four factors – composition, size, leadership, time for growth – is neglected. This is most likely to happen when the leadership of the team is poor and often during the stage of forming if the group is ignorant of normal team dynamics. When things go wrong the team can either carry on unsatisfactorily for an indefinite period or explode spectacularly with tremendous personal animosity. Team failure can be profoundly traumatic or simply a daily irritant.

Recognising behaviour in teams

There are basically two main groups of behaviour in teams: reasonable and unreasonable. Reasonable behaviours are seen in high performing teams. Teams which are guided poorly through the storming phase of development often continue to experience high levels of unreasonable behaviour. Such behaviour can cause a team to fail before it even starts. Unreasonable behaviour also commonly appears in response to external stress, which may then lead to a spiral of

Table 4.7   Behaviour in teams

Reasonable behaviours		Unreasonable behaviours
Task-directed (*Getting the job done*)	Maintenance-directed (*Keeping the team together*)	Egocentric
Initiating discussion	Setting standards	Dominating
Offering suggestions	Listening to others	Not listening/blocking suggestions
Elaborating ideas	Encouraging ideas	Sarcasm
Explaining points	Evaluating team working	Ganging-up
Giving/seeking information	Helping progress	Withholding facts/dishonesty
Seeking/giving opinions	Harmonising	Withdrawing
Clarifying points	Relieving tension	'Horsing around'
Summarising	Expressing group feelings	Sulking
Offering solutions	Diagnosing problems	Seeking sympathy
Seeking decisions	Facing conflict	Aggression
Seeking consensus	Compromising	Obstinacy

declining team performance irrespective of the course of the extrinsic event.

Reasonable behaviours are:

- Task-directed – getting the job done
- Team maintenance-directed – keeping the group together to get the job done.

Unreasonable behaviour is essentially egocentric, with an individual over-relying on whatever personality trait is most comfortable to them under stress, for example aggression, submission or avoidance. Examples of reasonable and unreasonable team behaviour are given in Table 4.7.

Table 4.8   Egocentric behaviour in team situations

Aggression		Submission		Avoidance	
Typical behaviours	Typical effects	Typical behaviours	Typical effects	Typical behaviours	Typical effects
Bulldozing	Short-term results	Indirect approach	Seen as ineffectual	Assumed agreement	Confused communication
Demanding	Lack of co-operation	Non-refusal of tasks	Overload with tasks	Facial gestures	Confused communication
Insisting	Minimal effort	Hold back requests	Shown scant consideration	Critical silence	
Authoritarian	Sabotage	Ingratiating	Seen as 'willing'	Manipulation	Feelings of being 'used'
Negative feedback	Demotivation	Under reacting	Victimised	Insincere flattery	Mistrust
Critical	Poor standard work	Hiding feelings	Taken for granted	False friendliness	Mistrust
Personality attack	Poor relationship	Embarrassment	Bullying	Ego boosting	
Blaming	Working to rule	Blame accepting	Martyrdom	Emotional blackmail	Retaliation
Hurting	Retaliation			Sarcasm	Anger
Spite	Avoidance/ignoring			Jokey put-downs	Avoidance Withholding information
				Hints of power	Embellished information Short-term results

Egocentric behaviour in team situations can be profoundly damaging to morale and fatal to team working. It is therefore worth being aware of the three main types of unreasonable behaviour which most commonly hamper effective group working and indeed human relationships more generally. Most types can easily be spotted in others, but we are usually less good at seeing our own failings. This is important as we are very rarely in a position to force another person to change behaviour, but we can always change our own.

Table 4.8 gives examples of each of the three main types of egocentric behaviour commonly seen in team situations. It has been laid out to indicate the effect which is likely to be produced by each example of unreasonable team behaviour. However, it is important to be aware that any of the behaviours listed can provoke any of the effects.

Summary

The organisational structure within which CHCNs work is complex and highly challenging, both personally and professionally. In principle, effective teamwork offers solutions to many of the problems facing primary care clinicians; however, the way the primary care sector his developed has raised significant obstacles. In particular, the status of GPs is unhelpful, as is the conflict of interest built into service development planning at practice level. A Griffiths-style review of the organisation of primary care is overdue.

Even under ideal circumstances effective teams do not form spontaneously. Although complex, team dynamics are *not* arbitrary and can be understood and moderated.

CHCNs must be diplomatic, assertive, sensitive to the implications of team dynamics and keenly self-aware if they are to help guide the group which they join towards high performance as a team in the interest of patients.

REFERENCES

Adams S 1953 Status congruence as a variable in small group performance. Social Forces 32:16–22

Andrews K 1987 Rehabilitation of the older adult. Edward Arnold, London

Ashton J, Seymour H 1988 The new public health. Open University Press, Milton Keynes

Bales R F, Borgatta E F 1956 Size of group as a factor in the interaction profile. In: Hare A P, Borgatta E F, Bales R F (eds) Small groups, Knopf, New York

Bales R F, Cohen S P 1979 SYMLOG: a system for multiple level observation of groups. Free Press, New York

Belbin R M 1981 Management teams. Heinemann, London

Belbin R M 1993 Team roles at work. Heinemann Butterworth, London

British Medical Association 1996 Medical taskforce – taskgroup report. BMA, London

Caplan R D 1972 Organisational stress and individual strain: a socio-psychological study of risk factors in CHD among administrators. engineers and scientists. Dissertation Abstracts International 32:6706b–6707b

Department of Health 1989 Caring for people. HMSO, London

Department of Health 1992 The health of the nation. HMSO, London

Department of Health and Social Security 1981 Care in the community. HMSO, London

Department of Health and Social Security 1986 Neighbourhood nursing – a focus for care. Report of the community nursing review (Cumberlege report). HMSO, London

Dowrick C 1992 Who will be 'caring for people'? British Journal of General Practice 42:2–3

Drury M 1988 Teamwork: the way forward. Practice Team 1(1):3

Hayden J 1996 Summative assessment – threat or opportunity? British Journal of General Practice 132–133

Iliffe S 1995 The retreat from equity: the implications of the shift towards a primary care-led NHS. Critical Public Health (6):3

McGrath J, Davies A 1992 Rehabilitation: where are we going and how do we get there? Clinical Rehabilitation 6:225–235

McWhinney I R 1989 A textbook of family medicine. Oxford University Press, New York

Marsh G N 1991 The future of general practice: caring for larger lists. British Medical Journal 303:1312–1316

Ministry of Health 1920 The Dawson report. HMSO, London

National Association of Health Authorities and Trusts 1994 Partners in learning: developing postgraduate training and continuing medical education for general practice. NAHAT, London

National Health Service and Community Care Act 1990 HMSO, London

NHS Management Executive 1995 Towards a primary care led NHS. HMSO, London

Salisbury C J 1989 How do people choose their doctor? British Medical Journal 299:608–610

Slater P F 1958 Contrasting correlates of group size. Sociometry 21:129–139

Starfield B 1994 Is primary care essential? Lancet 334:1129–1133

Thomas 1994 The nature of general medical practice. RCGP Report, London

Tuckman B 1965 Development sequence in small groups. Psychological Bulletin 63:384–399

Yetton P, Bottger P 1983 The relationship among group size, member ability, social decision scheme, and performance. Organisational Behaviour and Human Performance 32:145–159

FURTHER READING

French J R P Jr, Raven B 1960 The bases of social power. In: Cartwright D, Zander A F (eds) Group dynamics. 2nd edn. Row, Peterson, Evanston

Handy C Understanding organisations. Penguin, London

Mitchell T R, Larson J R In: People in organisations: an introduction to organisational behaviour. McGraw-Hill

2 Community health care nursing practice: individuals and families

5 Community health care nursing in primary health care: a shared future

Carmel Blackie

Once the community health care nurse has grasped the overall context and structure of primary health care, it is necessary to understand clearly exactly how nursing fits in to the system, how nursing care delivery is structured and the professional issues which affect the nurse's ability to deliver care. The basis is an holistic approach to caring for patients that respects both the professional and ethical principles of nursing and the rights and needs of the client. To this end, the community health care nurse must understand:

- The characteristics of community health care nursing
- Where it is practised
- The contribution of reflective practice and clinical supervision to nursing development
- The standards for continuing education
- The way in which specialist practitioners may develop the service in the future
- The standards that community health care nursing is expected to attain.

The major challenge in contemporary health care is to meet effectively the increasing and changing healthcare needs of the population in a way which is equitable, achieves maximum health gain and is affordable within limited national resources. Recent reforms of the NHS and the shift in emphasis from acute to primary and community care are an attempt to address this issue and, as a consequence, primary care has grown in importance and complexity. Primary health care

(PHC) teams based in general practice are pivotal to the planning and delivery of health care. Nurses form the largest single professional group within the health service (UKCC 1986) and represent a large financial and human resources investment. The organisation and role of nursing within PHC teams is at the heart of effective and efficient provision of health care.

Gregson et al (1991), Jarman & Cumberlege (1987), and Lawrence (1988) provide strong evidence that primary care is best provided for a population focused around a family doctor practice, where the needs of the population are assessed and met systematically by a team of doctors, nurses and other professionals working in partnership. This is the aim of the NHS reforms. The GP is a purchaser and provider of care as well as an employer of other professional groups. In the mid 1950s the only people working in general practice were doctors, secretary/receptionists and perhaps a nurse (Taylor 1954). In current general practice, a wide range of professional disciplines are represented. Some staff, such as practice nurses, are employed by the GP, others are attached to the practice from community trusts, and others are purchased as staff hours from primary care employment agencies, such as, Premier Health who provide integrated community nursing for Castlefields Health Centre in Cheshire. Providing the best possible health care for the client population means getting the best from the PHC team nursing workforce. To do this involves understanding the climate and issues which affect community health care (CHC) nursing in primary health care at the current time. Section 1 of this book deals with the NHS reforms and working in general practice settings.

COMMUNITY HEALTH CARE NURSING

CHC nursing is a client-centred, health-based profession committed to holistic caring (McFarlane 1982). This demands emotional, physical and intellectual attributes from the nurse and the effectiveness of nursing intervention depends upon the relationship between the client and the nurse (Haller 1976), and requires a complex knowledge base (Benner 1984, Rogers 1988, Schlotfeldt 1988, Gray & Forsstrom 1992, Miller 1992).

CHC nursing is a specialised branch of nursing which refers to the context of people's lives to attain and maintain health. It involves meeting simultaneously the healthcare needs of individuals, families and the community (McMurray 1993). There is a clinical focus as well as a public health element to the role (Williams 1986). The community health care nurse (CHCN) practises within a variety of settings and the client group has unique characteristics which impact upon practice goals and strategies. The boundaries of the CHCN's role are broad and include a range of activities carried out from an autonomous practice base. To be effective the CHCN must practise within the context of a multi-agency environment to offer complex and holistic primary health care.

The goals of practice are the promotion and maintenence of health and the prevention of illness through a continuous and proactive relationship with clients and colleagues. CHCNs practise in a climate of constant change. The NHS reforms have altered irrevocably the climate of care and the philosophy surrounding the way care is planned and organised. The NHS' internal market is constantly shaping itself (Holliday 1992) and CHCNs must adapt accordingly.

McMurray (1993) set out a framework for the characteristics of CHC nursing and the domains of practice (Boxes 5.1, 5.2) and others defined the nursing goals (Box 5.3).

In order to be most effective, nurses must work together in teams regardless of the patterns of their employment. CHCNs should develop co-operative and common goals and a philosophy which establishes integrated practice. For example, Sefton Health, Primary Educare and The Southport & Formby Community Trust Working Group On Community Nursing developed jointly a framework for integrating nursing teams based on a series of principles (Box 5.4).

Box 5.1 **The characteristics of CHC nursing (McMurray 1993)**

- Culturally appropriate practice
- Holistic practice
- Meets the needs of individual clients
- Meets the needs of subgroups as well as the main population
- Meets collective community needs
- Has an ecological approach (WHO 1992)
- Is client-based and health-focused

Box 5.2 **The domains of CHC nursing practice (McMurray 1993)**

- The management of client health and illness
- Monitoring and ensuring quality
- Organisational and work-related competencies
- The helping role
- Teaching function
- Consulting role

Box 5.3 **The nursing goals of the CHCN (Lee & Lancaster 1988)**

- Assessment
- Planning
- Implementation
- Evaluation

Box 5.4 **Principles for integrating CHC nursing teams in PHC**

- Unified commissioning of CHC nursing
- Unified CHC nursing caseloads
- Integrated CHC nursing teams based around a general practice population
- Integrated CHC nursing teams will be facilitated to identify the nursing needs of the practice population
- Needs assessment will inform skill mix and future commissioning
- Skill mix and future commissioning are directly linked to education and development provision and commissioning
- CHC nursing practice is evidence-based and takes account of national and local professional issues
- The quality of CHC nursing practice is integral to service and will be facilitated through clinical supervision and reflective practice
- Community Health care Nursing will make a contribution to PHC commissioning and the PHC-led NHS

CONSULTATION WITH CLIENTS

In each interaction with a client, the CHCN operates in a consultative role; each client contact offers an opportunity for therapeutic communication. Within the consultation, assessment leads to a nursing diagnosis, which has been defined by several authors (Gordon 1979, Bower 1989, Alfaro 1990, Atkinson & Murray 1990, Liss 1993). They emphasised that a nursing diagnosis should identify need, and requires cognitive ability, a broad knowledge base and intellectual capacity to ensure the integration and manipulation of several domains of knowledge simultaneously. It must also be distinct from a medical diagnosis. The collection of holistic data and the linkage of information is a core purpose of nursing diagnosis, and should allow practice to be appropriate to client need and encourage theory generation and autonomy (Zeigler 1986).

Diagnosis is traditionally associated with medical practice. Hamilton (1983) describes most approaches to medical diagnoses as involving the identification of a disease or pathology but states that nursing diagnosis involves the identification of issues which require 'nursing' intervention and have elements of primary prevention. Nursing diagnosis is distinct from medicine in that it is concerned with the client's ability to live a full life. This is a generalisation to which there are obvious exceptions, most notably general practice. The skill of diagnosis requires clinical and diagnostic reasoning ability. Alfaro (1990) outlined the diagnostic reasoning required in order for diagnosis to be made. This involves data collection, analysis and synthesis. The ability to solve problems has been identified as one of the salient hallmarks of specialist practice (Tanner et al 1987, Hurst 1991).

In a statement that encapsulates the benefits of nursing diagnosis to the client and to the profession, Jones (1988) says:

The emergence of professional nursing as a discrete and significant discipline in its own right rests on the competence of practising nurses to accurately define, with a high degree of specification, those areas of concern in health care for clients for which they, as nurses, are uniquely qualified to offer solutions. In making such definitions, a nurse will display a perspective towards the clients' problems which is distinct from those of other care team members with whom she shares a collaborative role in providing for the needs of society at large.

As nursing practice develops there are implications for nursing itself and for those with whom nurses interact. King (1967) identified several such issues within health care as a result of nurse diagnoses, which are still largely unresolved, having particular significance in a market-led health service. They include the following:

- The effect of nursing diagnosis upon the profession, e.g. education, accountability, role
- How other professions, notably medicine, view nursing diagnosis and the consequence of this upon teams and collaborative working.

Mason & Webb (1993) identify several models of nursing that examine nursing diagnosis (see Ch. 6 for nursing models). Applying a model to practice also aids evaluation by providing an obvious structure to the client interaction (Luker 1982, Philips 1987). Orem (1985) defined diagnosis as 'an investigative operation that enables nurses to make judgements about the existing health care situation and decisions about what should and can be done ... whilst encouraging self care'.

Consultation is an essential element of the role of the specialist CHCN. Studies of nurse practitioners in the USA indicate that consultation occupies between 40% and 69% of their time (ANA 1986). As CHCN specialist practice develops it is likely that a lot of the characteristics of autonomous nurse practitioners will be taken on by specialist nurses and consultation will become a more prominent feature of the specialist role. Wyers et al (1985) indicate that consultation ranks highly in the perception of nurse specialists in relation to their role and in the perception held of them by managers of the service. A consultation should be holistic and involves making a nursing diagnosis (Ingersoll 1992), which, ideally, helps the client avert crisis, or supports him through it. The process of consultation may be classified into stages which are documented by the practitioner, in partnership with the client. This also provides data for later reflection and

analysis of effectiveness and links everyday practice to clinical supervision and practice development. Edlund et al (1987) classified stages within a consultation as:

- entry to the system
- identification of the problem
- clarification of the consultee's situation
- identification of goals and desired outcomes
- data gathering
- development of the plan
- initiation of the plan
- follow up—to which should be added ...
- re-evaluation
- adaptation of care.

It has been shown that consultations sometimes fail because the client did not expect to take part in discussion. Clients usually already have an agenda and expectations of their own, particularly when they have initiated the contact, for example by interaction with a practice nurse, or where clients have a clear treatment goal, such as care given by district nurses, and are not amenable to extending it (Clarke 1986). Clarke also states that lack of clarity of purpose influences the success or failure of the consultation. The CHCN must have clear goals and a structure within which consultation takes place, but the structure must be flexible enough to allow clients to explain their own viewpoints and the CHCN to respond to this. Consultations tend to be more effective where the CHCN has built a previous relationship with a client as this influences the perception of competence held by the client in relation to the practitioner.

INDIVIDUAL AND FAMILY ASSESSMENT

As part of a consultation, all community nurses assess need. There are three levels to needs assessment:

- individual needs
- family health needs
- community health needs.

Family and individual needs are addressed in

this chapter, and community health needs are addressed in Ch. 9.

All needs assessment must be undertaken in partnership with the client. Assessment of individual and family needs identifies both actual and potential need. It is not solely concerned with problem identification, but this must play a part, as does identifying resources with which the individual or family unit can tackle their need. This necessitates understanding the concept of need.

Need

A human need is a condition to be fulfilled to maintain life or well-being. Bradshaw's *Taxonomy of Need* (1972) was developed for social work, but has significance for CHC nursing practice, which overlaps considerably. Need is categorised as:

- normative
- felt
- expressed
- comparative.

Normative need

Normative need is defined by an agreed standard that is laid down by an expert body, such as a government department, defining acceptable levels of poverty and linking this to welfare benefit calculations. If an individual falls short of the norm, a need is identified.

Felt need

Felt need is something that the individual wants. It is personal and may be subjective in nature. Often a client will state a felt need without necessarily taking action to achieve its fruition. Wants or wishes are not necessarily needs. Sometimes clients might not have insight into their own needs as seen by others, or their priorities might conflict with professional or social agendas.

Expressed need

Expressed need is a felt need translated into action. The client identifies his own need and consequently asks for, or demands, something from the system to meet that need. Collectively expressed need can turn into community action, such as lobbying for services.

Comparative need

Comparative need exists when two groups of people with the same condition receive unequal provision of services. If one group receives services but the other does not, a state of comparative need exists between the two groups.

Maslow (1943) identified a hierarchy of need represented as a pyramid. Each category, beginning with the base and working upwards, must be met in sequence to allow the others above it to be achieved (Fig. 5.1).

In assessing the health needs of individuals the CHCN must consider the following parameters:

- general health
- general mood
- specific issues/problems, e.g. rashes or pain
- past history
- family history
- medication
- allergies

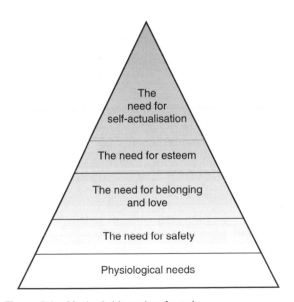

Figure 5.1   Maslow's hierarchy of needs.

- lifestyle
- occupation
- health-damaging behaviour
- gastrointestinal tract
- urogenital tract
- respiratory system
- infections
- immunisation status
- social circumstances
- housing
- stress
- alcohol
- diet.

Specialist themes within CHC nursing practice will emphasise some areas more than others.

In family assessment, all the factors which affect the individual are important, as well as the issues affecting each person and the whole family unit.

Factors influencing the health of an individual or family

The following factors influence the health of an individual or a family:

- physiological
- social policy
- environmental
- client/family medical history
- sociocultural
- client/family view of health
- intellectual
- emotional
- psychological.

These must be considered in parallel to other parameters within the assessment.

Action following the assessment

Assessment is a data-gathering exercise, which is a prelude to planning care, in partnership with the client and others (see Fig. 5.2).

A range of options arises from assessment, including the following:

- No need exists. Reassess later.
- Potential need. The client is given anticipatory

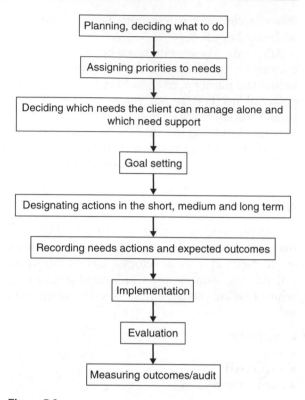

Figure 5.2

advice. This is the primary prevention phase.
- A need exists and is managed by the client. Reassess later to support the client.
- The client requires help, information or support, such as counselling or referral to other agencies.
- The client can't manage alone and requires intervention. This is the phase of secondary prevention.
- The client has long-term needs, and requires tertiary intervention.

The hallmarks of a CHC nursing assessment are that it:

- is holistic
- is not solely problem-centred
- looks at actual and potential need
- identifies resources
- helps clients and family articulate their own needs

- helps clients and family recognise professionally assessed needs
- makes sense of the information
- categorises needs, problems and resources
- balances needs against resources and competing demands.

DEVELOPING PRACTICE IN COMMUNITY HEALTH CARE NURSING

Reflective practice and clinical supervision

Reflection on and during practice (Benner 1984, 1991, Schon 1988) is the means by which an individual may revisit an experience, explore the event in context and link it to past experience and knowledge, apply evaluation and explicate meaning from it (Boud et al 1985). As a consequence new knowledge is synthesised and the individual and his or her practice are developed. The process is dynamic, and requires commitment to change and the application of intellectual rigour.

CHC nursing themes overlap between the functions of the practitioner groups; for example, between health visiting and practice nursing and between practice nursing and district nursing, as well as with other caring professions such as social work and medicine, in particular general practice. A real challenge for all concerned is therefore how to generate knowledge and apply this to practice from a diversity of perspectives. Between the domains of medicine and nursing a function exists which requires collaborative effort. This is the development ground for interdisciplinary practice and role sharing. Tackling areas of overlap within nursing, and between nursing and medicine, may require a move towards shared learning and a change in role and function for many of the groups involved with care. One way this can be achieved is through reflective practice (Schon 1988, Benner 1991).

Nursing in the NHS and world-wide is at a critical stage in its professional evolution (Watson 1993). CHCNs must develop appropriate knowledge and skills to allow the profession to achieve the autonomy enjoyed by other disciplines, notably medicine. Knowledge and theory generated through reflection structured within clinical supervision is the means to allow this to happen (Faugier 1994).

Clinical supervision has been defined by Butterworth (1992) as 'An exchange between practising professionals to enable the development of professional skills', and, more practically, by Wright (1989) as:

A meeting between two or more people who have a declared interest in examining a piece of work. The work is presented and they will together think about what was happening and why, what was done or said, and how it was handled – could it have been handled better or differently, and if so, how?

Many of the models of clinical supervision available to nursing derive from counselling, the most notable influence being Heron (1990). Several models exist such as that defined by Hawkins & Schoet (1991, 1992) who encourage structured, supervised reflection on observed practice using notes and a further reflective dimension in relation to the process of supervision itself. Guided, structured reflection and the ability to draw out knowledge embedded in practice have been shown to enhance practice (Paunonen 1991, Faugier & Butterworth 1994). Undertaking guided reflection requires a range of skills. Atkinson & Murphy (1994) identified these as:

- self-awareness
- accurate recollection
- identification of key issues
- critical analysis
- the ability to synthesise new knowledge.

Johns (1994) views guided reflection as a combination of several techniques which enable practitioners to apply hindsight to experience, reflect upon the situation, analyse and explicate meaning and synthesise a model for new experiences so developing practice (Box 5.5). The philosophy underpinning this view is that learning is integral to clinical development.

Knowing

Johns' (1994) model contains Carper's (1978) four

Box 5.5   Johns' model for structured reflection (1997) (Based on the 'Being available' template, Johns C 1977 Becoming an effective practitioner through guided reflection. PhD thesis, The Open University. Reproduced with kind permission from Christopher Johns.)

Write a description of the experience.
Consider: what are the significant issues I need to pay attention to?

Reflective cues

Aesthetics
● What was I trying to achieve?
● Why did I respond as I did?
● What were the consequences of that for:
  — the patient?
  — others?
  — myself?
● How was this person(s) feeling?
● How did I know this?

Personal
● How did I feel in this situation?
● What factors embodied within me or embedded within the environment were influencing me?

Ethics
● Did I act in accordance with my beliefs and for the best?
● If not, what factors made me act in incongruent ways?

Empirics
● What knowledge did or should have informed me?

Reflexivity
● How does this connect with my previous experiences?
● Could I handle this situation better in similar situations?
● What would the consequences of alternative actions be:
  — for the patient?
  — for others?
  — for myself?
● How do I *now* feel about this experience?
● Can I support myself and others better as a consequence?
● Am I now more 'available' to work with patients and families to help them meet their health needs?

ways of knowing and together they provide conceptual mapping through which reflection can take place. Carper (1978) described four fundamental patterns of knowing in relation to the knowledge required for nursing, which can be applied to any professional activity. These are aesthetics, personal knowing, ethics and empirical knowledge.

Aesthetic knowledge. This relates to the 'art' which the situation demands and includes empathy, understanding and perception. Carper (1978) considers this to be the ability to recognise subjectively and feel the situation through having experienced it, and to identify the essential nature of the situation, analyse it, make choices as to appropriate action and evaluate these choices in terms of effectiveness. Each situation is unique and so the aesthetic knowledge required is specific to the situation.

Ethical knowing. Also known as moral knowledge, this relates to the ability to respect and value individuals, maintaining their dignity throughout the process of care without compromising personal standards and integrity.

Personal knowing. Described by Carper (1978) as 'knowing, encountering and actualising of the concrete self', personal knowing involves making a conscious effort to know and understand oneself. The individual must gain insight into past cultural and life experiences, including any prejudices held, as well as having insight into professional socialisation and learning, and prevent them exerting undue influence on behaviour and decision making. Personal knowing encompasses subjective views as well as concrete knowledge as to how interpersonal processes evolve and influence events. It is existential and actively promotes wholeness and integrity.

Empirical knowledge. This relates to concrete factual theories which underpin practice; 'practice which is shorn of any theoretical foundations for growth is not a practice discipline, it is ritualised performance'.

Post Registration Education and Practice Project (PREPP)

The Post Registration Education and Practice Project (PREPP) was ratified by the United Kingdom Central Council For Nursing, Midwifery and Health Visiting (UKCC) on 23 February 1994 and gained Department of Health approval on 15 March 1995. It was enacted into law on 1 April 1995. It now applies to all registered and enrolled nurses and health visitors. Implementation will be phased: linked to periodic re-registration dates. The target date to include all nurses in the new arrangements is 1 April 2001.

Within PREP the UKCC has set new standards of practice and education for practice following registration, for all nurses, midwives and health visitors. The standards identified relate to the following areas:

- maintaining an effective registration
- post-registration education.

In order to maintain a valid registration the nurse, midwife or health visitor is required to:

- complete a minimum of 5 study days every 3 years
- complete a notification of practice form
- undertake and complete a return to practice programme if he has been out of practice for longer than 5 years
- compile and maintain a personal professional portfolio.

Post-registration education is rationalised and made more cost effective through a framework which matches client and service needs with flexible and responsive education. The new framework:

- reforms the existing range of post-registration provision
- reduces duplication and repetition of course content
- encourages shared learning of core knowledge and skills
- offers flexibility and responsiveness to service demands
- ensures common professional and academic standards across the UK and aims to allow transfer of credits
- clarifies language and terminology used in course prospectuses and curricula so that the information is accessible to all
- ensures teachers designing and running courses have clinical credibility through explicit practice-based links.

The PREP document is detailed and sets standards in a range of areas, including standards for practice, specialist practice, specialist community practice, midwifery, education and teaching. Transitional arrangements from the old to the new system are set out as are criteria for specialist nursing education and specialist community education. All nurses and health visitors should become familiar with the contents of the document. Of particular interest here are changes in relation to community education and practice.

There are various non-hierarchical levels of nursing practice which describe care offered at different stages of professional development post-registration.

Professional practice. This is the level of practice offered on achieving first level registration. The nurse is able to operate at a general level, supported by a framework of clinical supervision, in a broad spectrum of practice settings across acute and community areas. This level of practice is associated with diploma level study and qualification. It is designed to reflect the changes to nursing brought about by Project 2000.

Specialist practice. This is delivered after a period of consolidation and development and requires the practitioner to undertake further study in order to achieve knowledge and skills to address the complex health needs of client populations. CHC nursing is a recognised area of specialist practice and requires additional preparation post-registration. Within CHC nursing there are several categories or themes of expertise:

- general practice nursing
- community mental health nursing specialist
- community mental handicap nursing specialist
- community children's nursing specialist
- public health nursing specialist (health visiting)
- occupational health nursing specialist
- community nursing specialist in the home (district nursing)
- school nursing.

Specialist programmes

Specialist training programmes for CHC nursing practice commenced in September 1995. They replace traditional community courses, e.g. those leading to qualification as a district nurse or health visitor. Given the new structure of courses for CHCNs, it will be possible for practitioners to increase or complement their existing knowledge and skills by following additional units without repeating the core programmes, thus gaining more than one specialist qualification. For example, should a CHCN (general practice nursing) wish to practice as a CHCN (public health nursing specialist) or integrate aspects of this role into their current role within a practice, they could, in theory, follow the specialist public health units.

Programmes cover four broad areas, identified by the ENB as:

- clinical nursing practice
- care and programme management
- clinical practice development
- clinical practice leadership.

The categories are explained briefly below:

Clinical nursing practice. This offers a range of opportunities to allow the nurse to acquire additional knowledge and skills in order to meet the specialist clinical needs of patients and clients.

Care and programme management. This relates to individuals, families and communities within the care environment, enabling the practitioner to draw together relevant elements of acute and community provision. The focus is on health promotion and prevention of disease and emphasises the need for proactive management.

Clinical practice development. This relates to preparation of the practitioner to set standards of care for a high quality service and includes monitoring, evaluating and auditing care. Practitioners will develop a high level of expertise in their own field and are encouraged to identify appropriate research and contribute to practice-based research.

Clinical practice leadership. This part of the programme prepares the practitioner to lead and deliver services which are sensitive to consumer needs and to support and supervise other staff in practice. The specialist community practitioner will be able to oversee student placements, ensure staff development and provide clinical teaching.

General practice nursing

Practice nurse numbers increased dramatically as a result of the NHS reforms and the GP contract instituted in 1990, after which GPs employed nurses in order to meet the targets demanded in the contract (Woolnough 1990). As a consequence, the role of the practice nurse comprises duties for which the GP is responsible and which are delegated to the practice nurse (Atkin et al 1993).

Despite this rapid expansion, practice nursing is not new and nurses were working with family doctors as early as 1910 (Bowling & Stillwell 1990). Practice nursing has its roots in the implementation of a charter for family doctor services which allowed the doctor to employ two ancillary staff and receive 70% reimbursement for this. The majority of staff employed under this arrangement were reception staff although a few practice nurses were employed. In 1968 the Health Services and Public Health Act allowed district nurses to extend their role to offer care for patients on general practice premises and, as a consequence, the trend since the 1970s has been for community nurses employed by the health service to be aligned, if not attached, to GPs.

Now, GPs still receive 70% reimbursement, paying 30% of the costs themselves as a small business employer. As most practice nurses generate income for the practice through meeting practice targets, the 30% can be recovered by a well-organised practice, with a profit sometimes being made. Practice nurses employed by the GP are outside the NHS and are denied benefits enjoyed by other nurses, such as superannuation. In 1993 the Audit Commission found that many community nurses were concerned that a key element of their specialty was outside the main body of nursing.

Practice nurses may have difficulty with funding for attendance at specialist practice courses. Since the 1990 contract many practice nurses have undertaken study funded by the regional health authority and administered at local level by FHSAs (now merged with the DHA) through practice nurse advisors. This level of support has largely disappeared and many GPs do not require the practice nurse to work as a specialist, causing funding difficulties.

Role of the practice nurse following the 1990 GP contract

The role of the general practice nurse is to provide nursing care to clients within the context of a GP surgery. Practice nurses are usually the only CHCNs to be employed directly by a GP, although this could change as fundholding and other models of devolved budget broaden the scope for nurses to be employed by the GP.

The role of the practice nurse encompasses several elements:

Registration health check. This involves screening all new patients registering with the practice who are between the ages of 5 and 75. This should involve a full health profile assessment and consequent setting of priorities with the client to address issues which affect his health. It should also form the basis for forward planning of future health need. The GP can claim a fee for undertaking this service.

Adult health checks. This area of the contract has been dropped subsequently, but in the 1990 contract the GP was required to offer a health assessment to adult patients under 75 who had not been seen in the last 3 years.

Health promotion clinics. In the initial contract the practice could claim a fee for undertaking health promotion activity with patients. This included running clinics for chronic disease management in areas such as diabetes and asthma. In 1993 the fee was replaced by health promotion banding. The banding categories were abandoned in 1996 in favour of practice-selected, needs-based targets linked to local population need.

Minor surgery. The contract encouraged GPs to become accepted onto an approved list for minor surgery. The doctor can claim payment for a maximum of 15 minor surgical procedures in each financial quarter. Practice nurses often establish the infrastructure for minor surgery within the surgery and assist the GP in surgical procedures, taking responsibility for equipment and sterilisation, etc. In some instances the practice nurse/nurse practitioner may undertake minor procedures such as suturing.

Elderly screening. People over 75 years of age are offered an annual health check. If the person is mobile the check is carried out at the surgery. If not the client is visited at home.

Counselling. Some practice nurses offer a counselling service and can help clients adjusting to life traumas such as bereavement or the news of a chronic or terminal condition. Unfortunately, many practice nurses do not have the flexibility to manage their own caseload appointments due to the nature of their contract with the GP.

Administration. This involves the practice nurse in record keeping and general administration to support nursing within the practice. This could involve using computers to record episodes of care and the outcome of that care, audit, protocol or guideline development and supporting the GP in purchasing health care.

Treatment room work. This aspect of the role includes dressings, minor surgery, suturing, ear syringing, venepuncture, ECGs and a range of other activities.

Management of the practice nurse caseload. Management of the practice nurse caseload and making sure that all of the stocks required for clinical nursing care and treatment are available, such as sterile supplies and vaccines, constitute a major part of the practice nurse's role.

Community mental health nursing specialist

The first community psychiatric nurses were based at Warlingham Park Hospital, Surrey, in the mid 1950s. This innovation involved nurses working on the wards following patients to the home setting on discharge or during weekend leave, to monitor progress and support the client and the family. Other schemes followed and gradually throughout the 1960s the discipline developed.

The Seebohm report (1969), which reviewed local authority social service provision, recommended that social work teams should move from specialisms to a more generic role. Alongside the newly emerging psychiatric nurses, mental welfare officers from social services worked in parallel. When the Seebohm report was implemented in the early 1970s, the mental welfare officers joined generic teams and the void left was filled by increasing the workload and responsibility of psychiatric nurses in the community.

The number of psychiatric nurses in the community has increased steadily since. Research by White (1991) found that the spread of nurses across the country may not mirror actual need and that there should be a more needs-based approach to staffing allocations; for example, inner city areas may require higher levels of psychiatric nursing services than rural or less densely populated areas. This supports findings by Simmons & Brooker (1986). On average there are approximately 8.6 mental health nurses for every 100 000 people, ranging from 3 to 22 per 100 000 across the UK. This is clearly inequitable and not systematically needs-based. Many areas are attempting to produce a ratio of one nurse for every 10 000 people.

There is increasing pressure on community mental health services as the closure of psychiatric inpatient facilities continues and more clients are cared for and supervised in the community. A series of disturbing incidents, such as the unprovoked attack on and death of Jonathan Zito in 1992 by Christopher Clunis, who was being treated for a psychiatric illness in the community, has caused a wave of public and professional outrage. Many psychiatric nurses are based in health centres and around general practice, and there is an increasing number of referrals to the service from GPs and a decrease in the number of direct referrals from psychiatric hospital consultants.

Community mental handicap nursing specialist (learning disability)

Community mental handicap nursing or learning disability nursing developed in the late 1970s as a result of lobbying by families and carers of people with learning disability. Their aim was to achieve a more co-ordinated service for people with special needs, after the age of 19.

The aim of the nurse is to continue to co-ordinate care for clients and attempt to ensure a seamless service. The nurse offers a practical service to clients and carers as well as advice and education offered within the overall goals and philosophy of PHC and CHC nursing.

As more people are cared for in the community, the workload for learning disability nurses is increasing but the resources are in short supply, and so services for this vulnerable section of the population and their families and carers are relatively underdeveloped. The service has considerable overlap with social services as well as with other members of the CHC nursing team and GPs. The service may be compromised by the advent of GP fundholder purchasing of nursing services for the practice and other models of devolved budgeting. Some courses now offer a joint nursing and social work qualification in the area of learning disability.

As with nursing services for sick children, there are insufficient people with learning difficulties on any one practice list to merit the full time employment of a nurse. The future of the specialty, therefore, must lie with encouraging practices to purchase services as a consortium so that the nurse covers a larger area and population than one practice, or through closer links with social services.

Community children's nursing specialist

Children's nursing in the community, like practice nursing and school nursing, is a recently recognised aspect of the specialism and as such is developing its own body of knowledge. For many years the care of sick children in the community was undertaken by district nurses who primarily have an adult focus to their work. It has long been recognised that nursing children requires special skills and this has lately been reinforced by the NHSE report Child Health in the Community – a Guide to Good Practice, published in September 1996 (NHSE 1996).

The paediatric district nursing service has developed over several years and has usually taken one of the following forms:

- community-based initiative
- hospital-based initiative
- specialist nursing acting as a resource.

Most of the initiatives were linked to paediatric units in hospitals and offered outreach services. Establishing a community service for sick children is difficult. Again, there are insufficient sick children per GP practice to merit the attachment to practices. The NHS reforms mean that the onus is on fundholders or developed budget holders to purchase nursing. Paediatric district nursing services are not likely to be purchased unless in a collaborative venture between several practices to ensure that the practice population is large enough to merit a nursing team. Tatman (1994) in a publication entitled 'Wise Decisions: Developing Paediatric Home Care Schemes', contains excellent advice for those wishing to establish home care schemes, such as how to establish networks between primary and secondary care providers, and some of the pitfalls that may be encountered.

Public health nursing specialist (health visiting)

Of all of the community health care nursing themes, health visiting will probably be the most radically affected by the NHS reforms and the introduction of market features into commissioning and provision of health care. Public health nursing (health visiting) is the only CHC nursing theme which is a registerable qualification; the other themes and the specialty itself are recordable.

Health visiting orginated in the public health movement and developed at the turn of the century in Manchester in response to poor social and health conditions amongst working populations. Prompted by the awful conditions, the Ladies' Sanitary Reform Movement was founded in 1862. Middle class women were recruited to call at the homes of the poor to offer help and education in the care of infants and families (McCleary 1933). This initiative was reproduced in industri-

al cities throughout the country and overlapped to an extent with the work of women sanitary inspectors, who mixed public health inspection with education for mothers and home visiting. These women were keen to ensure that the advice element of their role was securely linked to the public health role, which at the time was thought to be unsuitable work for women. Later the two elements of the function were split and the 'health visitor' was created.

The role of the health visitor was seen to have less status than the public health role and was considered a suitable use of the skills and talents of women workers (Robinson 1982, Davies 1988). In its early days health visiting focused upon the welfare of mothers and children. At the time, the levels of maternal and childhood mortality and morbidity were high and as these fell, partly as a result of health visitor activity, partly as a result of better sanitary, welfare and medical care, the continued need for the health visiting service was questioned. At the inception of the NHS, the role of health visitors was set within the legislation as 'Giving advice as to the care of persons suffering from illness ... to expectant mothers and nursing mothers, and to mothers and others with the care of young children'.

The NHS Act stated that the health visitor should be concerned with the welfare of the whole family or 'the household as a whole', and should work in close co-operation with GPs, without further encroaching upon the role of other nurses. This set the 'hands off' approach of health visitors in relation to combining practical care with advice and support (MoH 1946). As the health service developed, legislation continued to reinforce the family focus of health visiting (MoH 1956), but health visitors themselves were defining aggressively their own role and this came to include public health in its widest sense, as well as being concerned with families (CETHV 1977).

In 1977, the Council for the Education and Training of Health Visitors (CETHV), set out the principles of health visiting. These have been adapted in the intervening years but remain relevant and have been absorbed into the core purpose of CHC nursing as a whole.

The principles of health visiting

The search for health needs. Health visitors proactively seek out health needs, both those acknowledged by clients, families and communities and those which are as yet unrecognised.

The stimulation of the awareness of health needs. Health visitors also work with clients as individuals, families and communities to encourage them to recognise the health needs which exist and to work to empower them to take control of the issues for themselves. They also have a role in encouraging awareness of identified health needs amongst professional colleagues.

The influence on policies affecting health. This area takes the health visitor into the political domain. The health visitor must work to influence the direction of public policy at local and national level as it influences health. In practice most health visitors do not engage individually in this activity, but the profession as a whole accepts the challenge of influencing policies.

The facilitation of health enhancing activities. The health visitor encourages clients to adopt healthy lifestyles. This is achieved through direct health education and health promotion activities in partnership with clients, aimed at promoting health through client empowerment. It also involves the health visitor in working with community groups, drawing on the need to influence policies to encourage supportive community infrastructures to encourage healthy lifestyle options.

The principles of health visiting are separated out here for ease of understanding and clarity, but each one influences the others and in practice they are are indivisible.

As a result of the NHS reforms, planning for health care begins with an assessment of health needs (DoH 1992). Health visitors are ideally placed to provide the input required to health authorities, public health departments and GPs to allow this to happen. It could be argued that health visiting has come full circle and is now back at its roots, merging the public health and educative roles with clients. The vision of CETHV in 1977 in setting out the principles of health visiting could finally be realised in the current market climate, or it could lose out completely to the commissioning process. The main focus of the health visitor is health promotion and prevention of ill health. The success of both of these endeavours is hard to quantify and contracts usually demand tangible health gain results.

Occupational health nursing specialist

Occupational health nursing takes PHC into industry and is newly absorbed into CHC nursing practice and education as a result of lobbying by the Health and Safety Executive in the early 1990s for its inclusion into nurse education programmes (Griffin 1992). It is concerned with maintaining the health of working people through application of the principles of CHC nursing practice and in doing this, takes a proactive approach to the effects of work and the workplace on health and the effects of health on productivity.

Occupational health nurses work with people in a range of occupations and environments from heavy industry to retail. Most people, even at times of high unemployment, spend the majority of their adult lives after they leave education as part of the workforce. The economic success of the nation rests upon the endeavours of people in the workforce being productive to maintain international competitiveness, and supporting this goal makes the nurse in occupational health a critical member of primary care services. Occupational health nurses aim to prevent ill health, promote health and safety at work, monitor the work environment, provide nursing care if required, manage the nursing workload and work within an ethical and legal framework (Forward Strategies Working Group 1991). They are employed outside the NHS by individual companies.

Community nursing specialist in the home (district nursing)

District nursing developed from the mid nineteenth century in response to the need for the urban poor to be cared for at home. The district nursing service was first offered in a systematic way in Liverpool under the direction of William Rathbone, building on the enthusiasm for structured nursing generated by Florence Nightingale. The first district nurse course was offered at Liverpool Royal Infirmary. In the period before the NHS, district nursing, like other aspects of health care, was not free at the point of delivery and the patient was required to pay the nurse for care. Some patients were employed and so had national insurance linked to their job whilst others, perhaps the majority during times such as the depression of the 1920s, were unemployed and outside the scheme. They had no means of assisted payment and were denied care.

A district nurse, as defined by James & Low (1990), is:

a qualified registered nurse who has been especially trained to promote health, provide skilled nursing and health care to people in their own homes, wherever this may be. She/he leads a team of nursing staff and ensures that this care is appropriately planned and delivered to those who need it while at the same time making sure that other family members receive the help and support they need.

The district nurse provides nursing care directly to individuals and groups through direct access from self-referral and also receives referral from other members of the healthcare system and PHC team. District nurses care mainly for people who are ill or who are recovering from illness and require physical, practical nursing care as well as psychological support. Some of the care of clients is offered by family or friends acting as carers (see Ch. 8 for information on informal care), in which case the district nurse teaches carers aspects of the care process so that they can undertake this alone. The district nurse has responsibility to the person receiving treatment as the primary client and also to any carers as secondary clients of the service.

Practical nursing at home is not the same as in a hospital setting. The balance of power is shifted to the client and back-up services and equipment are remote. Homes are often not adapted to nursing procedures and sometimes the environment may be unsuitable. The nurse, therefore, must adapt procedures in order to offer care at home.

Skill and flexibility are hallmarks of a district nurse.

The NHS reforms have started changes in the district nurse role. More clients are cared for in the community, there is more emphasis on day surgery and early discharge from hospital following surgery. The numbers of frail older people have increased as a direct result of the NHS and Community Care Act 1990 which increased the amount of support available to keep elderly people at home rather than in institutional care. There has also been a rise in the number of 'hospital at home' initiatives. Work which was previously the domain of hospital practitioners is devolving to the district nursing services in a way which mirrors the change in emphasis of the NHS reforms and the ascendancy of primary health care. The workload for the district nurse will continue to increase and clients are likely to be more ill than previously as early discharge from hospital and 'hospital at home' schemes become more popular. The district nurse will require new clinical skills in order to manage care. Many nurses see the shift in services as a positive challenge to the district nurse to develop new and innovative ways of working (Hancock 1991, Corbett et al 1993). This is not, however, a uniformly held point of view.

The situation is complicated by the advent of skill mix (Case study 5.1). In the past, most clients requiring district nursing care were seen by qualified district nurses, or experienced staff nurses waiting to go onto district nurse training programmes. Now, financial constraints have encouraged skill mix of the district nursing team. Under the direction of a qualified district nurse most of the physical care of clients is carried out by junior grade non-specialist nursing staff and healthcare support workers who may be employed by social services. Similarly, all assessment was undertaken previously by the qualified district nurses and aspects of the care decided upon were delegated to the team. Increasingly, registered general nurses are undertaking assessment and leading the case management with the qualified district nurse acting only as a named case holder (Hancock 1991, Firth & Bindless 1993). Additionally, some of the care previously

---

Case study 5.1   The 'Value for Money' report

A report by the University of York and the NHSME Value for Money (VFM) unit (1992) revealed that only 3.4% of a G grade district nurse's time was spent on appropriate duties such as assessment and evaluating the quality of care. Other time was spent in activities which could be carried out by developmental grades, for example, by Project 2000 qualifiers who are not specialists in community care but who can practise in that domain with supervision, or community qualified nurses employed in non-specialist grade posts lower than the current G grade. The report was challenged by district nurses and the RCN as being task oriented in its view of district nursing and therefore not grasping the complexity of the role of a G grade nurse or nursing sister. The 'Value for Money' report, as it became known, recommended a drastic shift in skill mix in district nursing. It recommended that the G/H grade nurses should constitute only 25% of the workforce and that the remaining 75% should be D/E grade nurses.

The research consisted of describing a district nurse's role as a series of tasks and then measuring the amount of time each task took to complete. In addition, a level of skill was assigned to each task and this was taken into consideration in the final analysis. The report was not well received and was criticised for its lack of depth. Its critics stated that it was nothing more than a time and motion study. The RCN (1993) produced a counter response, the thrust of which was that the VFM report:

- Did not recognise aspects of psychological or therapeutic care given by district nurses
- Did not recognise the concept of holistic care
- Did not recognise the team approach to offering care which is undertaken by district nurses
- Did not recognise achievements made by district nurses in relation to their clients.

---

offered by the district nurse as part of an holistic package is now undertaken by social services following the division of need into health and social care parameters. Many district nurses believe that this devalues their role and that coupled with other aspects of the NHS reforms and changes in nurse education and practice, it places their function under threat (Lawton 1994). This problem is accentuated by limited resources.

In Liverpool the North Mersey Community Trust attempted to implement the 'Value for Money' report. The Trust planned to reduce the G/H grade complement of district nurses from 82 to 57 and ensure that all other staff would have developmental grades up to E grade. This was resisted by the district nurses on the basis that it would delegate to qualified district nurses a more supervisory role which would be detrimental to overall quality of care. The nurses won the argument, and 74 posts were maintained, because they emphasised the clinical and holistic nature of the complex care they offer.

School nursing

The school nurse is concerned with offering health promotion and health surveillance to the school age population through school-based programmes of surveillance, screening and education which are integrated into the life of the school. The nurse links school concerns regarding the child to those of the family and GP practice and should be the link between the school, the family and the PHC team. There is currently much debate over the suitability of primary care provision to school children, particularly adolescents, and a more developed link between the school nursing service and practice-based community health care nursing would be of great value. School nurses are involved in a variety of areas:

- health screening of new entrants to the school
- school-based vaccination programmes
- health screening of the school population
- health promotion and education, both one-to-one and in the classroom
- involvement in the life of the school as a member of the school team
- support to teachers and others with regard to managing chronic conditions
- direct health advice to children and parents.

THE FUTURE OF COMMUNITY NURSING SERVICES

The shape of community nursing services has been the subject of review and discussion for some time. Debate has centred around potential options to achieve the best for the population from the existing resources.

The Cumberlege report (1986)

This report envisioned community nurses working in teams of mixed skills and experience to reflect the assessed needs of a defined and naturally occurring population. The teams of nurses would work together, serving the population in an area with approximately 10 000–25 000 people. The nursing teams were to be integrated and to liaise with general practice, but not to be attached to the practice, placing nursing, rather than medicine, at the forefront of primary health care provision. Cumberlege emphasised the need for partnership between all professionals impacting upon the health of the population within a neighbourhood. Cumberlege also envisioned community nurses overlapping more in their areas of responsibility and having a shared core training programme. At the time of publication many nurses were attached to general practitioners and the report highlights three limitations of this system (Cumberlege 1986):

We see district nurses, health visitors and school nurses, with their support staff, working together as an integrated nursing team. Individually they would still work closely together with General Practitioners, but, as part also of a nursing team, they could, we believe, become a major force for change and improvement in Community health services.

Apart from other benefits, which we will describe, the neighbourhood nursing service would bring school nursing in from the periphery of primary care: it would mean that the needs of a neighbourhood's children would be brought into much sharper focus and would make it easier to take a more integrated, family based approach to the health care of children and young people.

Having identified particular health needs in the community, the members of the neighbourhood nursing services would be able to bring relevant problems and ideas for solutions to their general practitioner colleagues for individual or joint action; at the same time, general practitioners would have access to more nursing skills than are normally available in a smaller primary health care team working alone.

At a time when health visiting was moving towards its roots in a community-oriented approach to practice, Cumberlege (1986) recognised that GP attachment might stifle this potential. Additionally, while GP attachment could work well if the practice was developed fully and a primary health care team existed, many practices could not support this type of working and so the potential benefits could be lost.

The Cumberlege report was not fully implemented. Opposition from GPs centred around the fact that, if the report was implemented, they would no longer employ nurses directly and would lose the reimbursement they currently received. Coupled with this perhaps was fear of loss of control with regard to the direction of nursing for the practice. The recommendations of the Cumberlege report are listed in Box 5.6.

As a result of the NHS reforms, which did not address nursing in detail, several factors now predominantly influence the development of nursing in the community. Factors resulting from the NHS and Community Care Act 1990 are:

- the operation of an internal market for health care
- the GP contract
- development of fundholding, or other devolved budgeting
- direct employment of nurses and purchasing of nursing services by the GP from community trusts
- the merger of the family health service authorities with the district health authorities.

Factors resulting from PREPP are:

- the introduction of the overarching concept of the specialist practitioner as a recordable qualification, termed 'community health care nurse'
- the introduction of sub-specialist themes within community health care nursing
- registerable status for public health nursing specialists (health visiting) and recordable status for other themes
- combined specialist training programmes.

The Roy report (1990)

Prior to the introduction of the NHS and Community Care Act 1990, the White Papers that preceded it were open to scrutiny. As nei-

---

Box 5.6 The recommendations of the Cumberlege report (Cumberlege 1986)

1. District health authorities should identify neighbourhoods within their areas for the purposes of planning, organising and providing nursing and related primary health care services.
2. Neighbourhood nursing services should be established in each area.
3. Each neighbourhood nursing service should be headed by a manager based in the neighbourhood and selected on the basis of management skills and leadership qualities.
4. Community midwives, psychiatric nurses and mental handicap nurses should ensure, through co-ordination between their managers and the neighbourhood managers, that their specialist contribution to care is coordinated with that of the neighbourhood nursing service.
5. All other specialist nurses (e.g. diabetes specialist nurses, breast care nurses) who work outside the hospital should be based in the community as part of the neighbourhood nursing service. Each specialist nurse should be assigned to one or more neighbourhood services and the time allocated to each neighbourhood should be specified.
6. Nurse practitioners should be introduced to, and adopted within, primary health care.
7. The government should agree a limited list of items and agents that can be prescribed by nurses as part of nursing care and should issue guidelines to enable nurses to control drug dosages in defined circumstances.
8. To establish and be recognised as a primary health care team, each general medical practice and the community nurses associated with it should come to an understanding of the team's objectives and individual roles within it. The

understanding should be incorporated into a written agreement which names the doctors and community nurses comprising the team and should guarantee the rights of individuals to be consulted regarding changes, signed by the practice partners and the neighbourhood nursing service acting for the relevant health authority. The agreement should constitute a basis for any incentive payments which may be introduced to help develop and improve quality in general practice services.
9. The health advisory service should take on responsibility for identifying and promoting good practice in primary health care.
10. Subsidies to GPs, linked to employment of nursing staff, should be phased out.
11. Within 2 years the UKCC and ENB should introduce a common training course for all first level nurses intending to practise outside the hospital setting in health visiting, school nursing and district nursing.
12. The provision of community nursing services should remain the responsibility of the district health authority. In due course consideration should be given to merging the family practitioner committees (later developed into family health service authorities) with the district health authorities in order to bring all of primary health care services under the influence of one body.
13. A short, but rigorous, practical (as opposed to academic) manpower planning exercise should be undertaken to ensure that the training and supply of community nurses is, and remains, at an appropriate level. This review should be supported by the NHS Management Board as a constituent of reviewing regional health authority planning.

---

ther Working for Patients (1989) nor Caring for People (1989) made much mention of nursing services there was concern that nursing could be radically altered without any recourse to the profession. As a response to this the Roy report (1990) was commissioned by the Minister of Health. The remit of the report was to consider the management of district nurses, health visitors, community midwives, community psychiatric nurses, community mental handicap nurses, school nurses and other community-based specialists, including general practice nurses employed by GPs. The report identified five models of organisational management (Box 5.7).

Future community nursing organisation

The most likely model for community nursing organisation is focused around a GP population. The debate of who should employ nurses in primary care is unresolved, but it is a major contributor to success or failure of PHC development and should be explored thoroughly. It is unlikely that, as CHCNs integrate with general practice and overlap in function with professional colleagues, the number of specialist nurses will remain as at present. In other words, there will be fewer G grade or equivalent posts. For instance, if all the CHCNs share a practice popu-

---

Box 5.7 Models of organisational management, Roy report (1990)

1. A stand-alone community trust or directly managed unit, which would be responsible for the management of all nurses within the community, offering these to GPs and others, including hospitals and the voluntary and private sectors, on a contractual basis.
2. Locality management or 'neighbourhood nursing'. Skill-mixed teams of community nurses would work and be managed in geographical areas, perhaps around a fundholder GP or a consortia of practices. The management of the nursing teams either would rest with the community trust or directly managed unit, or could be managed separately. GPs would continue to employ and manage practice nurses to work in parallel to the neighbourhood team.
3. An expanded FHSA model, where the FHSA would take on responsibility for the provision of community nursing services, providing the GP with access to a range of specialist skills, under the auspices of an agency arrangement, with the DHA as employer and provider of nurses. It was envisaged that in some circumstances the FHSA might directly employ community nurses rather than obtain them on contract. The GP would continue to employ the practice nurse.
4. Vertical integration/outreach model, where purchasing authorities would be encouraged to contract with directly managed units or trusts, in order to provide total packages of care, including discharge management. This model envisages combinations of acute and community unit integration, with either facet of the partnership acting in an outreach capacity to the other.
5. The primary health care team. This option envisaged community nursing services being brought under the direct control and management of GPs. The model centres round individual GPs or consortia groups acting together.

Box 5.8 Standards for community nursing practice (McMurray 1993)

The community health care nurse fulfils the obligations of the professional role:
- Complies with the UKCC Code of Conduct (1992a) and the Scope of Professional Practice (1992b) and is aware of his own professional competence
- Functions within the bounds of legislation and common law
- Promotes the client's rights
- Acts to empower the client
- Maintains safety

Ensures equitable, effective and efficient use of available resources:
- Regularly updates, evaluates and develops own and others' knowledge and competence
- Participates in research and applies research findings appropriately to the art and science of nursing
- Participates in healthcare planning and strategic development
- Fosters progress towards health for all within a culturally diverse community

Establishes and maintains enabling interactions in professional relationships:
- Uses and promotes effective communication
- Conducts empathetic and effective interpersonal communication
- Establishes and maintains effective communication with the PHC team
- Acts as a client advocate
- Creates and uses opportunities for learning
- Has effective and appropriate written communication skills

Provides effective and efficient holistic nursing care to clients and families, carers and the community:
- Acknowledges the individual as an holistic being and reflects this in nursing. Recognises the need for partnership with clients
- Practises within multidisciplinary primary health care
- Enables the client's full participation
- Encourages optimum self care and independence
- Identifies the needs of carers and significant others and attempts to meet these needs

Operates a nursing database:
- Analyses and interprets data in order to identify individuals' and communities' health strengths and resources and their potential expectations of care
- Formulates a care plan which addresses health strategies, concerns and expectations, includes a statement of expected outcomes, and includes nursing interventions and rationales
- Plans, implements and evaluates care in partnership

---

lation as a caseload and more nurses in the PHC team achieve multiple qualification, it is likely that one, perhaps two, CHCN specialist practitioners will assume responsibility for the overall nursing service to the practice population, supported by junior nurses. The resultant skill mix, therefore, must be needs-based and nursing skills must be matched to identified local health need. This begs several questions (Bryar 1994). What are the existing skills within community nursing? Do they match need? If skills do not match needs how can this be corrected? Are the skills required those of a specialist CHCN or can the tasks be undertaken, with supervision, by junior nurses or by non-nurses or carers? How can diverse and available nursing skills be blended to best effect giving individual clients and communities cost effective, evidence-based care and services which are measured against health outcomes?

Owing to the benefits of economy of scale, general practices are likely to be teamed with other practices for purchasing and strategic planning; this is beginning to happen as GP consortia develop. The Labour Party have stated that this model is their preferred option to replace fundholding. Ideally, the teamed practices would be similar in size to a social services patch which would facilitate planning, delivery and purchasing of community care. The total area would have an advanced practitioner public health nurse responsible for strategic planning for nursing, for nursing interface with social services and education and for nursing issues throughout the area. This aspect of nursing practice would be a new nursing role (Bryar 1994) building on the role and core skills of the public health nurse

(health visitor) and is pivotal. The model lends itself to community-based/oriented primary care rather than a medical model, frees up nurses to practise autonomously and releases doctors, expensively trained key professionals, to practise medicine.

McMurray (1993) sets out standards for CHC nursing practice which apply to core practice as well as discrete themes. They are set out in Box 5.8, adapted for UK practice, and could provide a framework for the future contribution of CHCNs to primary care.

Summary

Community health care nurses are practising and developing their specialist skills and carving a new niche within PHC in a climate of constant change. Flexibility and a clear concept of the goals and philosophy of the specialist are critical to success, as is an understanding of the political and social context within which health care is offered. The CHCNs of today are creating the services of the future as well as maintaining service to clients. The specialty demands skills and ability over and above the usual and the benefits to clients are potentially enormous.

REFERENCES

Alfaro R 1990 Applying nursing diagnosis and nursing process: a step by step guide, 2nd edn. Lippincott, New York

ANA 1974 Standards of community health nursing practice. In: Higgs Z, Gustafson D 1985 Community as client: assessment and diagnosis. Davis, New York Executive Committee & Standards Committee. Division On Community Health Nursing Practice. ANA, Kansas.

Atkin K, Lunt N, Parker G, Hirst M 1993 Nurses count: a national census of practice nurses. Social Policy Research Unit. University of York, York

Atkinson S, Murphy K 1994 Reflection: a review of the literature. Journal of Advanced Nursing. 18:1188–1192

Benner P 1984 From novice to expert. Addison Wesley, London

Benner P 1991 From novice to expert: excellence and power in clinical nursing practice. Addison Wesley, London

Boud D, Keogh R, Walker D 1985 Promoting reflection in learning: a model. In: Boud D, Keogh R, Walker D, Reflection: turning experience into learning. Kogan Page, London

Bowling A, Stillwell B 1990 The nurse in family practice. Scutari, London

Bradshaw J 1972 The concept of need. New Society 30: 640–643

Bryar R 1994 An examination of the need for new nursing roles in primary health care. Journal of Interprofessional Care. 8(1):73–84

Butterworth A, Faugier J 1992 Clinical supervision and mentoring in nursing. Chapman Hall, London

Carper B 1978 Fundamental patterns of knowing in nursing. Advances in Nursing Science 1(1):13–23

Clarke D 1986 Showing that it can be done. Health Service Journal 96(5019):1297

Clarke M 1984 Community nusing: health care for today and tomorrow. Reston Publishing, Reston

Corbett K, Meehan L, Sackey V A 1993 Strategy to enhance skills: developing IV therapy skills for community nursing. Professional Nurse 9(1):60–63

Council for the Education and Training of Health Visitors (CETHV) 1977 An investigation into the principles of health visiting. CETHV, London

Davies C 1988 The health visitor as mother's friend: a woman's place in public health, 1900–1914. The Social History Of Medicine 1:38–57

Department of Health 1989 Working for patients. White paper. Cm 555. HMSO, London

Department of Health 1989 Caring for people: community care in the next decade and beyond. Cm 849. HMSO, London

Department of Health 1990 National health service and community care act. HMSO, London

Department of Health 1990 The Roy report. HMSO, London

Department of Health 1992 Health of the nation: a strategy for health in England. HMSO, London

Department of Health and Social Security 1969 Report of the committee on local authority and allied personal social services (Seebohm report). Cm 3093. HMSO, London

Department of Health and Social Security (Cumberlege J) 1986 Neighbourhood nursing: a focus for care. HMSO, London

Faugier J 1994 Thin on the ground. Nursing Times 90(20):64–65

Faugier J, Butterworth T 1994 Clinical supervision: a position paper. University of Manchester, Manchester

Firth J, Bindless L 1993 Rally cry: or last post. Journal of Community Nursing 6(13):24

Forward Strategies Working Group 1991 Good health is good business. RCN, London

Gordon M 1979 The concept of nursing diagnosis. The Nursing Clinics of North America 14(3):487–496

Gray J, Forsstrom S 1992 Generating theory from practice: the reflective technique. In: Gray G, Pratt R Towards a discipline of nursing. Churchill Livingstone, Edinburgh

Gregson B, Cartlidge A, Bond J 1991 Interprofessional collaboration in primary health care organisations. Occasional Paper 32. Royal College of General Practitioners, London

Griffin N 1992 Occupational health advice as part of primary health care nursing. Health and Safety Executive, London

Haller L 1976 Clinical psychiatric supervision: process and problems – a method of teaching psychiatric concepts in nursing education. Perspectives in Psychiatric Care 14:115–129

Hancock C 1991 Community nursing: is there a future ? Senior Nurse 11(5):4–7

Hawkins P, Schoet R 1991 Supervision in the helping professions: an individual, group and organisational approach. Oxford University Press, Oxford

Heron J 1990 Helping the client. Sage Publications, London

Holliday I 1992 The NHS transformed. Baseline Books, Manchester

Hurst K 1991 The recognition and non-recognition of problem solving strategies in nursing practice. Journal of Advanced Nursing 16:1444–1455

James E, Low H 1990 The district nurse. RCN District Nurse Forum. Royal College of Nursing, London

Jarman B, Cumberlege J 1987 Developing primary health care. British Medical Journal 294:1005–1008

Johns C 1993 Note taking in guided reflection. Unpublished PhD thesis

Johns C 1994 Guided reflection. In: Palmer, Burns, Bulman. Reflective practice in nursing. Blackwell, Oxford

Johns C 1997 Model for structured reflection, 11th edn. Unpublished

Jones J 1988 Clinical reasoning in nursing. Journal of Advanced Nursing 13:185–192

King I S 1967 What is a diagnosis? Journal of The American Medical Association 202:714–717

Lawrence M 1988 All together now. Journal of The Royal College of General Practitioners 38:296–302

Lawton S 1994 Promoting district nursing skills. Journal of Community Nursing 8(6):8–10

Liss P E 1993 Health care need. Avebury, Aldershot

Luker K 1982 Evaluating health visiting practice. RCN, London

Maslow A 1943 A theory of human motivation. Psychological Review 50:370–396

Mason G, Webb C 1993 Nursing diagnosis: a review of the literature. Journal of Clinical Nursing 2:67–74

McCleary 1933 The early history of the infant welfare movement. Lewis, London

McFarlane J 1982 A charter for caring. Journal of Advanced Nursing

McMurray A 1993 Community health nursing: primary health care in practice, 2nd edn. Churchill Livingstone, Edinburgh

Miller S 1992 The cost of caring. Paediatric Nursing 4(9):25–26

Ministry of Health 1946 National Health Service Act. Health service to be provided by local health authorities under part 3 of the Act. Circ. 118/47. HMSO, London

Ministry of Health 1956 An enquiry into health visiting (Jameson Committee). HMSO, London

National Health Service Executive (NHSE) 1996 Child health in the community: a guide to good practice. HMSO, UK

National Health Service Management Executive 1992 The nursing skill mix in the district nursing service. NHSME, London

National Health Service Management Executive 1993 Nursing in primary health care: new world, new opportunities. HMSO, London

North N 1993 Empowerment in welfare markets. Journal of Health and Social Care in the Community. 1(3):129–137

Orem D 1985 Nursing: concepts of practice, 3rd edn. McGraw Hill, New York

Paunonen N 1991 Changes initiated by a nursing supervision programme: an analysis based on log-linear models. Journal of Advanced Nursing 16:982–986

Philips J R 1987 A critique of Parse's man-living-health theory. In: Nursing science, Parse R R (ed), Saunders, Philadelphia

Robinson J 1982 An evaluation of health visiting. Council for the Education and Training of Health Visitors, London

Rogers K 1988 Nursing science and art: a perspective. Nursing Science Quarterly 1:99–102

Royal College of Nursing 1993 District nurses and value for money: an RCN response. RCN, London

Schlotfeldt R M 1988 Structuring nursing knowledge: a priority for creating nursing's future. Nursing Science Quarterly 1:35–38

Schon D 1988 Educating the reflective practitioner. Jossey Bass, USA

Sefton Health, Primary Educare, Southport & Formby Community Trust 1996 Working group on community nursing. Sefton Health, Unpublished

Simmons S, Brooker C 1986 Community psychiatric nursing: a social perspective. Heinemann, London

Tanner C A, Benner P, Chesla C, Gordon D 1987 The phenomenology of knowing the patient. Image: Journal of Nursing Scholarship. 25(4):273–280

Tatman M 1994 Wise decisions: developing paediatric home care schemes. Scutari, London

Taylor S 1954 Good general practice. Oxford University Press, Oxford

UKCC 1992a Code of professional conduct. UKCC, London

UKCC 1992b The scope of professional practice. UKCC, London

UKCC 1994 The future of professional practice: the councils standards for education and practice following registration. UKCC, London

Watson J 1993 Advanced nursing practice and what might be. Keynote Paper, 3rd National Conference of Nurse Practitioners, Canada

White E 1991 The third quinquennial national community psychiatric nursing survey. Department of Nursing, University of Manchester, Manchester

Williams C 1986 Community health nursing: what is it? In: Spradley B Readings in community health nursing, 3rd edn. Little Brown, Boston

Woolnough F 1990 A crisis of identity. Practice Nurse 2:447–8, 454

Zeigler S M 1986 Nursing process, nursing diagnosis, nursing knowledge: avenues to autonomy. Appleton Century Crofts, New York

Conceptual models for practice

Ros Carnwell

Nurses have looked to models of practice to provide an organisational structure for patient care as well as a way to develop and advance practice. Community health care nurses should be able to understand the basic principles which underpin the construction of models of nursing practice and appraise them critically to decide whether a particular model is appropriate for their area practice. To do this successfully, community health care nurses must be able to:

- Distinguish between concepts, models and theories
- Discuss and interpret a variety of models
- Apply models to community health care nursing
- Attempt to develop a model relevant to the community health care nursing needs of their patients.

The nursing profession has shown increasing interest in conceptual models of practice in order to question the basis of that practice. This has led to a stronger research base and the development of theories and models which explain and guide nursing practice. The first nursing model was developed for mental health nursing by Peplau in 1952. Since then authors such as Comley (1994) have compared different models; others have discussed their use (Girot 1990, Kenny 1993); and still others have developed new models (Chalmers and Kristajanson 1989, Chalmers

1992). In spite of this interest in models and theories, few attempts have been made to apply models to community health settings. However, it is useful to consider the application of a variety of models to the different disciplines within community health care (CHC) nursing. The nurse should be able to distinguish between concepts, models and theories, be aware of the models which are appropriate to CHC nursing, and be able to apply a model.

CONCEPTS, THEORIES AND MODELS

DEFINITIONS

Concepts can be described as labels that are ascribed to images and objects. By labelling objects and images categories can be developed to try to make sense of experience. For example, race is a concept associated with certain images of culture, religion and skin colour. By categorising race in this way, the complexity of racial issues can be considered.

Concepts such as race can be grouped together with other concepts, such as gender and class, to form a model. Models are, therefore, groups of concepts which are interrelated. Relating concepts to each other is referred to as the propositional stage of theory development. For example, we can propose that the relationship between race, gender and social class results in inequality of access to health care. However, at the propositional stage we cannot be sure of this because the proposition has not been tested. Testing this proposition will result in the development of theory, which can be defined as the reality which is discovered by testing propositions and which is used to describe, predict and explain actions.

Another example illustrates the relationship between concepts and theories. Each individual has different concepts (personal beliefs) about health and health behaviour which may be related in some way and will influence health behaviour. The propositional statement would specify this relationship, which could then be tested so that a theory could be developed. For example,

if beliefs about health do influence health behaviour, then nursing practice should be directed at understanding and influencing individual beliefs. Theories are useful, therefore, because their underlying assumptions organise nursing knowledge and guide practice (Akinsanya et al 1994).

For Akinsanya et al (1994) nursing models describe, explain and predict nursing practice. However, nursing models are not just the business of theorists: community nurses also need to use different components of the nursing discipline to inform their practice. In drawing from nursing and other disciplines to formulate models to guide their practice, community nurses will explain and predict their actions. Fawcett (1992) argues that there is a reciprocal relationship between conceptual models and nursing practice; models guide practice and practice provides evidence for the credibility of the model. For example, credibility is maintained when patient outcomes match the model's expectations. Orem's (1987) model, which is based on assumptions about the individual's capacity for self-care, provides an example of this. Orem assumes that self-care deficits occur when people become ill, and that nurses provide some type of system to either compensate for this deficit, or to support and educate the patient. If this is found to be the case, that Orem's model 'matches' what happens in the real world, then the model will have credibility.

Models do not, however, only describe and explain nursing actions. According to McClymont et al (1991) they also help practitioners to organise their thoughts and justify what they do and how they achieve it. Some NHS trusts require community nurses to use a particular model which may cause them to have a 'blinkered' approach when assessing a client's needs. A more successful approach is to select a model which is appropriate to a particular situation rather than attempting to make situations 'fit' a prescribed model.

DEVELOPING THEORIES AND MODELS

There are two means by which theory can be

developed: deductive and inductive. Inductive reasoning is the first step in attaining knowledge, and assumes that there are no known facts concerning the particular subject. The task of inductive reasoning is, therefore, to bring knowledge into view for the first time. Deductive reasoning is the reverse of inductive reasoning because it uses existing facts and knowledge to generate new theories.

For example, the deductive approach to nursing theory involves nurses borrowing theories from other disciplines. An example of this is Neuman's systems model (1989), which is based on Selye's (1956) theory of stress. By using Selye's theory within the health context, the CHC nurse is validating the theory empirically, that is, through his own experience. Thus, by using a general theory of stress, Neuman predicted the effect this would have on patient care. Alternatively, an inductive approach to theory development may be appropriate, involving the CHCN in examining an area of practice, identifying relationships within the practice and then using research to test and validate the efficacy of that practice (Akinsanya et al 1994). Case study 6.1 shows how this can be applied to practice.

In Case study 6.1 the district nurse is developing general rules from specific observations concerning patient anxiety. This empirical validation of both deductive and inductive theory is of great importance. Girot (1990) cites several authors who express concern about the lack of scientific testing of nursing theories. Chin & Jacobs (1978) in particular, believe that it is hazardous to develop nursing theory without validating proposed relationships empirically.

Case study 6.1   **Inductive theory development**
A district nurse notices that patients appear less anxious when they are expecting her at the time she arrives. She decides to test this assumption by surveying patients before and after the implementation of an appointment visiting system to establish whether the intervention results in reduced anxiety and increased satisfaction in patients.

TYPES OF MODEL

Meleis (1985) argues that early nursing models were based on guiding paradigms, which are widely agreed patterns, such as:

- Systems models which assume that the individual is a system, divided into subsystems and influenced by both internal and external environmental stimuli to which the person must adapt.
- Developmental models which are concerned with needs arising from the developmental stages humans pass through.
- Interaction models which rely on the concept of symbolic interactionism. This assumes that humans use symbols to interact with others and base their interactions with others on the interpretation of these symbols. Interaction theories are concerned with how nurses interact with patients and clients, rather than what they do.

All nursing models, therefore, fit into one of these paradigms. In addition, nursing models embody four metaparadigms:

- Person
- Health
- Environment
- Nursing.

Metaparadigms are fundamental to all nursing models and illustrate the interrelationship between nursing, the person, the person's perception of health, and how that is influenced by the environment.

NURSING MODELS AND CHC NURSING

Where appropriate the models presented in this chapter will be evaluated using Fawcett's (1984) criteria, specified in Box 6.1

NEUMAN'S SYSTEMS MODEL

Neuman's model views the client as a 'dynamic composite of physiological, sociocultural, devel-

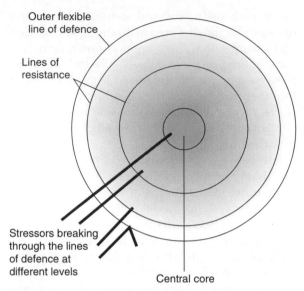

Figure 6.1   Neuman's defence circles.

opmental and spiritual variables' (Neuman 1989). The relationship between these variables can affect the ability of the individual to fight off stressors. According to Neuman, individuals have a defence system which is represented as a series of circles (Fig. 6.1.) The circles depict lines of defence which protect the central core from the effects of stressors. Stressors break through this normal line of defence when the outer flexible line of defence fails to protect the individual from stressors. When this occurs the internal lines of resistance attempt to re-stabilise the individual. The model is also based on assumptions concerning primary, secondary and tertiary prevention and their capacity to prevent stress. These assumptions are derived deductively from

a range of theories including general systems theory (Bertalanffy 1968), stress theory (Selye 1956) and levels of prevention theory (Caplan 1964). In addition, the model was inductively derived from Neuman's observations and experience in mental health nursing (Fawcett 1984). Case study 6.2 illustrates the use of Neuman's model in health visiting.

It shows how an holistic picture of the client's concerns can be built up using a model. The case study can also be used to illustrate the use of the four metaparadigms. The types of stressors evident in the case study correspond to the four nursing metaparadigms (Table 6.1).

It is also useful to note that Neuman's model also draws on Caplan's (1964) levels of prevention. Thus, the community health care nurse will use different levels of prevention in the identification of stressors. For example, in the case study, Sally would use primary prevention to educate Emily and her husband about the demands and responsibilities of parenthood. Secondary prevention would be used to identify stressors early so that intervention could be instigated, and tertiary prevention would involve support and counselling to prevent any further deterioration in Emily's emotional health.

Case study 6.2 **Using Neuman's model in health visiting**

John, aged 24 and his wife Emily, 22, had their first child, Sarah, 6 weeks ago. The delivery was normal and everything has progressed well. Sally is the health visitor and visits the family 6 weeks following the birth. She feels that everything is not well with Emily and decides to use Neuman's systems model because she feels that Emily's problems may be a result of stress. On discussion with Emily she discovers that Emily certainly does feel under a great deal of pressure. She says that although she is normally placid, for the past 2 weeks she has felt 'very low'. This could be likened to stressors permeating through the lines of resistance until they affect the internal core, thus creating negative feelings.

Sally believes that in order to help Emily to deal with her problems she will need to identify the causes. She therefore uses Neuman's model to explore with Emily the different types of stressors: intrapersonal, interpersonal and extrapersonal.

Intrapersonal stressors – these are stress factors that are present within Emily herself. Emily says that she has felt physically drained since the birth of Sarah and feels unable to function properly as a mother. This makes her feel guilty which then makes her feel more depressed and lethargic.

Interpersonal stressors – these are stress factors associated with relationships between two or more people. Emily says that her husband has a demanding job and works long hours. He has to get up early in the morning and therefore does not feed Sarah during the night. Because Sarah wakes several times each night and is difficult to settle, Emily is becoming more tired and feels resentful of her husband because he refuses to share in Sarah's care.

Extrapersonal stressors – these are stress factors outside the relationship in the wider environment. Emily states that their problems are compounded by the fact that the dividing walls between their house and the house next door are so thin that the neighbours have complained about Sarah's persistent crying.

Table 6.1 Relationship between metaparadigms and stressors

Metaparadigm	Type of stressor	Example
Physiological	Intrapersonal	Tiredness due to child birth and lack of sleep
	Interpersonal	Lethargy due to sole responsibility of child care
Psychological	Interpersonal	Arguments with husband about responsibility of child care
Sociocultural	Extrapersonal	Complaints from neighbours about baby crying
Developmental	Intrapersonal	Possibly post-natal depression due to hormonal changes

Evaluating Neuman's model

The four metaparadigms are clearly stated in Neuman's (1989) model. The person is viewed as a composite of physiological, psychological, sociocultural and developmental variables. Neuman (1974) stated that a stress reaction could be influenced by intra-, inter- and extrapersonal factors, that is within the individual, between individuals, and forces occurring outside the person.

This interaction between stressors within and outside the individual reflects the environment metaparadigm which holds that the environment is 'the internal and external forces surrounding man at any point in time' (Neuman 1982). The metaparadigm of health also draws on this notion of interaction since health is deemed to be a state of stability which occurs when the person's flexible line of defence has successfully prevented stressors from penetrating the normal line of defence (Neuman 1982). Fawcett (1984) suggests that Neuman's perception of variations of wellness determined by penetration of lines of resistance by stressors, is indicative of health as a continuum rather than a dichotomy of wellness or illness. The metaparadigm of nursing is summarised as attainment and maintenance of the client system stability (Neuman 1982). Nurses therefore, as indicated in Case study 6.2, intervene to reduce stressors penetrating the lines of resistance.

Neuman explains the assumptions concerning the four metaparadigms underlying the model – the impact of *stressors* and the *systems* approach (Fawcett 1984). She emphasises the need to consider both the client's and care giver's perceptions of stressors when negotiating goals with clients. Her choice of systems and her thinking views clients holistically within the context of their environment. These assumptions are particularly relevant to community nursing, since they reflect the dynamic nature of the individual emphasising equilibrium rather than illness. Nevertheless, Neuman assumes that nurse and client share common values on what constitutes equilibrium and harmony with the environment and, therefore, concepts of equilibrium and the normal range of responses are ambiguous for public health nursing (Haggart 1993).

Fawcett (1984) criticises the model on several counts. First, concepts of prevention, environment and health could be explained more fully. Second, the model is incongruent logically because it fails to acknowledge the person as well as the environment as a source of stress; this also challenges the classification of the model as a systems model. Third, this lack of two-way interaction between person and environment results in a closed rather than an open system (Fawcett 1992). In community nursing, because individuals are not seen as a source of stress, they are assumed to be passively reliant on nursing intervention to relieve stress. Recent emphasis on working in partnership with clients to empower them to make healthy choices and to take charge of their lives, suggests that they have the capacity to be more active in their control of stressors than is suggested by Neuman's model. In fact, Haggart (1993) suggests that community work aims to enable people to change the environment or situation rather than accept and adapt to it.

The social considerations evaluated by Fawcett (1984) comprise social congruence, social significance and social utility. In relation to social congruence, Fawcett claims that because primary prevention is not familiar to some consumers, it may not lead to important differences in health status. However, these criticisms are less applicable to community nursing in which primary prevention is widely practised. Using this model within an empowering relationship, for example through stress management groups and community participation, would probably result in a greater improvement in client health than is evident in hospital settings.

According to Fawcett (1984) the utility of the model is reflected in the literature, demonstrating its application in a variety of settings. Application of the model to public health nursing (Benedict & Behringer Sproles 1982), mental health, and community nursing (Beitler et al 1980) confirms its value to community settings. The ability of the model to generate and test theory remains questionable because concepts such as 'intervention' would need to be operationally defined before being empirically tested (Fawcett 1984). However, the contribution of Neuman's model to nursing knowledge is sufficiently diverse to be applicable to community nursing. Fawcett (1984) concludes that the model covers the total person; environmental influences on health; the feature of wellness; and clients' perceptions of stressors. These characteristics will appeal to all community nurses who view their clients holistically.

PEPLAU'S DEVELOPMENTAL MODEL

Peplau's (1952) model was the first attempt to base mental health nursing on theory. Like more recent models, it was derived from existing theories which Peplau used to understand the development of the nurse–patient relationship. Peplau referred to this relationship as 'psychodynamic nursing' because it was based on theories of psychoanalysis, social learning, motivation and personality (Comley 1994). The concept of psychodynamic nursing has been defined as 'being able to understand one's own behaviour to help others identify felt difficulties, and to apply principles of human relations to problems at all levels of experience' (Peplau 1952).

Peplau's model is a developmental model (Chin 1980) because it includes the notion of growth of the nurse and client through the development of the nurse–patient relationship (Simpson 1991). Simpson (1991) also asserts that the model possesses characteristics of an interaction model (Heiss 1976, Benoliel 1977), such as social acts, relationship building, role and self concept.

Peplau assumes that the kind of person the nurse becomes in the relationship with the client affects what the client learns from the experience of illness. She proposes that the nurse should confront interpersonal problems so that both the nurse and client learn, develop and mature through the mutual relationship. This maturity in the nurse allows clients greater opportunity to learn about and develop insight into their condition so that they gain greater control over their own actions in relation to their health problems.

This psychodynamic aspect of nursing seems appropriate to community settings, because CHC nursing normally requires practitioners to develop a closer relationship with clients and patients than is possible in hospital settings. The community nurse's behaviour and maturity are fundamental to developing a partnership with clients, empowering them to make positive choices so that successful outcomes can be achieved.

The phases of the nurse–patient relationship described by Peplau (1952) illustrate its application beyond mental health nursing, and are:

- Orientation
- Identification
- Exploitation
- Resolution.

Although these phases overlap, the relationship develops through the sequence described, during which Peplau suggests that nurses adopt certain roles:

- Stranger
- Resource person
- Teacher
- Leader
- Surrogate
- Counsellor.

Orientation phase. The orientation stage refers to the early stage of the nurse/client relationship which may be instigated by either the patient or the nurse. For example, a mental health nurse or district nurse may visit the client following referral from a GP, or a health visitor may visit either antenatally or following the birth of a baby. Alternatively, the client may instigate the relationship by seeking advice from the nurse.

The community nurse will need to work hard to develop trust during the orientation stage so that the client's needs can be accurately assessed. Although this model views the nurse–patient relationship as a means of solving the client's problems, a relationship may be established to prevent health problems and to promote good health. This would apply to health visiting and perhaps learning disability nurses who may be supporting families and promoting a healthy environment rather than solving problems.

The orientation stage, then, illustrates the importance of establishing a rapport with clients on their own terms. During this stage the community nurse will adopt the role of stranger initially, but will quickly become a resource person, teacher or leader. Roles of teacher and resource person are quite prevalent during the early stages of a relationship in which information is often given about the resources available, and the client may be educated about healthy lifestyles. It may take a considerable time before the relationship moves towards the identification stage.

Identification phase. During the identification stage the nurse adopts a counsellor role, allowing the client to explore feelings so that problems can be identified and positive forces in the personality can be strengthened. Although this stage is problem oriented, this need not be the case in community nursing. For example, a district nurse visiting a terminally ill patient may use the identification phase of the nurse–patient relationship to help the patient to draw on inner spiritual resources. This identification of inner resources also shows how the patient may gain full value from the nurse–patient relationship during the exploitation phase.

Exploitation stage. During the exploitation stage the nurse's role combines counselling with surrogacy. The district nurse may work with the patient and family to facilitate independence, although Peplau anticipated that the nurse–patient relationship would vacillate between dependence and independence during the exploitation stage. It is a particularly productive stage and a necessary precursor to the final stage.

Resolution stage. The fourth stage of the relationship, resolution, is demonstrated in relation to mental health nursing. The nurse may work through the stages of orientation, identification and exploitation with a client with depression; once problems are identified and the relationship has been exploited, goals would be set for the future which the client would be able to achieve with minimal input from the nurse. The role of leader is typical of this stage, as the mental health nurse works with other members of the primary health care (PHC) team such as the GP, practice nurse and health visitor, to instigate ongoing support for the client.

This example also demonstrates how the model can be used by various members of the PHC team, each working at a different developmental stage and adopting different roles in their relationship with the client. For example, the health visitor may work with a new mother and conclude at the identification stage that she is suffering from post-natal depression. Referral to a GP may confirm this diagnosis, although the relationship may not move beyond the orientation stage. The mental health nurse may take over the care of the client from the health visitor and would work through all the processes to the resolution stage. In Case study 6.3, the use of Peplau's model in district nursing is illustrated.

The development of the relationship between the district nurse and Mrs Green is examined in Table 6.2, which shows how different roles are exploited at different stages of the relationship.

Case study 6.3   Using Peplau's model in district nursing

Mrs Green is terminally ill following a diagnosis of leukaemia 10 months ago. She is 35 years old and has a husband and three school-age children. During her last hospital admission Mrs Green was told that she did not have long to live and decided that she would like to spend her final weeks at home.

Lynne was the district nurse who commenced visiting following discharge. Lynne realised immediately that the family were extremely distressed and that if she was to be of help to the whole family her relationship with them was crucial. She therefore decided to use Peplau's model to assess the family's needs and plan her care.

Table 6.2 Analysing Peplau's model in action

Phase	Role	Example
Orientation	Stranger Resource person Teacher Leader	Lynne enters the relationship as a stranger and orientates herself to the family's needs. She works hard to gain their trust by acting as a resource person in mobilising other resources. She also acts as teacher and leader by explaining to the family how Mrs Green's pain can be controlled
Identification	Counsellor	Lynne uses a counselling role to identify the feelings of the whole family. By using this role she is able to identify the family's religious beliefs and helps them to draw on their inner resources
Exploitation	Counsellor Surrogate	The benefits of the relationship are fully exploited at this stage as Lynne acts as counsellor and surrogate by allowing the family members to express their feelings freely
Resolution	Leader	During this stage Lynne prepares the family for the future. She supports the family in their quest to consider their future family life and acts as a leader by explaining about support facilities which will be available for the family

Evaluating Peplau's model

In relating Peplau's (1952) model to the four metaparadigms, the person is perceived as an organism living in an unstable environment. Environmental instability will affect health status; for example, poverty has clear links with ill health (Blackburn 1992) and environmental pollution may also affect well-being. Health is defined by Peplau (1952) as growth of personality towards creative, constructive, productive, personal and community living. She focuses on the maturing personality rather than physiological and biological aspects of health (Comley 1994). Although this conception of health is not holistic, it does reflect the need for constructive and productive community living which the nurse could facilitate even in unstable environmental conditions. Peplau perceives the environment as forces outside the individual but within the cultural context, which affect the interpersonal process. The goal of nursing is to have an impact on conditions that motivate natural, continuing tendencies in people. For health visitors this may include the influence of policies affecting health (CETHV 1977) at national, local and private levels.

Evaluation of Peplau's model using Fawcett's (1984) criteria indicates that the model has evolved from historical roots in psychology, the metaparadigm concepts being oriented towards interpersonal relationships. Although Comley (1994) criticises the model for a lack of holistic perspective, she recognises that it was developed before nurses realised the need for a holistic approach to client care. Relationships between concepts are relatively clear, as are the assumptions underpinning the model. The stages of the nurse–patient relationship specified are logical. The model could generate theories in nursing, particularly if applied to the nurse–patient relationship beyond mental health nursing in community settings. Theories could also be generated from this model in relation to multidisciplinary involvement with clients, which may include members of the PHC team and multi-agency participation in client care, each member operating at a different stage of relationship with the client.

OREM'S SELF-CARE MODEL

Orem's model is derived both inductively, from empirical conceptualisations arising from her observations of patients, and deductively from behavioural sciences and psychoanalysis (Comley 1994). From her empirical observations Orem (1971) concluded that people need nursing when their ability to care for themselves is limited (Marriner 1986). Although Meleis (1985) describes the model as needs-based, it could also be defined as a systems model with interactionist elements. Unlike other interactionist models, it focuses on coping strategies that have already been developed and therefore cannot be described as reductionist (Rourke 1991). Before considering the subdivisions of Orem's model and applying them to community nursing, it is worth considering her view of the metaparadigms and assumptions underpinning the model.

Orem views humans as biopsychosocial beings, capable of and willing to provide care for themselves but dependent on others. Self-care behaviour is initiated and performed on one's own behalf to maintain health, life and well-being. It is learned behaviour used to meet known needs (Comley 1994). Orem (1985) divides these needs into three groups of 'self care requisites':

- Universal requirements are those which all individuals need to maintain, regardless of their stage of life and development, such as air, food and water, elimination, exercise and rest, interaction and safety.
- Developmental life cycle factors are the requirements which promote growth and development and prevent conditions which adversely affect health.
- Health deviation requisites refer to the increased demands on an individual experiencing disease or illness resulting from structural, functional and genetic defects requiring intervention and treatment.

Orem divides her theory of nursing into three sub-theories:

- Self-care deficit
- Self-care
- Nursing systems.

Self-care deficit. The self-care deficit proposes

that nursing is used to enhance a person's own efforts when self-care is limited due to ill health. The deficit refers to the unequal relationship between capabilities (agency) of the adult and the required self-care demand; this deficit must exist for nursing care to be legitimate (Orem 1987). Nursing care may be minimal, however, when the self-care deficit is partial, but may be total when the self-care deficit is complete (Orem 1991).

Self-care. Self-care is based on presuppositions that self-care action varies by individual social experience and culture, and is a deliberate action in response to a known need (Hartweg 1991). Depending on factors such as culture or social experience, some individuals will choose deliberately to undertake self-care, and others will not be motivated to do so. Dependent care is required when individuals (such as infants or individuals with special needs) have not matured to the extent that they can engage in self-care.

Nursing systems. Orem (1987) defines her theory of nursing as a unifying theory since it subsumes the theories of self-care and self-care deficit. The central idea is that nurses use their abilities to determine whether nursing help is legitimate (Hartweg 1991). The nurse assesses the relationship between the client's ability to self-care and existing or potential self-care deficit and negotiates a plan of action to determine how the deficit will be met. The nurse is, therefore, empowering the client to meet self-care needs, rather than decreasing the demand for self-care.

Orem (1985) describes three systems of nursing which are adopted according to the client's self-care deficit:

- The wholly compensatory system involves total care for patients who are completely unable to care for themselves. District nurses, for example, will provide total care for clients who have severe physical disabilities.
- The partially compensatory system involves nurse and client working together to meet the self-care deficit. For example, learning disability nurses provide partial care when assisting clients towards independent living.

- The supportive–educative system is used when clients are able to engage in self-care. This system is used when the self-care deficit involves lack of knowledge which prevents the client from meeting healthcare needs. For example, nurses working in health education and health promotion provide information and support to empower the client to make appropriate choices to achieve self-care. Examples of this system include McClymont et al's (1991) application to health visiting older people, and Dean's (1991) use of the model to provide health visiting support to a family with a handicapped child.

The supportive–educative system is probably the nursing system most suited to a variety of community nursing disciplines. By educating people about their health and supporting them in their decisions, CHCNs empower people to meet their own self-care needs. Table 6.3 illustrates how these systems can be applied in different community nursing disciplines.

Evaluating Orem's model

Orem perceives the person as an integrated whole with inseparable physical, psychological and social aspects of health, and with the capacity for deliberate action. She describes the environment in terms of developmental, physical and psychosocial conditions that promote achievement of goals. Her view of nursing emphasises the different roles required by nurses determined by the level of compensation for self-care required. The four metaparadigms are, therefore, clearly specified in Orem's model in an holistic manner. Concepts within the model are logically related and defined. The model has proved useful in generating theory due to its application in nurse education and research (Hartweg 1991).

Rourke (1991) criticises the model for its presumption that patients know their own limitations or deficits, and may be unaware that their behaviour could be detrimental to health. If the ability to care for oneself is determined by education, culture and resources, then patients who are socially and intellectually disadvantaged may

Table 6.3 Applying Orem's systems of nursing

Nursing discipline	Example
District nurse	Advice to patients regarding an appropriate diet to facilitate healing. The partial compensatory system may have been used to enable the patient to engage in self-care activities but the nurse continues to monitor the patient's progress using a supportive– educative system
Mental health nurse	Used for severely depressed client who may lack self-determination. Counselling techniques used to increase the client's insight into her condition and hence the ability to meet self-care needs
School nurse	Teaching children about health and hygiene
Practice nurse	Teaching self-examination of the breast, or testicular self-examination
Occupational health nurse	Running stress management groups
Learning disability nurse	Teaching clients about personal relationships
Community children's nurse	Teaching parents how to care for and manage their child's illness in the home environment
Health visitor	Setting up a health stall in a market to deliver health messages to the public

not be able to maximise their potential (Rourke 1991). The supportive–educative system could then be maximised to enable people to reach their potential.

ROY'S ADAPTATION MODEL

Meleis (1985) describes Roy's (1984) model as an outcome model, concerned with maintaining balance and stability and enhancing harmony between the individual and the environment. Theories underpinning this conceptualisation are systems adaptation and developmental theories (Meleis 1985), their main focus being the outcome of care. Systems and adaptation theories are evident in her conception of the person as a biopsychosocial being who uses biological, psychological and social mechanisms in interacting

with and adapting to the environment. Each system within the person is motivated towards homeostasis and constancy of functioning (Roy 1984). (Homeostasis is a concept borrowed from biology, which refers to the tendency of the body to maintain itself at an optimal level (e.g. temperature) and to take corrective action if it departs from this.) Environmental changes require individuals to adapt to varying degrees depending on the level of environmental stimulus.

Physiological homeostasis is achieved by regulation of food and water and behavioural homeostasis is maintained by coping with new psychological or social experiences. Individuals strive for relative equilibrium, the adaptation required being unique to each individual. If new stimuli fall within this range of adaptation, it is more favourable for the individual than stimuli that fall outside this range. According to Roy (1984), adaptation is controlled by three sets of stimuli:

- Focal stimuli which are immediately present
- Contextual stimuli which occur alongside the focal stimuli
- Residual stimuli arising from past experience.

Also, four modes of adaptation influence behaviour:

- The physiological mode
- The self-concept mode
- The role-mastery mode,
- The interdependency mode.

A deficit or excess of resources relating to a mode of adaptation within the individual's environment requires nursing intervention to manipulate the relationship between environmental stimuli and the patient's adaptation level, so that the stimuli fall within the person's range of adaptations.

Applying modes and stimuli to CHC nursing practice

The physiological mode involves achieving homeostasis which relies on mutual working relationships between the different body systems and their interactions with each other (Akinsanya et al 1994). Physiological needs include exercise, rest, respiration and reproduction.

The self-concept model refers to self-understanding of behaviour and relationships with others. It includes beliefs and feelings arising from perceptions of internal and external environmental changes (Akinsanya et al 1994). Case studies 6.4 and 6.5 show the feelings which arise from maladaptation within self-concepts such as frustration, anxiety, anger, pride and fear. The immediate problem (focal), the context in which it occurs (contextual), and past experience (residual) influence the client's expression of self and hence the emotions experienced. In this way, Roy's model allows the nurse to gain a greater understanding of the individual's needs.

The role function mode refers to the sociological role played by a person such as wife or mother. Akinsanya et al (1994) suggest that this mode alerts us to possible tensions when demands upon a person's role fall outside the range of roles that they can accept. Maladaptation could occur in this mode due to ill health or adverse environmental conditions. The case studies indicate the roles

played, such as employee, wife and athlete, which are threatened by life events.

The interdependence mode refers to 'the close relationship of people that involves the willingness to love, respect and value others and to respond to love, respect and value given by others' (Roy & Andrews 1991). The conflict between a desire for independence and need for dependence is reflected in the Case studies 6.4 and 6.5.

Evaluating Roy's model

Roy's (1984) model helps the nurse to focus on the context of the problem, including the residual stimuli or past events affecting the client's perception of the problem and hence the level of adaptation achieved, rather than the problem on its own. In fact, this model can be used to focus on normal life events, such as the birth of a new baby, rather than problems. Crouch (1994) also demonstrates the use of the model by health visitors to develop a helping relationship with clients.

The model is holistic because of the modes of

Case study 6.4	**Roy's model applied in school nursing**			
Mode of adaptation	Problem	Focal	Contextual	Residual
Role function	Andrew wants to be a professional athlete but gets breathless.	Previously controlled asthma now out of control.	Worried about GCSEs. Parents have high expectations and want him to go to university. He wants to read sports studies, they want him to be a lawyer.	Has been a member of various sporting teams throughout school life. His friends are all successful in sport and less interested in academic work.
Interdependence	Andrew wishes to be independent of parents and enjoy social life with friends.	Frequently forgets to take inhaler to school and becomes breathless.	Parents very concerned about his health, a little over-protective.	His older sister died 3 years ago as a result of cystic fibrosis. He feels that his parents are too protective and limit his freedom.
Physiological	Andrew has had an asthma attack.	Asthma well controlled.	Taking GCSE examinations. Attack occurred after 10 minutes of writing.	Has suffered from asthma for 3 years. Normally uses inhaler but did not have inhaler with him during this attack.
Self-concept	Andrew does not like to use inhaler in front of friends.	Previously well controlled asthma now out of control.	Worried about GCSEs. Parents have high expectations and want him to go to university.	Resents the asthma for interfering with his social life. Has never really adjusted to suffering from asthma.

Case study 6.5	**Roy's model applied in practice nursing**			
Mode of adaptation	Problem	Focal	Contextual	Residual
Physiological	Sheila has a breast lump.	Attended routine appointment for smear test.	Has not noticed lump herself. Was more concerned about potential positive smear.	Her mother died from breast cancer 10 years ago.
Self-concept	Fear of mastectomy and the effect this would have on self-image.	Attended routine appointment for smear test.	Is an attractive and popular 32-year-old with no children. Is planning to get married next year.	Has always had an active social life. Always takes care of her appearance and works out three times per week to retain her figure.
Role function	Fears that her partner would find her less attractive if a mastectomy is required.	Breast lump found at routine appointment for smear test.	Has just started a new job as a company representative. Needs to look her best and meet the company targets.	Fears that she will lose her job due to sickness and has not worked there long enough to receive any benefits. Wants to save money for her wedding.
Interdependence	Does not want to subject her future husband to caring for her if she is terminally ill.	Worried that breast lump may be malignant.	Partner works as a marketing manager and is 'on his way to the top'. She does not want to ruin his chances of success.	She recalls the amount of care given to her mother during her terminal illness. Her father was required to take sick leave and ultimately lost his job.

adaptation and the different stimuli within these modes, combined with Roy's view of the person as a biopsychosocial being. Meleis (1985) criticises Roy's model for the lack of clarity of concepts which could be enhanced by 'theoretical distinctiveness, operational definitions, valid empirical referents and reliable data'.

The application of this model to a variety of nursing settings has demonstrated its ability to clarify practice, although the boundaries between some of the modes of adaptation are unclear (Meleis 1985). The model is time intensive due to its derivation from psychology, biology and sociology (Akinsanya et al 1994). Nevertheless, CHCNs wishing to understand the complexities of clients' needs in order to reflect on and enhance their practice, would find this model useful.

TOWARDS A MODEL OF CHC NURSING

In developing a model for CHC nursing some

existing models and theories should be examined. Elements of these theories, in addition to the concepts derived from the models discussed in this chapter, can be used to clarify and explain the role of the CHCN.

MODELS FOR COMMUNITY NURSING

Chalmers & Kristajanson (1989) compared three models of community nursing in order to examine its theoretical basis: the public health model, the community participation model, and the community change model. They point out that the public health model was developed in the nineteenth century to respond to threats to health such as communicable diseases and malnutrition. The model assumes that disease is determined by exposure of the host (the individual) to the agent, as well as the level of susceptibility of the host. This interaction between the individual and the environment is known as the host–agent environment interaction. The nurse intervenes in this relationship using primary and secondary prevention, thus protecting the health of the entire population by reducing the spread of disease. This was achieved by promotion of good nutrition to prevent the occurrence of disease (primary prevention), and screening the population for disease and immunisation (secondary prevention).

The community participation model involves the community in planning and delivering health services (Chalmers & Kristajanson 1989). The nurse assists communities in identifying their own problems and solutions, thus requiring a shift in power and control from professionals to community groups (Orr 1985). The community change model is an extension of this model, involving all sectors of the community in creating systems to work towards improving the community's health (Chalmers & Kristajanson 1989). It is more pervasive and political than the community participation model because it is based on Orr's (1985) belief that professional activities either confirm or challenge the dominant value system. This model assumes co-operative action from a united nursing body in order to 'influence policies affecting health' (CETHV 1977).

Theories of health visiting practice

Models and theories pertaining to health visiting include those developed by Chalmers (1992) and Robertson (1991). Although based in health visiting practice, both of these models could be applied to other community nursing disciplines.

Chalmers (1992) developed a theory of giving and receiving in health visiting which could be described as both interactive and developmental. It is interactive because of the psychosocial process of interaction between the client and health visitor which is regulated by the giving and receiving of information. The developmental nature of the model is determined by the management of the relationship through time, thus any community nurse who develops a relationship with clients and patients through time could find this model useful.

Chalmers identifies three phases of the health visitor/client relationship:

- The entry phase

- The health promotion phase
- The termination phase.

During the entry phase the health visitor gains access to the client within either an 'open context', that is, in response to an identified problem or need, or a 'closed context', that is, through 'routine' initiation by the health visitor. Depending on the context, the health visitor will either make a routine offer of information, or focus on needs identified by the client. In either case the client's perception of the value of the offer will determine whether it is received positively enough to progress to the health promotion phase. Advice and help is offered during this phase to promote health, its success again being determined by its value to the client. Help viewed positively will enable the client to share a range of health issues which can be addressed throughout the relationship.

Alternatively, the client may 'block' any offers not perceived as being of value. The interaction between the health visitor and client is, therefore, regulated by the type of offer made by the health visitor and the perception of its value by the client. The termination phase is characterised by either negotiated termination during which the client is prepared for the termination of visiting, or non-negotiation in which the visits are terminated without any input from the client.

Robertson (1991) developed a family health needs model for health visiting specifying four areas of health need:

- General environment
- Physical health
- Mental/emotional health
- Social aspects of health.

The health visitor reviews each of these areas of health need when assessing and planning care for individuals and families. Each area could be integrated with the other, allowing them to have an impact on each other. For example, damp housing conditions could contribute to chest infections and asthma, and a lack of play space could result in difficulties in managing child behaviour with an associated deterioration in mental health. Social aspects of health such as family support, friends and community facilities may, however, counteract environmental problems so that the worst physical and emotional effects may be avoided.

The holistic nature of this model will appeal to all community nurses. For example, a district nurse visiting an older person to administer monthly injections may be concerned that the physical environment and lack of income are contributing to poor health.

Robertson (1991) uses the health visiting cycle as the planning process, which equates to the nursing process, for the family health needs model. In operating the health visiting cycle, she distinguishes between different sources of information used in the assessment. These include knowledge gained from the locality, from records and other health professionals, from the client's viewpoint, from observations made during the visit and from a synthesis of information gleaned from previous visits to the family as well as information emerging from the visit. This planning process as well as the sources of information would apply equally to all community nursing disciplines.

A model for occupational health nursing

Rogers' (1990) model identifies the various components of occupational health nursing stating that its goal is to improve, protect, maintain and restore the health of the workforce within a legal/ethical framework. Thus, it is the context of practice – the workforce within a legal/ethical framework – that separates the goal of occupational health nurses from other nurses. Rogers suggests that occupational health nurse practice is influenced by conditions in the work setting such as availability of resources, corporate culture, work hazards and workforce characteristics. These influences operate within a framework of economic, population and health trends, legislation and politics and technology.

Rogers' model is underpinned by a philosophy of occupational health nursing practice and a definition of occupational health nursing. The model is useful for community health nursing because it emphasises the same macro-environmental influences that affect the goals of all community nurses, but also identifies work-based issues, which equate to the impact of the environment on the wider community. Thus, the wider role of the CHCN embraces the role of the occupational health nurse in promoting the health of the workforce.

Evaluating community health models

Using Fawcett's (1984) criteria to evaluate these models and theories, it can be seen that, with the exception of Robertson's (1991) family health needs model, the theories discussed are all based on existing theories. Chalmers & Kristajanson's (1989) theory of CHC nursing draws on biological theories of the host–agent environment and susceptibility, as well as assumptions about professional power, co-operation and political activity. Chalmers' (1992) model is based on theoretical concepts from symbolic interactionism (Mead 1934, Blumer 1969) because she argues that health visitor interactions with clients are influenced by the meaning that events have for them within the context of past experience. Exchange theory (Homans 1961, Blau 1964) is also used by Chalmers (1992), who suggests that health visitor/client interactions which do not provide any benefits or which create a sense of a lack of self-worth, or feelings of rejection or powerlessness, will be avoided. Rogers' (1990) occupational health nursing model identifies concepts concerning the context, philosophy and role of the occupational health nurse.

Chalmers & Kristajanson's (1989) theory is deductively derived from existing models. Chalmers (1992) model is both inductive, through its use of grounded theory, and deductive, because findings are substantiated by existing theory. Robertson's (1991) model again falls short here since the lack of theory to underpin it makes it neither inductive nor deductive. Concepts within the models are not clearly stated, although Chalmers (1992) and Rogers (1990) are most successful in this respect. None of the community models discussed specifies relationships between metaparadigms. The strength of the models lies in the specification of the areas of concern and their social considerations. Owing to the lack of propositional concepts they cannot be described as logically congruent.

THE DEVELOPMENT OF A MODEL FOR CHC NURSING

A DYNAMIC, ECLECTIC MODEL

The majority of the models discussed in this chapter focus on the individual and to a lesser extent the family. Other models focus only on the community (Chalmers & Kristajanson 1989). Moreover, Anderson & McFarlane (1988) discuss several community models, most of which focus on the community level and largely ignore the relationship between community and client.

The development of a unified model for CHC nursing is, therefore, problematic due to the diverse nature of the nursing task. The community nurse's role is determined largely by the nursing specialty which specifies the extent to which the nurse is involved in counselling, health promotion, treatment of conditions, caring, teaching, empowering clients or working with community groups. Such diverse tasks require a model which is sufficiently flexible to guide rather than constrain practice. This is consistent with Hardy's (1974) view which stresses the importance of multiple models rather than a single theory which rests on a naive view of the individual and his or her social surroundings.

The remainder of this chapter will draw on a number of models to try to develop a model for CHC nursing. The proposed eclectic model (Fig. 6.2) draws on systems theory, interaction theories and developmental theories. The model includes elements of models discussed in this chapter, such as the interaction between the individual and the environment (Roy 1984, Neuman 1989, Orem 1991); the development of the nurse/client relationship and the different roles adopted throughout these stages; and the extent and manner in which advice is received and acted upon (Peplau 1952, Chalmers 1992).

These elements reflect the nurse's role with the individual client. However, the goal of community nursing is also to work with families and communities. For this reason a model for community nursing must recognise the functioning of families and the relationships between family members. The model, therefore, relates the above elements to relationships within the family and draws on Friedmann's (1989) congruence model. The community dimension in the model, in addition to drawing on systems and interaction theories, also acknowledges the community participation and community change models (Chalmers & Kristajanson 1989).

It is important to consider the definitions and relationships between the four metaparadigms in the proposed model.

The nature of the person. The person is seen as a biopsychosocial being in constant interaction with and having an effect upon the environment. Individuals are considered to be in control of their environment, in terms of both the manner in which they negotiate relationships with other people, and the impact of the decisions they make on the ecological environment. Individuals are, therefore, viewed as powerful creators of their own destinies.

Environment. The environment is defined as both physical/ecological and human. Thus, the combination of ecological factors and human relationships will determine how individuals, families, groups and communities experience the environment. The relationship between individuals and their environment is dynamic, therefore the environment is affected by the decisions and behaviour of people, which in turn affects the people's experience of the environment. This view of the environment draws on systems theory and interactionism. The individual is seen as an open system in interaction with the environment. The ability of individuals to control their environment is fundamental to this model which is acknowledged by the different goals of different disciplines within CHC nursing.

Health. Health is viewed from two dimensions, reflecting individual experience and objective measures more suited to measuring community health needs. At an individual level health is considered to be a unique and variable experi-

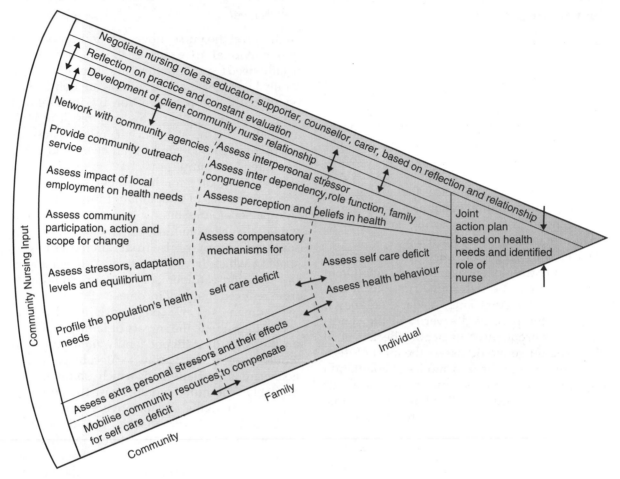

Figure 6.2   A dynamic, eclectic model for community health care nursing.

ence of contentment. At a community level health is defined as an equilibrium in which the community successfully adapts to change so that conditions such as poverty, poor housing, homelessness and crime remain within an acceptable range of community adaptation.

The goal of CHC nursing. The goal of CHC nursing is complex due to the nature of nursing within individual, family, work and community settings, which often coincide. The goal of community nursing is, therefore, to promote health and to maintain health at a level acceptable to the individual, family, workplace and community. Attaining this goal will include the use of primary, secondary and tertiary prevention

(Caplan 1964) to prevent the occurrence of disequilibrium, to detect disequilibrium at its earliest stage and to prevent further disequilibrium. The term 'disequilibrium' is preferred to 'illness' or 'disease' because disequilibrium can be equated with social, corporate or political, rather than biological, malfunctioning. For example, poor housing and poverty may contribute to a rise in crime in a particular community, which would result in disequilibrium and maladaptation within the community. Similarly, changes in employment practices may contribute to disequilibrium and stress in the workplace which may have an adverse effect on families and communities.

The role of CHCNs

Individual level

At this level the CHCN uses his relationship with the client to assess and diagnose individual health needs. The model draws on Peplau's (1952) view of the developing relationship between nurse and client. Peplau believes that the nurse matures throughout the relationship, thus enhancing the communication skills of the nurse and encouraging the development of trust and integrity. This will influence the giving and receiving of information (Chalmers 1992) and so the likelihood of the client acting on the advice and information given by the nurse.

During this stage the nurse will assess the client's capacity to engage in self-care (Orem 1991). This may be determined by social and psychological factors such as lack of knowledge, and the perceived severity of the condition and consequences of action (Becker et al 1974). The nurse would assess the level of disequilibrium within the four modes of adaptation (Roy 1984) as well as any inter-, intra-, or extrapersonal stressors (Neuman 1989). It must be stressed, however, that the professional role of the CHCN requires a level of judgement regarding which is the most appropriate tool for assessment, that is, the ability to self-care, modes of adaptation or stressors. Such decisions underpin the dynamic nature of the model and reflect the high level of skills and knowledge required by the CHCN.

Having assessed the nature of health needs, the nurse will determine his role as wholly or partially compensatory, as supporter, educator, counsellor, leader (Peplau 1952, Orem 1991), or as an intervener within the situation to alleviate the effects of stressors (Neuman 1989). This reflects the implementation phase of the nursing process during which roles and plans are negotiated between client and nurse. The evaluation phase requires the client and nurse to review the progress, including the effectiveness of the relationship, the advice offered and the assessment tools used. At this stage it may be necessary to change from using the elements of one model to using those of another.

Family level

At this level the nurse moves beyond concern for the individual to examine the impact of the health needs and nursing intervention at the family level. For example, a self-care deficit may be partially compensated for by intervention from a family member. This may result in maladaptation in the self-concept, role mastery or interdependency mode of both client and carer. The carer, for example, may have given up a high status job to care for his or her spouse, thus affecting modes of adaptation. Intra-, inter- and extrapersonal stressors for both client and carer would also be examined; for example, intrapersonal stressors may arise from differences in personality which have not proved problematic in the past, and extrapersonal stressors could arise from reduced financial income.

Friedmann's (1989) congruence model proves useful to evaluate the impact of family problems on the roles of different family members. This would require the family to decide on which goals are important and which solutions are available. The nurse would assist the family to draw on strengths and positive experiences to build a better future. Goals would need to acknowledge the needs of different family members in order to work towards congruence within the family. The evaluation stage of the nursing process would also require an evaluation of the impact of the nursing intervention for each family member as well as the family as a whole and within the wider community.

Community level

At this level the CHCN may adopt a community health approach with a focus on the people comprising the community or a public health approach emphasising whole populations or at risk groups within them (American Public Health Association 1991). Both of these approaches may involve the community nurse in assessing stressors within the community, examining the equilibrium within that community, and judging the capacity of the community to care for itself. However, the community health model would focus on the impact of community health as it affects individuals and families, whereas the public health model would focus on subgroups or at risk groups within populations.

Both approaches would use the nurse's expertise in profiling populations to identify health needs. Client involvement would be essential to confirm the health needs identified and to develop programmes to respond to health needs in the community setting. The community health orientation would reflect the community participation model, and the public health approach would reflect the community change model (Chalmers & Kristajanson 1989). The latter model would require CHCNs to collaborate to influence policy at national and local levels. Collaboration between nurse members of the PHC team and occupational health nurses would expose the impact of health needs on the workforce at the community level. Conversely, the nurse in primary health care would be able to plan services with the knowledge of the impact of local changes in employment. The three levels of prevention would be used at this stage to prevent, identify and improve the consequences of disequilibrium in the community.

The role of the different disciplines within community nursing is reflected in Figure 6.2. The cone shaped diagrammatic representation illustrates the importance of reflection in practice and the development of the client/community/nurse relationship in each dimension. The arrows indicate the interactive nature within the dimensions and the broken lines show how the community nurse will assess similar factors at different levels between the individual and the community. The long arrow beneath the model identifies the interactive nature of the community nurse's input and the joint action plan which would be the outcome of the assessment. Reflective practice and constant evaluation underpin the model so that, rather than being a continuous process, community nursing is a dynamic and cyclical process which is a product of joint collaboration at all levels.

Summary

The evaluation of models for nursing practice is an important skill for community health care nurses. A variety of models exist which may or may not be appropriate as a basis for the organisation of care delivery in one particular setting. It is the nurses' responsibility to decide which model, if any, is suitable for their work. It is important to recognise that the use of a single model could constrain nursing practice by neglecting to embrace the complexity of interaction between human beings and their environment. A dynamic, eclectic model is, therefore, recommended in which the nurse can move between the different dimensions of caring for an environment, to caring for the individual and families within it.

REFERENCES

Akinsanya J, Cox G, Crouch C, Fletcher L 1994 The Roy adaptation model in action. Macmillan, Basingstoke

American Public Health Association, Public Health Nursing Section 1991 The definition and role of public health nursing in the delivery of health care. A position paper. APHA Newsletter, London

Anderson E T, McFarlane J M 1988 Community as client. Application of the nursing process. Lippincott, Philadelphia

Becker M H, Drachman R H, Kirscht J P 1974 A new approach to explaining sick-role behaviour in low-income populations. American Journal of Public Health 64(3):205–216

Beitler B, Tkachuck B, Aamodt 1980 The Neuman model applied to mental health, community health and medical-surgical nursing. In: Riehl J P, Roy C (eds) Conceptual models for nursing practice, 2nd edn. Appleton-Century-Crofts, New York

Benedict M M, Behringer Sproles J 1982 Application of the Neuman model to public health nursing practice. In:

Neuman B (ed) Neuman systems model. Application to nursing education and practice. Appleton-Century-Crofts, East Norwalk, Connecticut

Benoliel J Q 1977 The interaction between theory and research. Nursing Outlook 25:108–113

Bertalanffy L 1968 General systems theory. George Braziller, New York

Blackburn C 1992 Improving health and welfare work with families in poverty. A handbook. OU Press, London

Blau P M 1964 Exchange and power in social life. Wiley, New York

Blumer H 1969 Symbolic interactionism: perspective and method. Prentice-Hall, Englewood Cliffs, New Jersey

Caplan G 1964 Principles of preventive psychiatry. Basic Books, New York

Chalmers K I 1992 Giving and receiving: an empirically derived theory on health visiting practice. Journal of Advanced Nursing 17:1317–1325

Chalmers K, Kristajanson L 1989 The theoretical basis of

nursing at the community level: a comparison of three models. Journal of Advanced Nursing 14:569–574

Chin R 1980 The utility of systems models and developmental models for practitioners. In: Riehl J P, Roy C (eds) Conceptual models for nursing practice. Appleton-Century-Crofts, New York

Chin P L, Jacobs M K 1978 A model of theory development in nursing. Advances in Nursing Science 1(1):1–11

Comley A L 1994 A comparative analysis of Orem's self-care model and Peplau's interpersonal theory. Journal of Advanced Nursing 20:755–760

Council for Education and Training of Health Visitors (CETHV) 1977 An investigation into the principles of health visiting. CETHV, London

Crouch C 1994 Applying the mode II. In: Akinsanya J, Cox G, Crouch C, Fletcher L 1994 The Roy adaptation model in action. Macmillan, Basingstoke

Dean S 1991 Health visiting support of a family with a handicapped child based on Orem's self-care model. In: While A (ed) Caring for children: towards partnership with families. Edward Arnold, London

Fawcett J 1984 Analysis and evaluation of conceptual models of nursing. Davis, Philadelphia

Fawcett J 1992 Conceptual models and nursing practice: the reciprocal relationship. Journal of Advanced Nursing 17:224–228

Friedmann M L 1989 Closing the gap between grand theory and mental health practice with families. Part 2: The control-congruence model for mental health nursing of families. Archives of Psychiatric Nursing 3:20–28

Girot E 1990 Discussing nursing theory. Senior Nurse 10:6

Haggart M 1993 A critical analysis of Neuman's systems model in relation to public health nursing. Journal of Advanced Nursing 18:1917–1922

Hartweg D L 1991 Dorothea Orem: self-care deficit theory. Notes on nursing theories 4. Sage, Newbury Park

Heiss J 1976 Family roles and interaction. Rand-McNally, Chicago

Homans G 1961 Social behaviour: its elementary forms. Harcourt Brace Jovanovich, New York

Kenny T 1993 Nursing models fail in practice. British Journal of Nursing 2, 2

McClymont M, Thomas S, Denham M J 1991 Health visiting and elderly people. A health promotion challenge. Churchill Livingstone, Edinburgh

Marriner A 1986 Nursing theorists and their work. Mosby, St Louis

Mead G H 1934 Mind, self, and society. University of Chicago Press, Chicago

Meleis A 1985 Theoretical nursing: development and progress. Lippincott, Philadelphia

Neuman B 1974 The Betty Neuman health-care systems model: a total person approach to patient problems. In: Riehl J P, Roy C Conceptual models for practice. Appleton-Century-Crofts, New York

Neuman B 1982 Neuman systems model. Application to nursing education and practice. Appleton-Century-Crofts, East Norwalk, Connecticut

Neuman B 1989 The Neuman systems model. Appleton & Lange, East Norwalk, Connecticut

Orem D E 1971 Nursing: concepts of practice. McGraw-Hill, New York

Orem D E 1985 Nursing: concepts of practice, 3rd edn. McGraw-Hill, New York

Orem D E 1987 Orem's general theory of nursing. In: Parse R (ed) Nursing science: major paradigms, theories and critiques. Saunders, Philadelphia

Orem D E 1991 Nursing: concepts of practice, 4th edn. Mosby-Year Book, St Louis

Orr J 1985 The community dimension In: Luker K, Orr J (eds) Health visiting. Blackwell Scientific, Oxford

Peplau H 1952 Interpersonal relations in nursing. Putman, New York

Robertson C 1991 Health visiting in practice. Churchill Livingstone, Edinburgh

Rogers B 1990 Conceptual model for occupational health nursing practice. American Association of Occupational Health Nurses 38(11):536–543

Rourke A M 1991 Self-care: chore or challenge. Journal of Advanced Nursing 16:223–241

Roy C 1984 Introduction to nursing – an adaptation model. Prentice-Hall, Englewood Cliffs, New Jersey

Roy C, Andrews H 1991 The Roy adaptation model, the definitive statement. Appleton & Lange, Norwalk, Connecticut

Selye H 1956 The stress of life. McGraw-Hill, New York

Simpson H 1991 Peplau's model in action. Macmillan, Basingstoke

FURTHER READING

Akinsanya J 1994 The Roy adaptation model in action. Macmillan, Basingstoke

Hardy M E 1974 Theories: components, development, evaluation. Nursing Research 23(2):100–107

McMurray A 1990 Community health nursing. Churchill Livingstone, Edinburgh

7

Managing change in the contract culture

Anne Robotham

CHAPTER CONTENTS

The reform of health service management and the emphasis placed on community health care mean that nurses and their professional colleagues must possess a broader range of knowledge than has previously been necessary. They are required to think critically beyond clinical issues to the structure, provision and management of services. The implications are that:

- They must be able to manage change
- They must promote their services in the NHS internal market
- They must understand the underlying philosophy and processes which govern GP fundholding
- They must be able to reflect on their practice and the way in which it is structured to be able to respond effectively to the changing needs of the client groups they serve.

As a result of the changes in the education and employment of community health care nurses (CHCNs) and health visitors in the 1990s, the requirements of their roles are far more demanding than for any other generation. To be able to cope with these demands the practitioner must be able to respond quickly and effectively to the many changes that are occurring. Additionally, the content of courses leading to a community health care (CHC) specialism must include an understanding of the practical aspects of management, especially in relation to change.

Criticism of the NHS in the 1960s showed the

organisation to be unable to adapt sufficiently quickly to the changing needs of the population. Reorganisation in 1974 resulted in a need for further examination of the NHS's problems, many of which centred around economic constraints. The NHS Management Inquiry (DoH 1983) was set up in order to 'review initiatives to improve the efficiency of the health service and to advise on the management action needed to secure the best value for money and the best possible service to patients'. The report is discussed in greater detail in Section 1 of this book.

To be able to understand new roles in this management climate, the nurse should be familiar with how organisations function and how they can be changed, as well as how roles are established. In many community units/trusts, management reorganisations continue to take place and an understanding of how to manage change is becoming essential.

MANAGING CHANGE IN THE COMMUNITY UNIT/TRUST

CURRENT PERSPECTIVES ON ORGANISATIONAL CHANGE

A balanced examination of organisational change offers two perspectives. The first is the theory perspective in which there is an objective discussion of the many theories that are found in current literature on organisational change. The second perspective is the practical perspective, which is a subjective analysis of how organisational change is represented in the minds of those individuals involved in the process of change. Spurgeon & Barwell (1991) draw on the work of Egan (1985) and Legge (1984) to diagnose change processes in terms of their theory and practicality and define two frameworks, 'descriptive' organisational change and 'prescriptive' organisational change. The former attempts to describe how and why organisational change actually takes place by modelling and analysing the dynamics of the process; the latter attempts to provide a specification of how best to achieve different future organisational states or outcomes.

Descriptive organisational change theory

According to this theory change can come about in several ways. First, it can occur as a result of an explosion within a structure or organisation which creates surprise and causes turbulence. It is due often to the perverse interaction of internal and external change systems in the business and its environment, for example, the development of GP fundholding and its relationships to community trusts.

Second, change can be an implosion in a structure or organisation which is due to the collapse of an internal system upon which the main structures depend and which leads to collapse of the organisation. For example, the change in ownership and management of internal organisations within a hospital, such as catering or laundry services, to the contractual purchase of private services can precipitate the process of change.

Third, strategic planning, which is the creation of long-term goals in order to anticipate and shape the future environment, can lead to strategic change. This is the reshaping of strategy, structure and culture of an organisation over time, by internal design, by external forces or by simple drift (Grundy 1993) as in, for example, the NHS reforms.

Prescriptive organisational change theory

Although some of this information relates to quality issues, it is also about change. There are several theories of organisational change that are useful in developing ideas from a prescriptive organisational viewpoint. Lewin (1951) was an early analyst of change theory and he describes three stages of planned change (Box 7.1). Employing these stages to organise change in a structured way can have significant benefits for all members of the organisation, as Case study 7.1 illustrates.

Clearly, any innovation will be more effective and create less anxiety if stability is allowed to occur and it must be remembered that continual communication throughout such initiatives is essential.

Box 7.1 Lewin's (1951) stages of planned change

Stage 1	Unfreezing	The need for change is established within the organisation or by the at-risk population.
Stage 2	Moving process	A change agent (or agents) emerges and problems are identified. Alternative ways are sought to solve the problems. A plan is devised and if necessary modified to suit the circumstances.
Stage 3	Refreezing	The planned change is implemented and the situation allowed to stabilise.

Case study 7.1 Applying Lewin's stages of planned change

The nurse executive director of a community trust is an experienced and forward-looking manager who has asked his senior community managers to meet for a discussion over a major change in the continuing development of field staff. He has decided to employ a lecturer practitioner to facilitate staff and student development, and to gradually withdraw the need for community practice teachers. The innovation had been under way for 6 months when one of the managers decided that more community practice teachers should be trained and accordingly set this in motion. There had been no discussion with the director, and this created considerable anxiety amongst both field staff and the lecturer practitioner.

If Lewin's planned change model had been successfully applied in this scenario then the following should have occurred:

Stage 1 The nurse executive director meets with his senior community managers to discuss his ideas and reasons for a major change. He gains their approval to employ a lecturer practitioner to facilitate staff and student development.

Stage 2 One of the managers is designated as project manager to employ the lecturer practitioner and agreement is reached over the length of the pilot stage of the project, following which there will be a review before any changes are made.

Stage 3 A review takes place and one of the managers puts forward her views on the need to continue to train community practice teachers. The new idea is discussed at the review and views are sought from the director, all the managers and the lecturer practitioner before any further decisions are made.

Bennis et al (1976) suggest that the strategies used in the change process could be grouped into three categories (Box 7.2).

The models which have been outlined are more about processes than structures and rely on the organisation's problem-solving ability rather than helping to solve one specific problem. In the early stages of Bennis et al's model, progress centres around communication/ intervention processes which rely on managers' ability to communicate and listen. Recently however, there has been a move away from the human intervention process towards the need to match the intervention strategy with the underlying causes of the organisation's difficulties. Pettigrew (1985) suggests that change often originates with a small subset of people in the organisation who have become aware of a mismatch between the demands of a changing environment and the current performance of the organisation. Pettigrew argues that it becomes essential for those who are pursuing the objectives of change to 'delegitimise' or undermine their opponents' ideas and actions in order to increase concern, energy and enthusiasm, which stimulates appropriate action for change.

It is interesting to note that Handy (1991) suggests that the organisations that change successfully are those with good resources, and these are not necessarily financial. A successful institution that is able to make changes often attracts people who in turn are attracted by change; they may, for example, see it as a good omen for promotion.

CULTURAL PERSPECTIVES AND CHANGE THEORY

There are many analyses of the meaning of culture within organisations which, for this discussion, is understood to mean shared understanding and common values within the organisation and to derive from sociological factors. For change to succeed, the manager is required to understand the culture that she is submerged in and to know how to use this understanding to initiate and manage change. Spurgeon & Barwell (1991), citing Plant (1987), argue that the learning process is

Box 7.2	Categories of change strategy (Bennis et al 1976)	
Category 1	Empirical–rational	This assumes that people will act in a rational way by demonstrating the benefits to be gained from adopting the innovation, and bringing knowledge to create awareness for those who do not have the knowledge.
Category 2	Normative–re-educative	This activates forces within the system to change it, improves the problem-solving capacity of the client system, and fosters an atmosphere in which people will be creative given a consensus between different interest groups.
Category 3	Power–coercive	This relies on power, using political, legal, administrative, economic and moral power. It is concerned with majority votes rather than changes in norms, roles or relationships.

the key to managing self-change and change within organisations. This learning process runs through a number of stages and the change agent can be either a stimulator or an educator.

In many instances, change from a cultural perspective is not so much about role alteration or job change, but more about altering ideas and attitudes to allow different approaches to be taken to the problems already identified. If clinicians are to be involved in managing and becoming accountable for their own actions, then they must be more motivated to take on a new set of organisational values and priorities.

CHANGE PROCESSES

Grundy (1993), examining varieties of change processes, identifies three, all of which are concerned with an equation involving time and rate. The change that most managers would aspire to is that of 'smooth incremental change' in which change takes place without setbacks and the rate is such that people involved can cope. As might be imagined, this requires a fairly steady state in market expansion or environmental reorganisation. Secondly, Grundy identifies 'bumpy incremental change' which is characterised by periods of relative tranquillity, punctuated by an acceleration in the pace of change perceived as 'overload'. It is often in a change of management organisation such as has been seen in community units/trusts that overload is described. Grundy's third change process is that of 'discontinuous change' which is marked by rapid shifts in strategy, structure or culture. It can occur because internal change has not kept up with external

change, such as managers in community units who have not understood the purchasing power of Health Authority Commissioners, or where a change in the markets has propelled the organisation into a radically new way of operating. An example of this is where health visitors who, despite education which covered working with age groups from the cradle to the grave, have traditionally practised by working with mothers and under-5s and are now being asked by purchasers – GPs – to work with other client groups. There has, however, always been regional variation in this aspect of organisation within the community.

As discontinuous change is commonly seen, it is likely that there is an underlying cause where change occurs as part of the main business of the organisation, the 'strategy' described above, or at change project level, the 'structure' described above, or finally, at the level of the individual, the 'culture' described above. It is also likely that these levels are interlinked through the structure and culture list (Fig. 7.1).

In Figure 7.1, strategy is determined by government policy, which, for example, lays down the methods by which the NHS should achieve outcomes to support policy. It is possible to pursue a variety of alternative methods providing they satisfy the overall policy. In many ways there is a close link between strategy and structure, because structure combines both methods and outcome and is clearly the planning and executive area in which senior management functions. The culture of the organisation is the way in which management actually carries out its policies in line with strategy and structure and

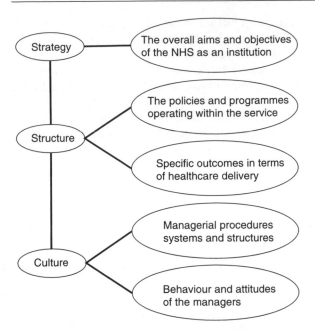

Figure 7.1   The structure underlying discontinuous change.

creates the climate in which the workforce functions.

An effective organisation taking on this model would expect all staff to have some say in structure and culture even if they cannot reach the strategy level. However, there is evidence that this can work among successful large companies in the private sector where all workers do have an opportunity to be involved at strategy level.

Change agents

Change agents can be both internal and external to the organisation. Where they are external they tend to be a set of circumstances, for example, change of regulations, competition, standards or technology. Internal change agents are usually the people who manage and are part of the chain of responsibility for the change. In reality, the 'change agent' in a large organisation such as a community unit/trust is embodied in more than one person. The change catalyst is usually the general manager of the unit, usually with an effective overview of the change process and a vision of the ultimate end of the process.

It is possible that the change agent is not the person who carries out the day to day moves and alterations; this may be left to the steering agent. The change agent and the steering agent usually work closely together. Both require some sort of vision of what is the intended outcome of change and the change agent relies to a certain extent on what the steering agent identifies during the organisational process. For example, the steering agent may identify a problem within one of the community teams which the two agents then discuss, and the mental image that the change agent has of the final model of the change structure will determine which small scale, internal mechanisms can be used to ease in the change.

One of the major problems experienced by senior managers is that when the change process involves the same people who have been involved in running and working in the organisation for some time, there is a tendency to become enthusiastic about the change process but for little actual change to occur at ground level. The assumption is that change is taking place but what is happening in reality is a state of 'dynamic conservatism' where no real progress is occurring (Schön 1971). Schön argues that all real change involves passing through zones of uncertainty, the situation of being all at sea, of being lost, of confronting more information than you can handle. This may be true, but it must be remembered that change is a process and not a single event, and that the total process from initiation to institutionalisation can be lengthy; even moderately complex changes can take from 3 to 5 years, while major restructuring events can take from 5 to 10 years.

Anybody can act as a change agent, although it is usually a manager, and move progress in a positive direction. It is probably natural to think of the general manager as an agent of change, but it could just as easily be a nurse, doctor or locality/neighbourhood manager who takes on this role. Change agents have certain skills which enable them to see how organisational factors may affect the performance of the individual or groups of individuals within the organisation. On the basis of this assessment the agent can positively and creatively challenge some of the assumptions traditionally made within the organisation. These agents will have clear views on the organisational framework model (Fig. 7.1.) and use various 'tools' or tactics to tackle aspects of change.

Change tools

There are a number of tools that managers may use to analyse change issues, plan and control the implementation of change, and educate and reinforce learning. Grundy (1993) suggests that four basic tools can prove to be effective in managing strategic change:

- Force field analysis
- Change systems
- Stakeholder analysis
- Change project management.

Force field analysis

Lewin (1935) first described force field analysis, stating that 'force field analysis is the diagnosis and evaluation enabling and restraining forces that have an impact on the change process'. Force field analysis is a tool which brings to the surface underlying factors which may advance a particular change, or which may prevent progress or even reverse the change process. However, forces cannot be identified individually before the change objective is set. The change objective is where the organisation wants to be or needs to be, which suggests that there is a gap between that and where the organisation is now. Of course, this change objective is linked in to the strategic vision for the organisation.

To begin this process a force field analysis should be undertaken by drawing a line down the centre of a piece of paper and writing enabling forces to the right of the line and constraining forces to the left. Care must be taken not to confuse force field analysis with cost–benefit analysis, because a force field analysis does not analyse whether the content of the change is of great value or not. There are a number of forces which can be seen as general to any analysis, and others that may be specific to the change objective alone. An example of a general force field analysis is contained in Figure 7.2.

The relative strength of each force is represented in the diagram by an arrowed line the length of which is proportionate to the relative strength of the force. In preparing the diagram, it is often most effective to list all the forces related to the change objective and then decide whether they are enabling or constraining forces. At this point, it may be useful to examine how force field analysis works in practice, and an example is given in Case study 7.2.

Grundy (1993) summarises the 'do's' and 'don'ts' of force field analysis (Box 7.3).

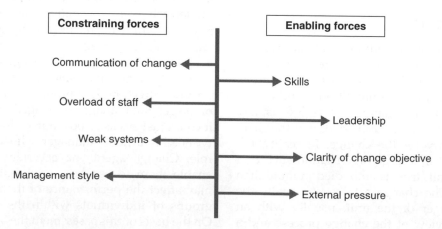

Figure 7.2 A general force field analysis.

Case study 7.2   Force field analysis in health visiting

The director of a community trust is concerned that the health visitors on her staff are becoming very disillusioned with their work. They are complaining that the measurement of their effectiveness is by the number of contacts only, and that this is increasingly related to the number of clinics they run, rather than any other form of client contact. Her objective is to introduce a system of workload definition based on a needs analysis of the caseload profile, and agreed between an individual health visitor and manager. The director thinks there may be opposition from a number of managers and field staff.

As an experienced manager the director knows that this proposed change will require careful and well planned introduction. She needs to understand which forces will influence this change and prepares a force field analysis accordingly. Initially the director is unsure of the strength of some of the forces and simply prepares a list of those she sees as enabling and those as constraining. The prepared list looks like this:

Constraining forces

1. Difficulty in communicating personally with all staff at the same time.
2. With long-term sickness there are a number of staff covering for colleagues.
3. Staff are saying they have insufficient time to extend their work in any way.
4. The data collection system is based on the needs of the public health department and is designed for quantitative analysis.
5. The small number of managers at locality level do not always have a community nursing background and have difficulty in understanding qualitative analysis measures.

Enabling forces

1. Recently qualified health visitors have shown that they are well able to plan care programmes based on health needs of their target population.
2. There are a number of community practice teachers who are frustrated by some of the traditional practice they see amongst their colleagues and are interested in developing new protocols.
3. A new locality manager has shown charisma and creativity in her dealings with her staff.
4. The district nursing service has shown considerable advancement in its ability to practise in an innovative way.
5. The change objective is based on the professional health visitor using her skills to bring a better service to her clients.
6. Many health visitors, concerned about the need to run developmental screening clinics in catchment populations, will always seek advice if they are concerned about any aspect of a child's progress.

Having drawn up her list of forces, the director now has to decide whether she has placed the forces in the correct columns – is the force an 'enabler' or a 'constraint', and in any case, what is the strength of the force? Relative strengths have been evaluated using two methods: scoring the force as 'high', 'medium' or 'low' impact; scoring each force numerically on a scale of 1 to 5.

The director decides that it is at this stage that she must share her thoughts with the locality managers in order to determine whether there are any other forces that she has not identified, and what strength they would score for those that have been identified. The managers feel that the forces are correct, but one manager in particular sees the whole exercise as subjective. The director decides that to respond to this criticism they should consider three questions:

1. Why is the force an enabler or a constraint?
2. How important an influence is it on the change process (and when)?
3. What underlying factors does it depend upon in turn?

These questions highlight the fact that any force field analysis is dependent on several assumptions, many of which will have been implicit.

Box 7.3   The 'do's' and 'don'ts' of force field analysis

Do:

- Brainstorm all the key tangible and less tangible forces impacting on the change process.
- Test your judgements by questioning why a force is strong or weak by reference to the change objective and by thinking about its constraints within the change process.
- Do the initial force field analysis on an 'as is' basis – show the warts and prepare to be provocative.
- Where a major constraint exists, draw this in as a stopper to draw attention to its role in impeding the change process.
- Use the tool throughout the change process as the change forces will alter over time.
- Involve others to provide the input analysis and to test your views.

Do not:

- Confuse force field analysis with simple cost–benefit analysis. Benefits should only be included as a force if they are perceived by and owned by key stakeholders. Often, these benefits are in the eye of the change initiator and are neutral in driving the change process forward.
- Use force field analysis as a tool just to describe the current position. Force field analysis should be used actively to reshape your change plan to optimise the effect of enabling forces and to neutralise or flip over the constraining forces to become enablers.
- Get bogged down in attempts to rate the forces precisely – force field analysis is an imprecise science.

In considering the force field analysis for Case study 7.2, the director and the managers made a series of decisions. In relation to the constraining forces, they decided that:

- Difficulty in communication to all the staff at the same time was a low impact consideration
- Covering for sick colleagues was a medium impact consideration
- Staff concerns over work time was a medium impact consideration
- The data collection system was a high impact consideration
- The lack of 'discipline specific' managers was a high impact consideration.

In relation to enabling forces, they decided that:

- The numbers of newly qualified health visitors and community practice teachers (CPTs) together came to almost a fifth of the health visiting workforce and were thus seen as a medium impact consideration
- The recently appointed manager was seen as a high impact consideration especially when she could draw on the notion of the professional health visitor determining her own work programmes
- The influence of the changed pattern of work from within the district nursing service was

seen as low impact in relation to this change project
- The fact that some health visitors see themselves as performing unnecessary tasks was seen as a high impact consideration.

How these decisions translated into the composition of the force field analysis diagram is shown in Figure 7.3.

Change systems

Grundy described a tool for change systems incorporating strategy, structure, skills, systems and style. This is an extension of the strategy, structure and culture diagram and provides information for the decision of where to start the intervention. If one starts at the tangible end with systems and structures, then change is open and visible and benefits can be felt early in the process. If one starts at the skills and style end, then there may be some time-lag before effects are felt and people may become quickly disillusioned. A change systems model may appear as illustrated in Figure 7.4.

The philosophy behind such a model is that it is driven (or led) by strategy, but to be more effective the 'tangible' factors of systems and structure are seen to be moving parallel to the intangible factors of skills and style (style in this

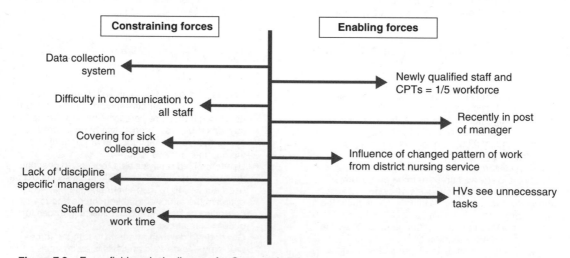

Figure 7.3   Force field analysis diagram for Case study 7.2.

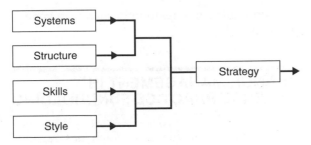

Figure 7.4   A change systems model.

instance refers to the style of management). The use of such a model strengthens the value of a force field analysis.

This tool can be related to Case study 7.2. The director and the managers discussed the need to ensure that the intangible factors of skills and style were addressed early. In this case, it was clear that although the health visitors were all able to undertake caseload profiles, they were less able to determine a personal work programme based on the health needs of their profile, and to evaluate the effectiveness of the interventions that they had determined. In addition, they were concerned that the GPs who were their purchasers would not want them to work in any way other than the one to which they were accustomed.

In connection with the factors of structure and systems there were a number of difficulties; not least was the need to persuade the public health department that the number of contacts made by health visitors was not necessarily indicative of public health status within the trust. Thus, there would be a need to examine just what information it was that the system was collecting, and to link this with the need to satisfy Department of Health requests with the Chief Executive's annual plan.

The director and the staff now needed to consider a further change tool, stakeholder analysis.

Stakeholder analysis

This tool involves the systematic identification of key stakeholders and the appraisal of their influence and opinion of the change. The potential behaviour in the change process of these stakeholders may be indicated by their general level of influence in the organisation.

The questions that then need to be asked about stakeholders relate to how they should be handled.

- Should new stakeholders be brought in to shift the balance between positive and negative behaviours?
- Is it possible to boost the influence of stakeholders who are currently in favour of change?
- Is it possible to reduce the influence of antagonistic stakeholders?
- Can positive coalitions be achieved?
- Can negative coalitions be prevented?
- Can the change itself, in appearance or substance, be reformulated to diffuse hostility to the change?
- Can negative stakeholders be persuaded to become positive by incorporating one of their prized ideas in the process?

Relating these issues and questions to the health visiting case study, the director and her managers considered that the key stakeholders in the proposed change were the staff themselves, the director of public health and the community paediatric physician. In analysing the influence that each individual/group held it was felt that the staff had the greatest influence, whilst the director of public health and the community paediatric physician held medium influence. The director and the managers felt that the way to cope with the stakeholders was to set up one or two working parties amongst the staff to look at key issues of concern and to include both the director of public health and the community paediatric physician in the discussions. It was made quite clear that all parties involved had equal status and that the medical profession representatives were there simply as group members in the initial meetings. Group members were then asked to prepare criteria for implementation of the project.

Before these initial meetings were allowed to move events forward, the director made use of a fourth tool for change, change project management.

Change project management

Change project management is the focusing of change into one or more discrete projects to reach a preplanned result within a specified time and cost whilst managing interdependencies with other projects (Grundy 1993).

This change tool does not necessarily come last in the change process and may well be used before stakeholder analysis.

The most effective management of change has change projects as a management process, and these:

- Help managers to perform diagnosis and planning of the change process more thoroughly and define a clear objective for change
- Provide a vehicle for control
- Can help identify the key stakeholders in the project
- Provide clear ownership for the change
- Enable necessary resources to be highlighted so that they can be mobilised in good time.

For the director and the managers in the case study, the use of these change tools enabled them to set up the change project management team which had clear goals and objectives. This team determined a timescale for the various objectives to be achieved or reviewed. Into this timescale was built an allowance for further force field analyses as the project moved forward. The planning subgroups were made up of a member of staff who could be identified as a steering agent, one or two key stakeholders and a small group of field staff made up of newly qualified health visitors, some health visitors who had been in practice for several years and a few community practice teachers. The make-up of these planning subgroups was such that they recruited staff from various sectors within the trust, were not too large as to be unwieldy, and clearly felt that they would have ownership of the final project once it was up and running.

This case study has raised a number of discussion points in relation to managing change within the community unit/trust and it is worth considering them in relation to change in general practice.

CHANGE MANAGEMENT IN GENERAL PRACTICE FUNDHOLDING

One of the major changes which has resulted from GP fundholding is the notion of the practice 'purchasing' CHC staff from the 'provider' unit – the community unit/trust. Prior to the institution of fundholding, district nurses, health visitors, community mental health nurses, community midwives and others, either attached or aligned to a practice, tended to make the practice population their caseload. Their work was agreed between the various community managers and the GP, but their main working focus was that of the unit/trust rather than the GP practice.

However, GP fundholding has produced a contract culture whereby the GP fundholder may purchase CHC nursing practitioners appropriate for the needs of the practice population. Initial purchasing has been on the basis of the knowledge held of traditional individual specialists' practice, in the hope that these will meet the practice's targets. It has become increasingly obvious, however, that many GPs are not aware of the desire of community health care practitioners to move away from traditional practice in order to become more innovative and cost effective. Initially, GPs felt that they knew the type of care they wished to purchase from district nurses, community mental health nurses and community midwives, but were less aware of what could be offered by health visitors.

THE HEALTH VISITOR MARKETING PROJECT

The Health Visitor Marketing Project (NHSME 1994) was commissioned by the NHS Executive from Coopers and Lybrand in the light of a perceived need for health visitors to consider more carefully the needs of purchasers and to enable health visitors to demonstrate that they have skills which are needed to meet identified health needs of the practice population. At the same time, concerns have been expressed by GPs and health visitors in a number of areas that there is insufficient health visitor time provided to meet the needs of the practice population. Although the project was originally intended for health visiting its messages are applicable to all CHCNs.

A survey was conducted in 108 trusts/units of their existing market activity. Subsequently, health visitors from 40 trusts around England participated in workshops to develop marketing skills and so align their service provision more closely with purchaser objectives. Finally, interviews were conducted with staff in 25 district health authorities and with 100 GP fundholders.

Few CHCNs have any understanding or experience of planning and promoting their services to purchasers. At best, they assume that GPs know what they do, at worst they act entirely as the GP's assistant.

One of the most important principles underpinning the functioning of the primary health care (PHC) team is the need to define the concept of teamwork, which is considered in greater detail in Chapter 4. The dictionary definition states that it is 'work performed by several persons in collaboration; the ability of a group to collaborate harmoniously'. Using this definition as a basis for the work of the PHC team it is clear that a team is not a hierarchical body, dependent on the instructions of the purchaser (in this case the GP), but a vibrant group of highly qualified individuals who have the delivery of health care as their prime aim and similar objectives. In the contract culture of the 1990s, there is a clear need to prioritise health needs and promotional opportunities in accordance with Health of the Nation (DoH 1990) targets. This means that not only health visitors but all members of the PHC team should understand the principles of marketing and should be able to construct a marketing plan. It is important that the team is seen to have a co-ordinator, although this person is not necessarily the leader and in particular is not likely to be the GP. If the GP sees herself as the leader then it is likely that a medical model of practice will dominate and if this is so, then the various disciplines that operate on a social model

of health will be hindered by the medical model. It could be argued that a medical model already dominates as a result of the NHS reforms. Using the Health Visitor Marketing Project (DoH 1994) as a guideline, it is suggested that individual disciplines among CHC workers or the PHC team should devise their own marketing plan.

Developing a marketing plan

There are seven stages which can be followed to structure the development of a plan.

Stage 1: Understanding the principles. It is necessary, at the start of the process, to be aware of and understand the fundamental activities of marketing, and these are described in Box 7.4.

Stage 2: Identifying the issues. The next stage involves examining the issues involved in marketing and what is on offer to the target customer. This can be done effectively in brainstorming sessions (Box 7.5).

The issues defined in these sessions will form the basis for the direction of the marketing action plan, and will need to be referred to at stage 6.

Box 7.4   The fundamental activities of marketing

Define	Define markets or customer groups which fall within your capability to serve (e.g. GPs, purchasers).
Understand	Find out what each of these groups wants or might want in the future.
Segment	If the groups in the market want different things from one discipline, group them into categories according to what they seek (e.g. client requirements are likely to differ from GP requirements).
Focus	Select those groups whose needs and wants can best be met by your services.
Design	Determine what you will offer these customers (e.g. what services).
Distribute	Make the service available.
Inform	Communicate with customers to inform them about the service, its key benefits and how it may be obtained.
Change	Decide on a continuous basis what services to add, subtract, modify or upgrade to meet changing customer needs and wants.

Box 7.5   How to brainstorm the issues

Step 1	A discipline group	Gather a group of one discipline together. This helps to provide a variety of perspectives and stimulates ideas.
Step 2	Brainstorm the issues	Think about all the issues you are currently facing. Examples of broad issues to think about and build upon include: • understanding and developing relationships with GPs • understanding and influencing the purchasing process • relationship with management • changes within the NHS and the impact on your discipline • clarify your role. There are likely to be a series of issues under each of these broad headings for you to identify.
Step 3	Discipline group	Having developed a long list of issues you need to decide which are the most important and which will have the most impact once they are addressed.

Stage 3: Understanding your customers. Use a questionnaire to interview your customers (district purchaser or GP) to discover their perspective. You will then be in an improved position to understand your customers' needs and identify the most effective way to communicate the service being offered to meet those needs, that is, develop a marketing plan.

The interview with the GPs/purchasers must be handled carefully. An appointment, allowing half an hour, should be made with a clear explana-tion of the objectives of the interview – to understand their priorities and key requirements from the interviewing group (health visitors, district nurses and so on) and how they would like to see the role develop in the future. This is a listening exercise and judging or commenting on the responses should be avoided. The questions should be relevant to the status of the interviewee and might include the examples given in Box 7.6.

Stage 4: Understanding your current position. Using a SWOT analysis (strengths, weaknesses,

---

Box 7.6   Examples of marketing questionnaire items

For district purchasers
• How many GP practices are in the area?
• How many of these are fundholders?
• How many (your discipline group e.g. health visitors) do you deal with?

For GPs
• Size of practice? How many GPs?
• Description of practice area.
• Which community health providers are attached to the practice?

For GP/district purchasers
• What changes have occurred in patient needs, practice management and your practice priorities over the past 4 years – which affect your use of CHC services?
• What do you see as the main services provided by the CHC disciplines?*
• Do you regard all of these services as equally valuable? Are some services seen to have a higher priority than others?*

• Do you feel that there are other types of services which may be appropriate for the CHC disciplines to provide? How would you like to see these services extended?*
• What are your key requirements when 'purchasing' CHC services? Which one of these requirements is most important when deciding to use one provider of care over another provider of care?*
• What do you see as the main strengths or weaknesses of the CHC disciplines?*
• Do you see (your discipline group, e.g. district nurses) as having special skills which distinguish them from other providers of care in the community? What are these particular skills?*
• How can we (your discipline group, e.g. community psychiatric nurses) improve the way we communicate with you so we can best meet your needs?

The questions marked with an asterisk* are the most important and in many cases you can complete the earlier ones from your own knowledge.

opportunities, threats), you can evaluate the strengths and weaknesses of your services. You can use the information from the questionnaire to see how your services are perceived by the customers, you can examine what opportunities exist for new services or consolidating existing services, and finally, you can consider the potential threats in developing or consolidating existing services. A typical SWOT analysis tool is shown in Box 7.7.

Stage 5: Clearly define the services you offer. The process of defining the services being offered has four steps: identify services; prioritise services; read the following service definition example which has been made out for HV service definition; and finally, complete your service profile using the same kind of tool as the example (Box 7.8.).

Each discipline will need to adapt the tool to match their own perspective.

Stage 6: Establish the specialist practitioner position and set objectives. It is important to find out what the gap is between what the specialist practitioner desires and what is reality. This is done using a gap analysis. Active steps must be taken to reduce any gap, and this process should be carried out in steps in order to be effective.

- Step 1 – Choose one of the issues identified at Stage 2.
- Step 2 – What is your current position in relation to this issue?
  – Why is it an issue?
- Step 3 – How do you want things to be in relation to this issue?
- Step 4 – What is your objective to close the gap between the current and desired position?
  – Objectives must follow the SMART principles – SPECIFIC, MEASURABLE, ACHIEVABLE, RELEVANT, TIMELY (DoH 1994).
- Step 5 – Repeat this exercise with another issue.
- Step 6 – Prioritise objectives to be developed into an action plan.
  – Identify the objectives which will be the easiest to achieve and have the

Box 7.7 **A SWOT analysis tool**	
Strengths	Weaknesses
Opportunities	Threats

Box 7.8 **Service definition tool from the health visiting perspective**	
Service need	What is the problem/symptom?
Clients	Who are they?
Your solution	How do you provide the services now (e.g. clinic, home visit)?
Resource implications of solution	What will it cost the purchaser – will they need to forego a service to buy a new service?
	What resources will you need to provide the service?
Benefits of your solutions	Outline the benefits (maybe for both GP and client) to persuade customers this is a service worth providing
Outcome measures	Decreased demand on GP service
	Impact on client
	Impact on demand for other services
	Improved relations
Why use HV services?	Why is the HV required to provide this service?
	Draw on key strengths of HVs
What are the current purchaser alternatives?	Where else could customers go for these services?
How will the purchaser be influenced?	Meeting of targets
	For GP – income, workload, call outs, etc.
Other considerations	Public view
	Media

greatest impact, and start with these.
– Continue to focus on the objectives which will have the greatest impact when achieved.

The information for the gap analysis generated by following these steps can be collated and compared under three headings: current position; desired position; and objectives for closing the gap.

Stage 7: Developing the marketing action plan. The final stage involves synthesising the data collected into the actual marketing action plan, and again, this is achieved most effectively in steps.

- Step 1 – Transfer the top priority objective set during the gap analysis onto the action plan sheet.
- Step 2 – Identify the specific tasks which will need to be done to achieve this objective.
  – Write them in the order in which they will need to be performed.
  – Be very specific and detailed about the tasks.
- Step 3 – What will be the direct output once you have completed the task (e.g. if your task was to set up a meeting, the direct output is the meeting date and time)?
- Step 4 – For each task identified, determine the time frame in which it must happen.
- Step 5 – For each task identified, determine who will be responsible for completing this task (this may be an individual or a group of people).

The decisions made during this process can be grouped under five appropriate headings: objective; key tasks; output; timescale; who?

Assembling the plan

At the end of the seven stages the plan will need to be formulated using the information from the tools to influence the planning process and produce, finally, a written plan with provision for reviewing it in the future (Fig. 7.5).

Although this plan was originally designed for health visitors the basic principles of marketing are very clearly set out and will allow any CHC worker to adopt them for her own use. The most

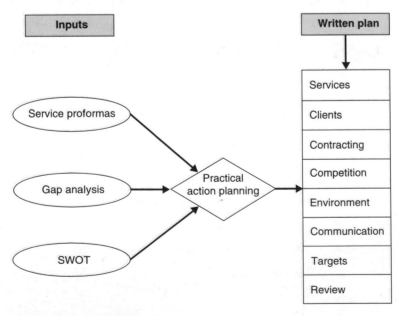

Figure 7.5 Assembling the plan.

important resource for the development of a marketing plan is a comprehensive health profile of the population because it is principally from this overview of the community's health and need that innovative practice can be developed.

Most healthcare professionals working in the community have used a community profile, which of necessity features aspects of their own discipline. However, since the publication of Health of the Nation (DoH 1990) and the use of the term 'public health awareness' as part of the United Kingdom Central Council for Nursing, Midwifery and Health Visiting (UKCC) proposals for characteristics of all CHC workers, the traditional profile takes little account of the 'public health'. Most healthcare professionals profile their working area and caseload, but a comprehensive profile should contain the profile from each specialist practitioner to give an overall view of the health status of the community. Profiles will therefore need to be altered to accommodate the information necessary to inform the 'public health'.

There are differences between the community health profile as described by Orr (1985), which takes a wide overview drawing on knowledge from sociology, psychology, epidemiology and social policy, and a caseload profile which may be an analysis of the health needs and characteristics of the records held by the practitioner, as described by the English National Board in their health visitor supervised practice assessment form (ENB 1987). Other approaches have been described by Blackburn (1991) and Tinson (1995) and these are worth studying in addition to Orr (1985). Billingham (1991) also discussed a useful approach to profiling. With the need to embrace fully the public health aspect of the specialist practitioner in community health care, the health profile described in the next section is an appropriate tool for change in community health care.

RESOURCES FOR CHANGE

THE HEALTH PROFILE

It has now become standard practice for CHCNs

to undertake a caseload profile and to update it annually. There are a number of ways in which profiles can be undertaken but for their use as a resource for change, the end result has to be a profile against which practice can be managed, measured and evaluated. This means that the PHC team, based in a GP practice, must be flexible and responsive to the profile, and be prepared to alter the focus of practice accordingly.

It is important that the validity of the community and practice profile is established and much thought should be given to how health status is established. If health is viewed from the perspective of a medical model only, then the data used most frequently by public health departments and GPs tends to become the basis for the profile, using statistics such as mortality and morbidity rates on which to base health input. The Black report (DHSS 1980), although initially suppressed, nevertheless raised awareness amongst health and social workers of the need to use a number of indicators to identify health status. Research undertaken in the last 20 years provided the basis for the indicators used currently to establish the link between health and social status. Subjective elements which are part of the social climate were shown by Moos (1976) to be clear influences on the quality of life, and other researchers concentrated on social indicators to measure changes in the socio-economic conditions of life (Carlisle 1972, Hatch & Sherrat 1973, Chen et al 1975, Land & McMillan 1978).

Inequalities in health

There is a constant need for research and data collection to:

- Uncover the most important determinants of health
- Demonstrate how inequity is related to health inequalities
- Establish the need for reliable, cheap and easy-to-apply methods of assessing health status and health determinants at small area level
- Establish the need for interpretative– qualitative, ethnographic and case study research on how people experience

inequalities in health and inequalities in their ability to obtain the basic determinants of health.

An example of one research focus that has been of great value to community nurses is that undertaken by Hunt (1987) who carried out a double-blind study of 300 local authority housing occupants using a face-to-face health survey, then a conditions survey with particular reference to the presence of damp and visible mould growth. Hunt found that the presence of damp was largely confined to certain streets and was related to building structure making it impossible to attribute dampness to individual behaviour. There were strong and statistically significant links between the presence of damp and emotional distress in women, and reports of respiratory and gastrointestinal problems and infections in children. The results were independent of smoking, income, unemployment and other relevant variables.

A larger second study was undertaken in Glasgow (Martin et al 1987). There were close–response relationships between mould in the air and on the walls and the extent and type of symptoms in children, and these findings were independent of smoking in the household, unemployment, income, household composition, the presence of pets and type of cooking facilities.

This type of research is critical to accurate profiling and does mean that the community health profile is an essential resource for the delivery of effective health care. However, when undertaking health needs analysis, all perspectives must be considered.

A pilot survey was undertaken in Nottingham by health visitors (Hunt 1986) to establish health needs from the client perspective. Survey forms were distributed by 19 health visitors, managed by 3 managers, to 450 clients who were asked to give half an hour to complete the forms which were part of the public health survey. The answers gave a clear indication of client priorities over health visiting service demands. The design of the survey is shown in Box 7.9.

Although the Nottingham survey was carried

Box 7.9 Health needs survey questionnaire (Hunt 1986)

1. Do you have worries about the health of anyone in your family?
Think about each person in turn including yourself and write your answer adding any further details
Family illness/inherited illness   ....
Disability/handicap   ....
Illness   ....
Women's health   ....
Family planning   ....
Depression or anxiety   ....
Allergy   ....
Anything else?   ....

2. Is there anything that you think makes you or your family unhealthy?
Tick if concerned
Food   ....   Drugs ....
Alcohol   ....   Lack of exercise ....
Smoking   ....   Unemployment or work ....
Money   ....   Stress ....
Relationships with children .... parents .... partner ....
Anything else?

3. How do you feel about where you live? Tick if you are concerned about:
Housing ....
Facilities, e.g. parks .... shops .... libraries ....
Leisure provision ....
Pollution (e.g. noise, smells, water, air) ....
Crime ....
Harassment ....
Neighbours/local area ....
Safety (in and outside the home) ....
Anything else? ....

4. Are there any recent changes in your life affecting your health?
e.g.   New baby
Change of job/house/partner
Money
Loneliness
Bereavement
Loss of confidence
New neighbours, etc.

5. Summary of family   Family to do   Health visitor
health needs   to do
_____
_____
_____
_____

The final question was designed to be negotiated between health visitor and client to determine the way forward in responding to the identified health needs.

out by health visitors, it can be adapted for use by any member of the PHC team.

What the results certainly showed was the difference between the health needs assumed by the healthcare professionals and those identified by the clients. It was also interesting that the health visitors felt angry about the focus on client perspective, concerned that their job focus might change and vulnerable in the face of a different type of client demand. The clients' response to being asked their opinions ranged between positive, negative and indifferent. The exercise showed clearly the different skills required by the healthcare professionals to identify need in this way; they needed to improve listening skills, acknowledge the problems rather than be defensive, and learn how to empower clients to identify their own health needs. Data collection in this way requires very different abilities from simply understanding social theories, epidemiology and data analysis. However, as indicated, to be most effective the profile needs input from the PHC team, which will now be examined as a focus for change.

THE PHC TEAM AS FOCUS FOR CHANGE

The fundholding GP practice in many cases has a readily identifiable team made up of district nurses, practice nurses, health visitors, midwives, mental health nurses, as well as speech and language therapists, physiotherapists and possibly a social worker. (The structure of the PHC team is discussed in greater detail in Chapter 4.)

Depending on the size of the practice there may be one or more members of each discipline contracted to the GP on a full- or part-time basis. Each of these professionals, although employed by the community unit or trust, works wholly or partially for the practice and is thus purchased by the GP, although practice nurses are often employed directly by the GP.

This is a major change in the organisation of community health care nurses and came about as a direct result of Working for Patients

(DoH 1989). How the team is organised often depends on how the GP views the team. Many more GP practices are now developing self-managed PHC teams.

Successful self-managed teams are likely to be the way forward for the future. If one starts with the premise that all nurses who work in the community are managers, albeit self-managers, then the notion of self-managed PHC teams becomes commonplace. McMurray (1990), drawing on the work of Sullivan & Decker (1985), highlights the essential ingredients of self-management. These range from self-awareness skills using reflective processes, mature interpersonal skills and sensitivity, highly developed sense of ethical and professional accountability, good time management and personal commitment, vision and creativity, a developed sense of awareness of the abilities and skills of the other members of the team, to finally, the skill to be a good team member.

Members of a newly formed PHC team will not possess uniformly well-developed personal management skills unless the team has been in place for some time. What is more likely is that individual members from different disciplines will have experience of a variety of management structures including acute units and have had limited opportunity to work alongside different disciplines in the practice team. The result is that the PHC team may take some time to co-ordinate its work, and much depends on how the team manages itself. Most self-managed teams elect their own team leader; in some cases the GP will identify the team leader as a member of his own employed staff, for example the practice nurse. In other cases the team elects a leader itself.

With the majority of the PHC team being employed by the community unit/trust, a management structure supplied by the unit/trust may be required. In many cases, however, the GP may not be happy about purchasing practitioners with their managers included. There is evidence to show that in some units/trusts, such as Premier Health, South East Staffordshire, this problem has been overcome by creative management, using a nursing development unit to provide education and staff development support for the effective running of the team. The team is thus left to manage itself under the umbrella of the nursing development unit.

An effective self-managed PHC team will have a team leader who acts as a co-ordinator for all the activities of the team. She will hold a small budget to be used as the team decides, and in several instances this means that bank staff hours can be purchased to support, for example, a team member who successfully bids to undertake a course or attend a conference.

The important fact about team leaders is that they are not in a management role and, therefore, are not responsible for individual team members. Their responsibility lies in their leadership skills which inevitably focus on interpersonal, interdisciplinary, intervention processes. In many cases the team leader will be the person who is experienced and will have developed academic as well as particular practical skills. The development of academic skills is very much the aim of the professional practitioner educated under the UKCC PREP (UKCC 1994) guidelines, and there is much evidence to show that practitioners who are academically able are also those who are more flexible, think more broadly and are able listeners (Fish & Parr 1991).

The benefits of self-managed PHC team organisation have yet to be fully evaluated, but practitioners who belong to one that is working well feel comfortable and confident in their practice. It is important that the team makes its own decisions over the philosophy behind the team function. Team members need to be able to cope with peer review for individual performance evaluation and recognise that there is not the cushion of management to fall back on when individual performance is found wanting. The onus is placed on the team to solve individual performer deficiencies.

One of the major benefits of the PHC team approach to community practice is the ability of the team to set up its own quality circle to identify and resolve relevant local healthcare problems. Methods would include the use of data analysis to identify the extent of the problem, and an emphasis on interpersonal skills and techniques for group problem solving and decision making. The role of the team leader is crucial to ensure maximum participation amongst members, maximum creativity in the production of ideas and problem solving, and minimum conflict.

In the early part of the discussion about the primary health care team mention was made of reflection as part of the learning experience of individual team members, and a reflective framework for change is an important feature of the whole change process.

A REFLECTIVE FRAMEWORK FOR CHANGE

Reflection has emerged as a key concept in nursing, midwifery and health visiting literature (Jarvis 1992, Palmer et al 1994). The outcomes of reflection depend on the capacity of the individual to explore her experiences and Boud et al (1985) argue that the success or otherwise of the individual adopting a reflective approach depends on the context in which the individual is working and the level of support, encouragement and facilitative intervention she receives. The capacity of the team to become the focus of facilitative intervention depends to a great extent on the leadership and teamwork of the PHC team. Practitioners have to deal with what Lewin (1952) calls the 'wholeness' of the problem and it is suggested that being a member of the PHC team heightens awareness of the 'wholeness' of problems. Argyris & Schön (1974) explored theories of action across a variety of different professional groups to develop a theory of competent interpersonal practice and to explore how individuals learn in practice situations. They concluded that theories of action underpin and shape human interactions. They constructed two levels of theories of action which were underpinned by espoused theory and theory-in-use. Of the theories-in-use, Argyris & Schön identified two models, one of which, Model II is the most valuable for the self-managing PHC team because it incorporates shared knowledge and information, shared task control and bilateral protection of self and others.

Model II contains governing variables for action:

- Maximisation of valid information
- Maximisation of free and informed choice
- Maximisation of internal commitment to decisions made.

The self-managing PHC team is in a unique position to put into practice these variables and to recognise the value of the integrated approach to solving the 'wholeness' of problems as well as learning by the experience of reflection in the process. Argyris & Schön (1974) describe the learning environment which should be created in this situation and suggest the following action strategies to maintain it:

- Shared design and management of the environment
- Shared task control
- Bilateral protection of self and others.

In such a context, knowledge and information is shared, people are free to discuss ideas and agree common goals, express and think about their own views and question those of others. An open commitment to learning enhances personal and professional development and increases the effectiveness of practice, as demonstrated in Case study 7.3.

In order to understand the processes involved in reflective practice, it is necessary to read and think about the meaning of reflection. This is a particularly important process in becoming a valuable team member and when teaching students. It has been argued (Boyd & Fales 1983, Kitchener & King 1990, Saylor 1990) that the analysis of self is fundamental to reflection. Boyd & Fales (1983), discussing knowledge and learning, considered learning by experience and argue that research on learning from experience has tended to focus on the outcomes of such learning rather than the process involved. They contend that a concept of the process of experiential learning must be developed and that most of this type of learning occurs without the support of structured learning environments, much of it is unin-

---

Case study 7.3   Reflective practice

The W family are well known to the Donaldson Practice and the PHC team members. Susan W is married to David and has three children, Mary, Ben and Jonathan. Jonathan is 9 and has asthma and attends the practice asthma clinic, Mary, aged 16, is pregnant. Susan W's mother, aged 60, lives with the family and suffers from Parkinson's disease. Susan always seems to be in a state of agitation about each member of the family and various members of the PHC team are involved; the practice nurse with Jonathan at the asthma clinic where he never seems to be able to use his inhaler without his mother's help; the health visitor is working with Mary to help support her through this unplanned pregnancy; and the district nurse with Susan's mother who is becoming increasingly unable to look after herself.

At the regular PHC team meeting the district nurse shares with colleagues increasing irritation with Susan, who seems to be constantly agitated and often seems set on undoing any work that the district nurse is undertaking with her mother. The district nurse feels guilty at feeling so irritated with Susan. As soon as this subject is raised it transpires that the health visitor, practice nurse and GP all admit to this sense of guilt over their feelings about Susan's behaviour.

The team then begins to reflect on the events as they have occurred and their feelings in relation to these. The team leader suggests that each member who comes into contact with Susan stops to think about the reflective questions: 'How is this woman making me feel now? How am I responding to her? What interventions shall I use now?' In this way the staff become increasingly sensitive to themselves and to their practice and begin to reflect-in-action (Schön 1987), or in other words to frame the problem and search for appropriate interventions whilst in the situation. They become better able to understand how Susan must be feeling trapped in the situation and can empathise with her. Each of the practitioners feels happier in the practice situation because they can begin to understand and control their experience.

Susan begins to feel better, because she is no longer being rejected and feels that someone is trying to understand and respond to her feelings. As time goes on the PHC team staff recognise that the process of reflection has begun to enhance their practice.

---

tentional and some of it is even unconscious. The main advantage in the relationship between practitioners and students is that the environment is structured to a greater or lesser extent, and for this reason the student may learn more quickly from

Defining reflecting	Being more aware of own process	Controlling the process	Facilitating the process for others	Utilising the concept as a new perspective

Figure 7.6 The progression of reflection.

experiential learning, particularly when there is active reflection through the debriefing process.

Reflective learning is the process of learning and is the core difference between whether a person repeats the same experience several times, becoming highly proficient at one behaviour, or learns from experience in such a way that she is cognitively or affectively changed. To explore the process of learning how to reflect, Boyd & Fales (1983) used qualified counsellors who were accepted by their peers as 'reflective persons'. In repeated interviews with nine counsellors, Boyd & Fales showed a progression of focus shifts within reflection on the process of reflection (Fig. 7.6).

The first focus, 'defining reflecting', explores initially the parameters of reflection. The greatest difficulty is pinning down what is meant by reflection. The second focus is influenced by the first; the person analysing the process of reflection is now more conscious of reflecting even if she is not sure what it is. It may be that it is self-revealing, that really it is about ourselves and our responses in relation to the situation. In the third focus, Boyd & Fales' group found that with this emphasis on reflection they were able actively to control decision making, and that the reflective and process enabled them to speed up active thinking. They did, however, feel the need to control the process and if they were stuck, to stop going round in circles. Interestingly, the counsellors felt that at times the focus was

unwelcome and they had to learn how to turn it off, to distract themselves. The fourth focus created some excitement in the counsellors, enabling them to allow the client/student to become more aware of what she was doing and letting her come to her own conclusions. In the final focus, the study group found that they had utilised reflecting as a concept to enhance existing knowledge and understanding.

As a result of this initial study, Boyd & Fales were able to construct a set of components of the process of reflection based on an analysis of self (Table 7.1). Their application can be understood if considered in relation to Case study 7.3.

Summary

Community health care nurses must be aware of the continuous process of change that affects their working environment and the people they care for. Analysis of tools of management is equally important to both managers in the community and the CHCNs who actually provide the care. To meet the demands inherent in the role, nurses must have the knowledge and the tools to be able to structure and change the services they offer according to the needs of all client groups. For PHC teams to be able to practise with confidence and introduce innovations where appropriate a mechanism to allow nurses to work in partnership with professionals from other disciplines, such as GPs, is necessary. If they are to practise their own specialism, but integrate their skills into the combined skills of the team, then a high level of skill in developing and advancing practice through reflection will be required.

Table 7.1 Components of the reflection process (Boyd & Fales 1983)

Stages of reflection	Process descriptors
1. A sense of inner discomfort	Awareness that something doesn't 'fit' A feeling as though we have 'forgotten' something
2. Identification or clarification of the concern	A key characteristic appears to be that unlike thinking or problem solving, the reflective process is conceptualised in relation to self
3. Openness to new information from internal and external sources, with ability to observe and take in from a variety of perspectives	Openness taking the form of reviewing past experience, foregoing the need for immediate closure on the issue (i.e. forming a conclusion), intentionally structured lateral thinking, intentionally setting aside the problem. For the CPT/counsellor this is a useful intervention stage, enabling the collecting of this information but avoiding forcing it into a pattern
4. Resolution, expressed as 'integration', 'coming together', 'acceptance of self-reality' and 'creative synthesis'	This is the 'eureka' stage of reflection when insight is gained and at which point people experience themselves as changed, having learned, or having come to a satisfactory point of closure in relation to the issue (i.e. reached a satisfactory end-point or conclusion)
5. Establishing continuity of self with past, present and future	There is a recognition in terms of similar solutions from past experience, reviewing past values in relation to the changed perspective, evaluating the change as better for self, applying the new perspective to a variety of additional issues in the present self-structure, planning for future behaviour consistent with the changed perspective, or examining the implications of the change for future behaviour
6. Deciding whether to act on the outcome of the reflective process	The change or resolution is evaluated in terms of the individual's own subjective criteria, the intensity of the subjective sense of the rightness of the resolution, its consistency with the individual's existing or aspired value structure, and with other desired goals of the self. The need to test one's self-changes against the mirror of others is an essential component of all growth

REFERENCES

Argyris C, Schön D 1974 Theory in practice: increasing professional effectiveness. Jossey-Bass, San Francisco

Bennis W, Benne K, Chin R eds 1976 The planning of change, 3rd edn. Holt, Rinehart & Winston, London

Billingham K 1991 Community health profiling. Unpublished paper. Nottingham Community Unit, Nottingham

Blackburn C 1991 Poverty and health: working with families. Open University Press, Milton Keynes

Boud D, Keogh R, Walker D (eds) 1985 Reflection: turning experience into learning. Kogan Page, London

Boyd E, Fales A W 1983 Reflective learning. Journal of Humanistic Psychology 23(2):99–117

Carlisle E 1972 The conceptual structure of social indicators. In: Schonfield A, Shaw S (eds) Social indicators and social policy. Heinemann, London

Chen M, Bush J, Patrick D 1975 Social indicators for health planning and policy analysis. Policy Sciences 6:71–89

Department of Health 1983 NHS management enquiry. (The Griffiths report.) HMSO, London

Department of Health 1989 Working for patients: the health service in the 1990s. Cmd 555. HMSO, London

Department of Health 1990 Health of the nation. HMSO, London

Department of Health and Social Security 1980 Inequalities in health (Black report) HMSO, London

Egan G 1985 Change agent skills in helping and human service setting. Brooks/Cole, San Diego

ENB 1987 Regulations and guidelines for the approval of a course leading to the health visiting qualification and entry on Part II of the register. ENB, London

Fish D, Parr B 1991 An evaluation of practice-based learning in continuing professional education in nursing, midwifery and health visiting. (Report) ENB, London

Grundy T 1993 Implementing strategic change – a practical guide for business. Kogan Page, London

Handy C 1991 The age of unreason. Business Books, London

Hatch S, Sherrat R 1973 Positive discrimination and the distribution of deprivations. In: Luker K, Orr J (eds) Health visiting. Blackwell Scientific, London

Hunt S M 1986 Measuring health in clinical care and clinical trials. In: Teeling-Smith G (ed) Measuring health: a practical approach. John Wiley, Chichester

Hunt S 1987 Emotional distress and bad housing. Health and Hygiene 11:72–79

Jarvis P 1992 Reflective practice and nursing. Nurse Education Today 12:174–175

Kitchener K S, King P M 1990 The reflective judgement model: transforming assumptions about knowing. In: Mezirow J et al (eds) Fostering critical reflection in adulthood. Jossey-Bass, San Francisco

Land K, McMillan M 1978 Demographic data and social indicators. Cited in: Luker K, Orr J (eds) 1992 Health visiting, 2nd edn. Blackwell Scientific, Oxford

Legge K 1984 Evaluating planned organisational change. Academic Press, London

Lewin K 1935 A dynamic theory of personality. McGraw Hill New York

Lewin K 1951 Field theory in social science. Harper & Row, New York

Martin C N, Platt S D, Hunt S M 1987 Housing conditions and ill health. British Medical Journal 294:1125–1127

McMurray A 1990 Community health nursing. Churchill Livingstone, Melbourne

Moos R H 1976 The human context: environmental determinants of behaviour. Cited in: Luker K, Orr J (eds) 1992 Health visiting, 2nd edn. Blackwell Scientific, Oxford

NHS Management Executive 1994 Health visitor marketing project. NHS Management Executive, Leeds

NHS Management Inquiry 1983 Report (The Griffiths report). HMSO, London

Orr J 1985 In: Luker K, Orr J 1992 Health visiting. Blackwell Scientific Press, Oxford

Palmer A, Burns S, Bulman C (eds) 1994 Reflective practice in nursing: the growth of the professional practitioner. Blackwell Science, Oxford

Pettigrew A 1985 The awakening giant: contingency and change in ICI. Blackwell, London

Plant R 1987 Managing change and making it stick. Fontana, London

Saylor C R 1990 Reflection and professional education: art, science, and competency. Nurse Educator 15(2):8–11

Schön D A 1971 Beyond the stable state: public and private learning in a changing society. M T Smith, London

Schön D A 1987 Educating the reflective practitioner. Jossey-Bass, San Francisco

Spurgeon P, Barwell F 1991 Implementing change in the NHS: a guide for general managers. Chapman and Hall, London

Sullivan E, Decker P 1985 Effective management. Cited in: McMurray A 1990 Community health nursing. Churchill Livingstone, Melbourne

Tinson S 1995 Assessing health need: a community perspective. Cited in: Cain P, Hyde V, Hawkins E 1995 Community nursing: dimensions and dilemmas. Edward Arnold, London

UKCC 1994 The future of professional practice: the Council's standards for education and practice following registration. HMSO, London

FURTHER READING

Bolt E, Powell J 1993 Becoming reflective. Distance Learning Centre, South Bank University, London

Cain P, Hyde V, Hawkins E 1995 Community nursing dimensions and dilemmas. Edward Arnold, London

Hawkins E 1995 Community nursing: dimensions and dilemmas. Edward Arnold, London

Luker K, Orr J 1992 Health visiting – towards community health nursing, 2nd edn. Blackwell Scientific, Oxford

Oakley P, Greaves E 1995 Restructuring the organisation. Health Service Journal 105:30–31

8

Clients and carers: the needs of individuals and families

Penny Reid

Any discussion on informal care should be linked with formal community care (see Ch. 3), but community health care nurses must understand the background to informal care and how caring patterns are changing to meet the needs of altered family arrangements. The needs of carers must be analysed so that community health care nurses can take them into consideration and combine them with the care they offer to patients. Community health care nurses must also be aware of the needs of multicultural groups and how their beliefs and traditions affect their attitudes to informal caring. To inform this process, community health care nurses should be able to:

- Define what is meant by the term 'informal carer'
- Discuss the role of women as carers
- Discuss the types of cost incurred by carers in carrying out their roles
- Identify the help that is available to informal carers through voluntary and statutory agencies
- Explain the joint assessment process.

STRUCTURES OF INFORMAL CARING

DEFINITIONS

The word 'caring' has many different meanings, so it is worth defining at the start of this discussion what it means in the context of care given by non-professional individuals and family and friends. Here, it is taken to mean the role carried out by one of these groups when supporting someone to allow him to remain in his own home rather than being cared for in an institution.

Considerable confusion and uncertainty has surrounded the meaning and aims of 'community care' and this is discussed in detail in Chapter 1. The term is often used by health authorities to refer to any care given outside the hospital setting. It is helpful to distinguish between care 'by' the community in terms of care given by family, neighbours and voluntary groups and care 'in' the community provided by formal services including residential provision. The term 'informal carers' should also be clarified: it is not an ideal term, implying perhaps that care not provided by professional carers is in some way less skilled or inferior. However, to use the term 'family carers' would exclude all those who provide care as neighbour or friend. The term 'informal carers' will therefore be used to describe those friends, neighbours and relatives who provide care which would otherwise need to be provided by the statutory and voluntary sectors.

INFORMAL CARE

Informal carers are not always free to choose whether or not they undertake the role. Many have little or no option because of a lack of satisfactory, realistic alternatives: either the dependent person's condition is not sufficiently advanced or severe to warrant residential care or admission to hospital, or community services are inadequate or insufficiently developed to meet the need. Consequently, the duty of care rests on friends or, more usually, family. In effect, this duty of care has fallen traditionally on women.

There can be no doubt that caring, whether informal or formal, voluntary or paid, is seriously undervalued in society. It is carried out chiefly by women and is largely taken for granted. Furthermore, if it is paid it is usually poorly paid, but it is often unpaid. This results in a low status

for carers and is manifested in the absence of resources and support available for informal caring needs. The relatively low salaries of paid carers – nurses and social workers, domiciliary day care and healthcare workers – compared with other professions, also signals the low status of caring (Nissel & Bonnerjea 1982).

In the past 10 years, the Conservative government made clear its commitment to community care, particularly since the publication of the White Paper Caring for People (Department of Health 1989a) which brought about major changes in the organisation and delivery of community care. Whilst health authorities retain responsibility for people requiring nursing care, the government states in the White Paper (Department of Health 1989) that 'It is essential that the caring services should work effectively together, each recognising and respecting the other's contribution and responsibility... there is no room in community care for a narrow view of individuals' needs, nor ways of meeting them'. It is important, therefore, to respect and support the contribution of carers, including informal carers who save the country money. Research carried out to ascertain the level of understanding amongst professionals in relation to the White Paper shows they believe its two most important functions to be promoting independent living (51%) and providing relief for carers (Caldock 1994).

The Carer's Act (1996)

The Carer's Recognition and Services Act, known as the Carer's Act, came into being on 1 April 1996 (Box 8.1).

While the White Paper Caring for People made support for carers one of the six principles underpinning the community care reforms, there was no mention of carers in the subsequent legislation.

The Carer's Act should provide real benefits for many carers without significant financial implications, and enshrines the good practices of many authorities. Those facing the greatest costs in implementing the Act will therefore be those who are not already providing appropriate carer support.

Box 8.1 Carer's Act

The Act entitles carers to their own assessment.

Guidance following the Act advised that in general, carers should be given the option of having their assessment interview in private, for example, in the absence of the person being cared for.

There is no right to a 'free standing' assessment; a carer is only entitled to an assessment when the person for whom he or she is caring is being assessed. A review of a person's care plan constitutes an assessment at law.

Only carers who provide, or intend to provide, 'a substantial amount of care on a regular basis' are entitled to an assessment. The term 'substantial' is obviously subjective but local authorities should take into account the personal characteristics of the carer.

The age of the carer is immaterial. Young carers (under 18 years old), parent carers (who care for their disabled children) and adult carers (one adult caring for another) are all covered by the Act.

The duty to assess a carer only arises if the carer requests the assessment.

The assessment carried out is of the carer's 'ability to provide and continue to provide care for the relevant person'.

The Act gives carers no right to any community care services but merely obliges social services to take into account the carer's assessment when deciding what services the disabled person needs. (Adapted from Clements 1996.)

Social trends affecting caring

Changes in family life over the last 20 years have disrupted its continuity, although many still try to follow the traditional pattern. Individuals who have a series of marriages during their lifetime have less opportunity, and tend to be less able, to develop emotional ties with older generations.

Women as principal carers

The family has traditionally had the responsibility of caring for the elderly, the infirm and the disabled. The welfare state and voluntary sector have acted as a combined safety net when the family failed or was unable to fulfil this role. It has been postulated that without the support provided by informal carers, total government expenditure on health and social services would be doubled (Land 1991). Despite the growing role of the welfare state during the 1970s and early 1980s, the family is still seen as having the

ultimate responsibility for 'caring', and the enactment of the NHS and Community Care Act (1990), which endorsed the Griffiths report (Department of Health 1989a) has emphasised the fact that family, friends and neighbours are the cornerstone of care.

In its original form, community care policy advocated a significant role for public services in maintaining highly dependent people outside large institutions. By the late 1970s, this was less clearly the case. Under the twin pressures of fiscal crisis and an ideologically driven commitment to reducing the role of the state in service provision, the original vision was replaced by a much stronger emphasis on the provision of care by the community itself (Parker 1990). It was at this time that gender emerged as a key variable in the analysis of community care policy (Finch & Groves 1983). Finch & Groves' paper transformed the contemporary debate on community care in two ways. They argued that community care was essentially about the care provided by women in the home, and discussed the effects of caring on women's equality of opportunity with men in life.

The authors argued that community care as policy stood would intensify the inequalities experienced by women by virtue of the care they provided both for children and for other relatives with physical or mental disabilities. The demanding and continuous nature of this work, and the fact that it was unpaid, meant that women's access to time and money of their own was much less than that of the men in their families (Finch & Groves 1983). Caring responsibilities also reduced women's opportunities for entering the labour force on an equal footing. Policy in the field of community care was based on the assumption that such exploitation would continue and indeed increase. The debate has continued, particularly in the light of feminist research in social policy (Twigg et al 1991, Glendinning 1992), and remains unresolved.

Informal care shares many of the characteristics of the work that women undertake in both the paid and unpaid sectors. It tends to be flexible and performed without relation to status or training. It often involves responsiveness to the needs of others, in ways that override the subject's own interests. Caring is often repetitive and carried out over long hours. Indeed, there are usually no limits circumscribing its performance; the obligations are continuous and open-ended. To a degree then, caring is best understood in the context of all the work women do in holding together their families, the economy and society. Often involving physical contact of an intimate character, the dominant cultural perception of caring sees it as involving essentially female qualities. This perception, which is shared by many women, is used to explain and justify the gendered division of caring. It therefore appears more appropriate for women to be the ones who wash, toilet, feed and care for people who are ill or frail (Finch & Groves 1983).

Families are now smaller, so fewer young people are available to take on a caring role. In the past, families moved around the country less frequently, so patterns of extended kinship in local areas were the norm even though the nuclear family household prevailed; the duty of care was more apparent and more easily managed by sharing it with a greater 'pool' of family members. Nowadays, the search for employment often leads families to leave the area of their upbringing, putting pressure on family relationships. This trend shows no sign of reversing and is likely to lead to severe difficulties in providing long-term care.

Changes in roles within families also have an impact on the availability of carers. Of women with children under 5, 50% now work outside the home (Bradshaw & Millar 1991). Women have now achieved greater financial independence and a certain amount of equality in the workplace. They are understandably reluctant, even unable, to relinquish this in order to care for relatives.

In the case of mentally handicapped children, Wilkin (1979) found that when it came to caring, most mothers were left to get on with it on their own. Fathers would help with childminding rather than child care, and with child care rather than household chores. In the case of physically disabled people, Blaxter (1976) found that elderly men could generally rely on their spouse who was not employed, but elderly women who sur-

vived their husbands had much greater difficulty in finding a relative to fulfil the caring role. Ungerson (1983) suggests that there is consistent evidence that however much men share in lifting, playtime and childminding, the strength of resistance to nappy changing is evidence of a deep-seated taboo as regards dealing with the bodily functions of others, and this is possibly even stronger in the case of physical care by men for older or disabled relatives of the opposite sex.

In a more recent set of case studies of the roles and responses of carers of elderly people in families (Twigg et al 1991), the significance of gender roles in caring has been explored. Virtually all those cared for had already deteriorated beyond the point at which they would have been considered appropriate applicants for accommodation in housing with an on-site warden.

The predominance of certain patterns for older people is quite clear. Elderly couples tend to remain in their own homes. Although wives tend to care for husbands who die before them, the only cases of men providing physical care for women were those of husbands for their wives. Of these, retired professional men had adapted most successfully by adopting a work-like approach to their tasks and by negotiating with the relevant agencies for the services they or their wives needed. The great majority of carers were wives of elderly husbands, and daughters with dependent parents, usually a widowed mother or mother-in-law. In no cases were their husbands sharing more than a few of the tasks of caring, and it was common for these informal female carers to feel torn between the attention they felt obliged to give their elderly relative, even the husband's parent, and a feeling of guilt about the relative neglect of their husbands or children. In fact husbands were considered very supportive if they talked to the older people and did not complain about their wives' preoccupation with their care.

If the actual social roles that people perform are so established and not just attitudinal stereotypes, they are most likely to be unamenable to change, even when so many men are stuck at home as a result of unemployment. In fact, any general assumption that unemployment will swell the ranks of informal carers or ease the burden on women fulfilling these duties is misplaced; it is more likely to exacerbate the tribulation of being unemployed. One could argue that social policy should be directed to providing an adequate recompense for the work these women do rather than seeking to generalise the burden by attempting to change gender roles.

Trends in caring

The General Household Survey first researched the numbers of carers in 1985 (Green 1988) and this was repeated in 1990. These two sets of figures can be used to compare trends in caring over the 5-year period. In 1985, 6 million people were carers, and by 1990 this had risen to 6.8 million people. In 1990 15% of people over 16 were carers compared to 14% in 1985. Therefore, 1 in 7 people had some kind of caring role in 1990. Also in 1990, 13% of men and 17% of women said they were carers; of the 6.8 million carers, 2.9 million were men and 3.9 million were women. What this does not show, however, is the extent of caring activities undertaken by the male and female respondents in this research.

The General Household Survey (Green 1988) examined people over the age of 16; however, there is growing awareness of the numbers of even younger people who are carers and it is important to consider other research. Surveys carried out in Thameside and Sandwell by Carers National Association (DoH 1989b) suggest there may be well over 10 000 children acting as primary carers nationwide. Typically, these are children from single parent families where the parent develops a disabling illness, or they may be living with an ageing grandparent. Some are children needed to help with a disabled sibling. The heavy responsibility can have serious effects on a child's personal and educational development. As well as the physical side of caring – washing, dressing, feeding – there is evidence that emotional pressures can lead to difficulties in forming social relationships. Poor school attendance is also common. The problem is exacerbated if they come to the attention of social services; they often feel guilty that they are letting down the person they are caring for.

24% of people in the age range 45–64 said they had caring responsibilities, this being the peak age group for caring. This compares to 8% of those aged 16–29, 15% of those aged 30–44, and 13% of those aged 65+ (DoH 1990). People were usually caring for parents. A range of services was provided:

- 22% of carers were involved in personal care tasks such as washing
- 16% administered medications
- 79% gave other practical help.

In 1990, 23% of carers spent more than 20 hours a week caring, and 11% were spending more than 50 hours per week caring. Most people looked after just one person, though 3% of adults were caring for more than one. The study also examined the reasons for caring:

- 71% of carers looked after someone with a physical disability
- 5% looked after someone with a mental disability
- 17% with both physical and mental disabilities
- Most carers looked after elderly people – 79% of those cared for were over 65 and 20% were 80 or over, an increase of 5% since 1985.

Giving long-term care to someone can have a direct effect on both the socio-economic circumstances of the carer and also on her health. The Carers National Association (1995) carried out a survey of its members to find out what it was like to be a carer:

- 47% had experienced financial difficulty since becoming a carer
- 65% said their own health had suffered
- 20% had never had a break
- 33% had got no help or support with their caring roles.

Many carers identified problems with being a carer, but some stressed the benefits they felt they gained from the close relationship they achieved with the person they were caring for. They also identified a sense of satisfaction from the work which came from the feeling of doing something really worthwhile, something highly valued by the person they were caring for.

Gender role research. This shift, from caring as a taken-for-granted and unquantified aspect of women's lives to its identification as problematic, warranting conceptual analysis and empirical investigation, resulted from the debate generated by the women's movement of the early 1970s. Liberal feminists had earlier studied the position of women in society generally, leaving the relations of men and women within families largely unquestioned. For the new wave of feminists, these relations and their connection to women's oppression in the wider society were a primary focus. The sexual division of labour within the family was the fulcrum around which analysis of gender relations swung. Crucially, the definition of women's unpaid activity within the home as work opened the way for critical appraisal of the relations between women and men, within both the family and the public sphere. A pioneering stream of research by Oakley (1974), Pahl (1980) and others rigorously analysed what went on in the domestic sphere, raising and answering questions about who did what and for whom, to whose benefit and to whose cost. A parallel stream of work in social policy highlighted the connections between these domestic divisions of labour and government policies, notably those promoting the care of elderly and disabled people in the community.

Help available to carers

The extent of the role of the state in the provision of care for the elderly and chronically sick can be examined by looking at the proportion of the population in institutional care. This appears to have been stable over this century, despite the growth of the welfare state. Since 1911 less than 5% of elderly people in England and Wales have been resident in institutions at the time of decennial census and the rate of institutionalisation in the general population has been consistently below 2% (Moroney 1976). In the case of those with learning difficulties there has been some increase in residential care compared with earlier this century. Even so, substantial numbers of those with severe learning difficulties (IQ below 50) were living outside institutions, many of them requiring considerable supervision and assistance.

Large numbers of dependent people are therefore being cared for at home by family members. In their study of the family care of elderly people, Nissel and Bonnerjea (1982) state:

While the family, where it exists, still cares for its elderly relatives within the family, it is wives, daughters, daughters-in-law and other female relatives who shoulder the main burden of responsibility. Moreover, once the carer has taken on the burden she is likely to receive little practical support from other relatives.

This is also the case with statutory services, which tend to assist elderly people on their own and help men caring for women at home, but do less if there is a female carer in the home. With local authority finance at a premium, Webb & Wistow (1987) found that despite attempts to maintain the volume of community services, the tendency was to spread them more thinly over the increasing numbers of people in need of them. The Audit Commission (1986) confirmed this in their analysis of trends in the balance of care for those aged over 75.

It is important to distinguish overall numbers, which may have increased, from provision for the population at risk or in need. Standing still in terms of provision will actually represent a decline if this population is increasing. The only sizeable increases are in private nursing and residential homes, because these lie outside government cash limits on the public sector and are directly funded from supplementary benefits as cases arise and apply. Even day centre places have barely kept pace with demand, although they represent a major form of relief to carers and delay the point of admission to residential care or even hospital. The number of meals taken to people at home has been greatly reduced, a trend more marked in recent years. For example, in 1986–1987 there was considerable protest in Buckinghamshire against a proposed cut in financial support for the voluntary Crossroad Care home attendant support scheme. This led to the services being retained. A project, initially with joint finance from the NHS, was subsequently accepted as a means of developing this service.

Financial aspects of caring

Financial help

The only benefit specifically available for carers is the disability allowance, which offers £34.50 a week for a 35-hour week, less than £1 an hour: some carers work a 50-hour week or more. The benefit is not available to those who become carers after they are 65. In fact, because of the strict rules only about 17.5% of carers receive disability allowance.

The earnings that carers have to forgo as the main provider of support to someone else are described as an 'opportunity cost'. Although some carers sacrifice a lot more than their potential money earnings, the cash they would have earned were they not carers is a crucial component of the opportunity cost of their unpaid work.

The recipients of care are generally members of the family, and the degree of care they receive varies enormously, from the round-the-clock attendance required by a severely disabled person to the weekly shopping needed by an elderly person. The degree to which caring interferes with a person's capacity to earn depends not only on the level of dependency of those they care for, but also on the extent to which their care is shared by other people, paid and unpaid. Expenditure on commodities such as domestic machinery, pre-cooked food, lifting devices and washing facilities can make a multiple role easier to perform well.

Costs incurred by carers

Comparing the cash that carers actually receive with what they might have earned is not to deny that caring activity does have material and emotional compensations, and that its value to the giver and receiver is sometimes beyond price. Neither is it suggested that 'labours of love' could be remunerated by wages in exact compensation. However, informal carers do need to receive recognition, appreciation and above all support, rather than being taken for granted (Finch & Groves 1983). It was only as recently as 1986 that married women became eligible to

apply for Invalid Care Allowance thus applying the idea of opportunity cost. When this benefit was introduced to help compensate people for having to give up employment to care for the infirm the presumption was that such costs were not incurred by married women.

Glendinning & Millar (1987) suggest that applying an alternative approach to costing unpaid care would be to value it at replacement cost, that is, what it would cost to pay somebody to do everything the unpaid carer does. This approach is particularly suited to the debate about policy on community care of the infirm and elderly (Henwood & Wicks 1984). It is not, however, necessarily appropriate when considering the personal financial sacrifices which carers make, because estimating replacement costs raises some practical difficulties in observing the tasks performed and the time they take or the time they would take someone who did not also live in the home, and in putting a price on the hours required.

Nissel & Bonnerjea (1982) estimate that the time taken to provide the care needed by a handicapped elderly person ranges from 24 to 35 hours per week; they tentatively suggest valuing these tasks at the market rate for domestic work, £1.80 per hour in 1980. Henwood & Wicks (1984) suggest using the official rate for local authority home helps, £2.90 in 1982–83. Clearly this has increased in the intervening years and will vary from area to area. Either rate may be well below the market value of some of the nursing skills involved and, as Nissel & Bonnerjea (1982) show, well below what the carer might have been able to earn in their occupation.

The equation of opportunity costs with forgone earnings is not the complete story because it makes no allowance for the free time which may be diverted into caring for others. Neither does it take into account the social and psychological benefits of avoiding isolation in the home. However, it has the advantage that it is possible to identify and quantify the cash opportunity cost of caring by observing what people do in the public domain of paid employment. The amount of paid work that people with domestic responsibilities manage to do is clearly less than that which those without domestic responsibilities manage to do. This approach is followed here in order to examine how caring affects carers' labour market participation and their hours of paid work, and their pay both in the short term and the long term.

The most difficult caring situations are relatively uncommon among women under 60. Only 14% of the women in the Women and Employment Survey reported that they had responsibility for someone needing care. Of these, a quarter were actually providing constant attention. Among those cared for were handicapped children and invalid husbands; some of the others, mainly elderly people, were living in separate households. The existence of these varied caring responsibilities lowered the employment rate on average. Caring responsibilities for the disabled are often combined, like maternal responsibilities, with some employment. Detailed studies of their situation stress the emotional as well as the financial benefits of the carer having another role outside of the home (Parker 1990). As the physical dependency of a disabled child is prolonged, mothers of children with special needs are less likely to manage the part-time employment that typifies mothers of healthy school children.

CARING AND LEARNING DIFFICULTIES

CARING FOR CHILDREN WITH LEARNING DIFFICULTIES

The framework of care and support by the statutory and voluntary sectors in relation to children and their carers comes under the NHS and Community Care Act (DoH 1990), the Children Act (1989) and the Education Act (1980).

Some families may be unable able to cope with the unexpected extra demands and strain created by the arrival of a child with learning difficulties or with a physical disability. Marriages may break down, possibly resulting in either the child being received into care, or one of the parents, usually the mother, being left with the sole responsibility for the child's upbringing. Most parents, however, react positively to their situation and strive to provide their child with all the love and attention he needs. In reality they have little choice, and although their task is not entirely devoid of many of the essential joys of child-rearing, it is often an isolating and debilitating struggle. Society's reluctance to share the responsibility means that the parents face a demanding future without respite.

Those who are parents of a child with learning difficulties need to make huge emotional adjustments as they endeavour to come to terms with the feelings brought about by a sense of overwhelming disappointment and loss. They may be counselled against having more children in case they conceive another child with special needs. They may worry too about the emotional stresses that having such a child might have on any siblings. Parents may experience a sense of guilt or shame at having produced a child with special needs because it is not seen as perfect by the rest of society. The situation is more difficult for families within some communities where having a disabled child, regardless of the disability, represents a divine punishment; and so the family will have to carry added stigma. Having a child with learning difficulties may mean that the family will be excluded from engaging in many of their hitherto cherished activities. Parents of children with learning difficulties need the support of friends and relatives more than most families, yet they are more likely to be isolated in this respect. For various reasons, including their own embarrassment, awkwardness and ignorance, friends and neighbours may be reluctant to visit or help out in a situation with which they are not familiar.

Social provision, such as financial benefits, home conversion grants, special school arrangements and respite care facilities, is available, to a varying degree, for families with children with physical or learning difficulties. However, such provision is often inadequate; it varies from region to region and is not always available from birth, and strict eligibility criteria exclude some families. The situation is obviously exacerbated when local authorities and voluntary organisations are forced to cut back on expenditure.

As children grow older the difficulties for parents increase; the children become heavier and physically more difficult to manage, and they need support in coping with the changes brought about by puberty and adolescence. Whilst the child is at school he is cared for. When he gets beyond school age, however, the responsibility for full-time care goes back to the parents. In some cases residential care is necessary, but for many families this is not appropriate. The Wagner report (Residential Care – a Positive Choice) recommends that 'Education and training for people with mental handicap should aim at enabling them to live with support in ordinary housing'. Until appropriate provision is made for young people, parents will continue to be plagued by their major concern, 'Who is going to look after him when I'm gone?'

CARING FOR ADULTS WITH LEARNING DIFFICULTIES

Once people with learning difficulties leave school, their parents face their most difficult times. Educational provision is statutory, but after the age of 19 people with learning difficulties have to compete with other adults requiring support. The reality is that, while provision should exist, it is severely limited. The Disabled Persons Act 1986 recommends, but does not insist, that local authorities should define need and provide for it. Without continuity of support the chances are that any progress and development made in childhood may be lost as the condition of people with learning difficulties deteriorates or they lose their confidence. Very few are able to find work directly; some may be able to obtain a place on a further education course, although these are not always available; some will remain at home; others will seek places at social services day centres, but again only where places are available.

JOINT ASSESSMENT FOR COMMUNITY CARE

The community care reforms (see Ch. 3) implemented as a result of the Griffiths report (DoH 1989a) put users and carers in the spotlight, and introduced needs-led rather than services-led assessment. The aim was to offer greater choice, so that users could stay at home with flexible health and social care support, thus maintaining their independence, rather than entering residential care. The meteoric rise in private residential home-care costs, from £10 million to £100 million over the period 1979–89 was a major factor, driving the government to initiate legislation to reduce the costs, in the belief that enabling people to remain in their homes would be more economic.

Social services departments are required to assess anyone who appears to be in need of services. The aim of assessment is to identify people who can be looked after at home, rather than in residential care, and to respond by providing appropriate services.

The expectations of carers were raised by the proposals of the new Act, under which every local authority was obliged to respond to those needing help, assess their need and draw up a plan for their care. However, the government felt that to implement the community care part of the Act, along with the changes being initiated in the NHS, would be too disruptive so these changes did not come into force until 1990. The delay prompted newspaper comment: 'Yet again, as with so many previous governments, the old and the disabled are being relegated to the bottom of the waiting lists' (Observer 22 July 1990 p. 11). As might be expected, reactions to the Health and Community Care Act proposals were mixed. The fact that overall administration of care was to remain with local authorities was received positively. It was felt to be a good thing that care packages or programmes are individually based and that client choice and the wishes of clients should be central to the whole exercise. Good practice would clearly be enhanced through more rigorous assessment and care management procedures. However, the needs of carers were only taken into account under the Disabled Persons Act 1986, which required social services departments to take into account the carers' health and their ability to continue caring when they decide what services are needed. This has since been addressed by the Carers Recognition and Services Act (1996) which ensures that carers also have a right to their own individual assessment. The sorts of services that can be offered include:

- A home-help – to help with either shopping or personal care
- A place at a day centre and transport to get there
- A hot meal at midday
- Respite care – perhaps a week at a residential home every few weeks to give the carer a break.

Once the services are recorded in the assessment, the carer has a legal right to them, and if for some reason they cannot be provided then the council must find some alternative that is acceptable to both the client and the carer. However, a research report from the Carers National Association (1995) found that amongst its members only 13% of carers surveyed had received an assessment in their own right, 91% thought carers should have a legal right to respite care, and 79% thought that community care had made a difference to them.

MULTICULTURAL GROUPS

In today's multicultural society there exist a range of family structures and an equally large number of beliefs about illness, disability and old age, all of which affect ability to provide care and the likelihood of care being provided within the family.

It is easy to stereotype cultural groups, believing, for example, that there is an extended family network willing and ready to carry out the caring role when needed. For some, this may be true, but not for all and each case should be assessed individually. The immigration process may have fragmented the family. In addition, all of the fac-

tors affecting families in the UK currently, also affect immigrant families, weakening their capacity to provide support and care for their family members. Indeed, the effects of racism may actually worsen their situation in relation to housing provision and employment. These difficulties often mean that parents become separated from their adult children; few houses or flats can readily accommodate more than two generations living together.

Access to services and advice may be severely limited due to language difficulties and to lack of awareness about what is available to them; community staff need to ensure that information is freely available to those who need it in a form they can understand. The way in which services are provided must take into account the diversity of carers' needs and the realities of their lives, including discrimination and racism.

Black and ethnic minority carers have similar needs to all other carers; they too need information, respite care and practical help. The issues that arise are often concerned with securing equal access to these services and equal treatment. New services must also take into account the diversity of language, culture and experience. The level of unmet need is difficult to identify. Some carers and their families may live in close-knit communities which provide their own support, and therefore do not need help from the statutory services. There are many others, however, whose experience of trying to obtain and receiving help from those agencies has been extremely traumatic. Clearly, improved access to services needs to be given some priority.

The King's Fund (1988) has identified five areas that require development in order to improve services for carers from ethnic minority groups.

Information giving. This should take into account the language difficulties which may isolate carers from the services available. Many arriving in this country do not expect benefits or services to be available to them as they do not exist in their country of origin, so it is important that service providers make a concerted effort to remember to tell carers what is available.

Recognition of racism. People who regularly experience discrimination in their everyday dealings with statutory services will remain sceptical about their access to services and to professionals' willingness to help them. Patronising or dismissive attitudes on the part of professionals or 'gatekeepers' can leave an enduring reluctance to seek the help needed.

Sensitivity and responsiveness. Service providers need to give attention to each family's circumstances when planning the services to be provided. For some families it will be critical to ensure that staff are from the same cultural group as themselves. Greater consultation with black and ethnic minority carers may be needed as well as continual monitoring and review to ensure that services remain appropriate.

Special services. There are a growing number of groups throughout the country which not only deal with the specific problem of the person being cared for but also focus on the particular cultural group, for instance, groups for Asian parents of children with learning difficulties.

Positive policies. Sometimes positive discrimination is needed so that more resources are directed at specific cultural and ethnic groups in an effort to meet their needs. More staff are being trained and recruited who reflect the needs of the community they serve, and who therefore have special insight into their needs, and can also make services more acceptable to the carers. Such people also need to be involved at the planning, purchasing and evaluation levels so that services can be made more appropriate and accessible to black and ethnic minority carers.

RESPITE CARE

Respite care has traditionally been inconsistent and depends on the resources of the local health authority. People requiring respite care may find that the facilities offered are not suited to their particular needs and are often offered 'care of the elderly' beds in general hospitals. There is also often a long wait before admission because of pressure on beds. The problem is that respite care is not usually planned; it is often needed at short notice due to sudden illness of the carer or to some crisis situation at home requiring an instant response. Carers frequently find that they lose

their own identity so they are often overlooked and receive little care themselves.

The Princess Royal Trust Carers' Centres are being developed across the UK, offering information, support and counselling for carers. The Trust operates as a charity receiving monetary support from donations received from large companies and individuals and recently from local authorities. The Trust was started in 1991 and it seeks to raise the necessary funds to provide information, counselling, help and support to carers and to raise public awareness of carers' needs and their contribution to society. They also offer emotional support by providing opportunities for carers to share their problems with volunteers and professional staff who understand their situation, thus helping to alleviate isolation and stress. The centres are also of practical help with such things as shopping, transport and laundry. They provide access to existing care attendance schemes or voluntary sitting services and mutual support by providing facilities for the development of self-help carer support groups and by providing an informal meeting place for carers. Staff also offer advice to carers, advocacy services at tribunals, assessments and are available whenever a carer needs a reliable friend or support.

Nurses supporting carers

Unlike carers, nurses have chosen to enter and develop the caring practice of nursing. However, both nurses and carers must avoid dominating and encouraging dependency in the person they care for. Instead they should, after assessment, offer support and encourage self-care. Such an approach aims to empower clients, giving them freedom to make informed choices. Nurses need to develop the skills to recognise the strains that carers are under, including emotional, physical, psychological and financial, and to provide both physical and psychological support.

Community nurses often work with scarce resources and acute care of the client tends to take priority over the needs of the carer, which are fitted in after the acute care obligations have been met.

SUMMARY

Caring (both formal and informal) has enormous power to help people and yet, as we have seen during this chapter, it tends to be undervalued by policy makers and by society in general. It is important that nursing recognises this power and that nurses use an holistic approach to looking after clients and their carers. The reform of the old health care system offers many opportunities for carers and for the incorporation of their needs and interests into service delivery. The carer issue has become an increasingly prominent one. The documentation relating to the new community care refers to carers extensively, and it is increasingly common for policy documents at local as well as national level to describe their needs as part of the legit-imate concerns of service provision. How far the new community care will in fact embody a radically different approach to service delivery is still unclear; much remains to be clarified, particularly in relation to patterns of funding. Changes in other sectors, notably the acute medical sector, though also in the structure of local government, may force the pace of change; but they may also, ironically, inhibit real change. Where carers will fit into this is similarly unclear. What remains clear, however, is that they will continue to provide the majority of care and how they are perceived by service providers will continue to determine the level and pattern of help they will receive in doing so.

REFERENCES

Audit Commission 1986 Making a reality of community care. HMSO, London

Blaxter M 1976 The meaning of disability. Heinemann, London

Bradshaw J, Millar J 1991 Lone parents in the UK. HMSO, London

Caldock K 1994 Policy and practice. Fundamental contradictions in the conceptualisation of community care for elderly people. Health and Social Care in the Community 2:133–141

Carers National Association 1995 Community care: just a fairy tale? Research report. Carers National Association, London

Carers Recognition and Services Act 1996 HMSO, London

Children Act 1989 HMSO, London

Clements L 1996 A real act of care. Community Care Vol. 14: 21–22

Department of Health 1989a Caring for people (Griffiths report). HMSO, London

Department of Health 1989b Sandwell caring for carers evaluation. HMSO, London

Department of Health 1990 General household survey. HMSO, London

Disabled Persons Act 1983 HMSO, London

Education Act 1980 HMSO, London

Finch J, Groves D (eds) 1983 A labour of love: women, work and caring. Routledge & Kegan Paul, London

Glendinning C 1992 The costs of informal care: looking inside the household. Social Policy Studies Unit, HMSO, London

Glendinning C, Millar J 1987 Women and poverty in Britain. Wheatsheaf Books, Brighton

Green H 1988 General household survey 1985–1986. HMSO, London

Henwood M, Wicks M 1984 The forgotten army: family care and elderly people. Family Policy Studies Unit, London

King's Fund Informal Carers Programme 1988 Action for carers: a guide to multi-disciplinary support at local level. King's Fund, London

Land H 1991 Time to care. In: Maclean M, Groves D (eds) Women's issues and social policy. Routledge, London

Moroney R 1976 The family and the state. Longman, London

NHS and Community Care Act 1990 HMSO, London

Nissel M, Bonnerjea L 1982 Family care of the handicapped elderly: who pays? Policy Studies Institute, London

Oakley A 1974 Women confined. Martin Robinson, Oxford

Pahl R 1980 Divisions of labour. Blackwell, Oxford

Parker G 1990 Whose care? Whose costs? Whose benefits? A critical review of research in case management. Ageing and Society 10

Parker R 1990 Care and the private sector. In: Sinclair I, Parker R, Leat D, Williams J (eds) The kaleidoscope of care. HMSO, London

Twigg J, Atkin K, Ungerson C 1991 Carers and service: a review of the research. HMSO, London

Ungerson C 1983 Women and caring: skills, tasks and taboos in the public and the private. In: Garmanikow D, Purvis J, Taylorson D (eds) Heinemann, London

Webb A, Wistow G 1987 Social work, social care and social planning: the personal social services since Seebohm.

Wilkin D 1979 Caring for the mentally handicapped child. Croom Helm, London

FURTHER READING

Bond J 1992 The politics of care giving: the professionalisation of informal care. Ageing and Society 12:15–21.

Bornat J, Pereira C, Pilgrim D, William F 1993 Community care: a reader. Open University in association with Macmillan Press, Basingstoke

Daley C 1988 Ideologies of caring: rethinking community and collectivism. Macmillan, London

Department of Health and Social Security 1971 Better services for the mentally handicapped. HMSO, London

Department of Health and Social Security 1975 Better services for the mentally ill. HMSO, London

Graham H 1983 A labour of love. In: Finch J, Groves D (eds) A labour of love: women, work and caring. Routledge & Kegan Paul, London

Graham H, Lewin E (eds) 1985 Women, health and healing. Tavistock, London

Green H 1985 Informal carers: a study. OPCS, London

Guardian 1992 Carers made ill by strains of editorial duties. 22/5/92: 4

Keith L 1990 Caring partnership. Community Care 2(2):90

Langan M 1992 Who cares? Women in the mixed economy of care. In: Langan M, Day L (eds) Oppression and social work. Routledge, London

Richardson A, Unell J 1989 A new deal for carers. King's Fund Informal Caring Support Unit, London

Taylor S, Field D 1993 Sociology of health and health care. Blackwell Science, Bodmin

Toynbee P 1990 Observer 22.7.90: 11

Ungerson C (ed) 1991 Gender and caring: work and welfare in Britain and Scandinavia. Harvester Wheatsheaf, London

Wagner G 1988 Residential care: a positive choice. Report of the independent review of residential care. HMSO, London

Webb R Tol D 1991 Social issues for carers: a community care perspective. Hodder & Stoughton, Bury St Edmunds

Webb A, Wistow G 1983 Public expenditure and policy implementation: the case of community care. Public Administration 61(1):21–24

9

Assessing community health needs

Carmel Blackie

Information derived from community health needs assessment forms the basis for the planning and delivery of care. It is essential, therefore, that the community health care nurse possesses the knowledge to participate actively in the process as an equal partner with professionals from other disciplines, to ensure that the nursing component of care is delivered according to the needs of the population. In order to fulfil this aspect of their role, community health care nurses must be able to:

- Understand the rationale for community health needs assessment focused (normally) on a general practice population
- Be aware of a range of strategies to carry this out
- Be aware of a range of data sources to inform the practice profile
- Consider the link between health profiling and primary care-led purchasing
- Understand the multidisciplinary nature of a community profile
- Understand the importance of involving the community in the process and have strategies to enable this to take place
- Recognise the concept of a community and the community as client
- Understand the concept of health gain
- Be able to identify groups in the community who are outside the general practice remit.

The assessment of and response to the health

care (CHC) needs of the general practice population by the multidisciplinary primary health care (PHC) team is the likely future for CHC nursing practice. It is at this level that local control and budgets will be based. However, CHC nurses (CHCNs) have always had a wide perspective and by selecting a general practice population as the focus of assessment, they should not lose sight of the needs of some vulnerable members of the population outside the registered practice list. They too have needs, many urgent, and PHC teams should consider outreach strategies and means of obtaining funding for these in order to work with at-risk populations. CHCNs are well placed to work in partnership with GPs to identify and meet local needs; 80% of direct care is given by nurses, midwives and health visitors and the nursing service currently costs 25% of the NHS budget. Health visitors in particular have a long tradition of community-based practice and can bring the public health perspective to the PHC team.

THE COMMUNITY AS CLIENT

The notion of the community as a client is a fundamental concept within CHC nursing practice. In planning and managing care with an individual client and carer or for a family, most CHCNs can comprehend the concept of assessment. Assessment of community needs in relation to health and health care is harder to understand but this must be the starting point for health care planning and strategy and for any intervention affecting a community. Community needs assessment involves knowledge and skills derived from blending nursing and public health. Together both dimensions give the CHCN the legitimate breadth and depth for practice within the context and philosophy of PHC practice. CHC nursing practice is concerned with the interaction between the individual, family and community in relation to determining, maintaining and promoting health.

PUBLIC HEALTH

Hilleboe & Larimore (1966) defined public health

as 'the science and art of applying knowledge and skills from medicine and allied sciences in an organised community effort to maintain and improve the health of groups of individuals'.

Another definition which originated in the 1920s (Higgs & Gustafson 1985) states that public health is the science and art of 'preventing disease, prolonging life, promoting health, through organised community effort and enabling every citizen to realise their birthright of health and longevity'.

The focus of public health practice is, therefore, the needs of the wider community, to be met for the greater good of the whole community and the individuals within it. Public health practice gives the data required for planning healthcare strategy on three levels; the individual, the family and the community. In practice, it means working with groups representing community interests in an holistic way which serves to empower the community to take action.

In taking the community to be the client, the CHCN must work collaboratively with other disciplines in order to identify the needs of the population. This enables the CHCN to identify groups and subgroups within the community and it is at these that practice intervention is aimed. The impact of intervention within groups and subgroups influences the health of the whole population.

The relationship between public health and CHC nursing practice is made clear by the American Nurses Association (1974):

Community health nursing is a synthesis of nursing practice and public health practice applied to promoting and preserving the health of populations. The nature of this practice is general and comprehensive. It is not limited to a particular age or diagnostic group. It is continuing, not episodic. The dominant responsibility is to the population as a whole. Therefore, nursing directed to individuals, families or groups contributes to the health of the total population. Health promotion, health maintenance, health education, co-ordination and continuity of care are utilised in an holistic approach to the family, group and community. The nurse's actions acknowledge the need for comprehensive health planning, recognise the influences of social and ecological issues, give attention to populations at risk and utilise the dynamic forces which influence change.

Public health data forms a large part of any community health needs assessment. It is freely available and is used as the basis for national policy and target setting; a recent example of the use of public health data in this way is the Health of the Nation (Department of Health 1992). Public health data must be combined in community needs assessment with other data sources. It can be criticised if used alone as a basis for decision making because:

- Public health data concentrates on normative needs and comparative needs
- It omits felt needs and expressed needs and so denies the community a voice and perspective
- The data gathered is from a large geographical area which might not reflect exactly the boundaries of a general practice population.

It is important to undertake needs assessment even if the needs identified cannot be met in the short term. This is because:

- The information gives a starting point for service development in the mid to longer term.
- The data can be used to assess how service delivery is currently organised and whether this is to the best possible effect.
- A base line for the measurement of future health gain is established. Without this starting point it is impossible to measure or prove anything.

The way that the health status of the population is reflected through public health data is described in Box 9.1.

The list is not exhaustive and serves to indicate

Box 9.1   Types of public health data

- Mortality rates, e.g. from coronary heart disease, cancers, neonatal death, suicide
- Morbidity rates, e.g. diabetes, asthma, disability
- Accident rates, e.g. the type of accident, age of the people involved, place of occurrence
- Children at risk or cause for concern, e.g. failure to thrive, frequent attendance at A&E, known family history of abuse or violence
- Stress factors, e.g. poverty levels, poor housing, unemployment and crime

---

only the avenues which might be explored. The more creative CHCNs are in seeking data sources, the richer and more holistic the picture of the population and the prevalent issues and health needs will be.

Data sources can be split into the following categories:

- Epidemiological, e.g. high mortality and morbidity, stress related illness, HIV and AIDS, alcohol and drug abuse
- Environmental issues, e.g. green space available, leisure facilities, pollution, urban or rural area, traffic patterns and so on
- Reasons for attending primary health care and A&E, e.g. traffic trauma, burns, wound injury, poisonings, medical emergency, chronic conditions, unexplained injury.

Other health status indices, used in conjunction with public health data, include:

- Health service indicators. The Department of Health has produced comparative data relating to the health service since 1983
- Community services data, e.g. child health, nursing returns and activity, audits data.

THE COMMUNITY

It is necessary for the CHCN to understand and have a working definition of what constitutes a community. There are many types and structures of 'community' and a precise definition is therefore difficult to achieve. There are, however, some key factors, identified by Connor (1969) and summarised by Higgs & Gustafson (1985), which serve to characterise a community and make it stand out as a unit in its own right.

- All communities include individuals variously referred to as a group (of any size), or a social group (indicating some type of interaction).
- All communities include people who, as members of a social group, interact with each other formally and informally within some type of organisational structure.

Examples of such communities are people who live in the same street or block of flats or people who work together. The boundaries and organisation between people within a certain community may be loosely defined or may be strictly regulated.

People who are members of a community tend to have a group perspective on issues, which makes them stand out from other groups or communities. The identity of the group or community can arise from many perspectives and influences (Box 9.2).

Box 9.2 Factors creating group identity

- Culture
- Ethnicity
- Race
- Religion
- Socio-economic background
- Education
- Occupation
- Area of residence/region of the country
- Language spoken
- Past experience
- Unemployment
- The law specific to the country where the community exists

Examples of communities which have developed from the factors highlighted in Box 9.2 can be seen throughout the UK. For instance, large cities such as London or Manchester contain populations/communities within the overall population which stand out because of particular characteristics; the Chinese community, the Jewish community, areas of the city which are 'middle class', and other areas which are predominantly 'working class'. There are both benefits and disadvantages in the formation of such communities. For example, the community can act as a source of collective support for individual members and reinforce cultural and other beliefs and practices. However, alienation of the wider population and the formation of geographical areas from which those not belonging to the main community are excluded can occur, as can social division.

Subgroups form within communities. These can include groups such as adolescents, the elderly, young families or people who suffer from a particular chronic disease, such as asthma or diabetes. These groups are often formed for the purpose of needs assessment by professionals in that area. In this case the 'group' members might never know that others similar to them exist or may not realise that they are categorised in this way. Sometimes the group forms of its own volition to meet a need for support.

If a community is identified simply by where the people are resident then they are usually known as a neighbourhood or locality. In primary health care the population unit is increasingly the population registered with a particular GP.

ASSESSING THE NEEDS OF THE COMMUNITY

The major challenge for the health service is how to make best use of available resources in a way which is equitable and maximises health gain for the population. Making best use of resources cannot be achieved without comprehensive knowledge of what need exists within the population and a consideration of the services required to meet the identified need. In the reformed NHS, general practice and the PHC team are the main focus of activity. The members of the team, through their association with general practice, have a statutory duty to provide health care for the practice population, and to assess need within the population in order to deliver care and shape strategically the service offered. The PHC team has several advantages which allow it to undertake this responsibility.

- 99% of the population are registered with a GP.
- 90% of clients registered with the practice will be seen by a member of the PHC team within a 3-year period.
- 90% of all concerns raised by clients are dealt with by members of the PHC team in the primary health care setting.
- The GP and other members of the PHC team are informed of the majority of other contacts

which clients have with other aspects of the health service, for example attendance at A&E. There are exceptions to this, e.g. genitourinary medicine clinics, but in general the exceptions are few and not highly significant.

- The PHC team, because it is multidisciplinary in nature, has the diversity of skills and experience required to examine needs holistically.
- The PHC team can bring an holistic approach to planning and implementing future services.

Community needs assessment is a high priority within the NHS. It is, however, a conceptually muddled and technically difficult concept to articulate and to put into practice (Stevens & Gabbay 1991). In part this is due to a confusion about what constitutes a definition of need. In relation to an assessment of health needs in the community, it must be remembered that the World Health Organization's definition of need (see Ch. 1) includes an holistic approach to the physical, social and emotional well-being of individuals and communities, not just the absence of disease or infirmity. Health is seen as a positive resource which individuals and communities can utilise to realise their potential. The needs of a community and the individuals within the community are complex; this is reflected in the multidisciplinary nature of primary health care philosophy, organisation and provision of care. In this sense then, health needs assessment must include data on a range of factors affecting health (Box 9.3).

Box 9.3 **Factors to be included in needs assessment**

- Health
- Education
- Social needs
- Social policy and the effect of this on health
- Social services provision
- Housing
- Leisure
- The environment

IDENTIFYING HEALTH NEEDS IN THE COMMUNITY

The identification of health needs in the community is required because:

1. It is essential to obtain an accurate holistic assessment of the services required by the population.
2. It is essential to obtain an accurate assessment of the quality and range of services currently offered.
3. Health needs are central to local and national policy making.
4. Identifying needs and matching these to services highlights gaps in service and in patterns of service, and so informs strategic planning.

Nurses are used to assessing need, including physical, intellectual, emotional and social needs, as a means of making a nursing diagnosis and action plan.

Assessment of need in a population group is challenging. What is need and who defines these needs? Is the clients' perspective dominant or is the professional perspective seen as more important? Where is the power in the relationship and how does this affect rationing of services? Assessment of needs is about making sure that services and resources are targeted most effectively. In a straitened economic climate, this will lead to the rationing or prioritising of services.

To meet identified needs the PHC team should:

- Set shared objectives
- Purchase services in relation to need
- Target services to greatest need
- Audit and evaluate progress regularly so that objectives can be set and purchasing decisions made for the next year.

Health needs and social needs. Health and social needs are interdependent. For example, there is a relationship between poverty and ill health and between poor housing and ill health (Townsend 1988).

Health and deprivation. In 1991 the census recorded data on long-standing illness and socio-economic status. The link between poverty and ill health has been recognised for some time, notably in the Black report (Townsend & Davidson 1988). There are many indices to show deprivation; the most commonly used are the Jarman index and the Townsend score. Both of these measures of deprivation are calculated by electoral ward. An electoral ward contains approximately 8000 people and may contain several general practices. It is also true that a general practice may have clients from more than one electoral ward and so the data for each may not be identical.

The Jarman index. The Jarman index links population status to the need for general practice services. Originally, GPs were asked to link data collected by the census to their workload patterns. From this original data Jarman developed eight variables (Box 9.4).

Box 9.4   Jarman's eight variables influencing need

- Single parent households
- Children under 5 years old
- Elderly people living alone
- Unemployed people
- Unskilled people
- Mobility of the population
- Overcrowded housing
- Ethnic minorities

The Townsend score. The Townsend score, like the Jarman index, is based on linking census data to mortality and morbidity rates. The Townsend score also considers variables as important indices of the need for health care:

- % of unemployed people
- % of households without a car
- % of overcrowded households
- % of households which are not owner occupied

The ACORN classification. A further method of looking at socio-economic status and health in a general practice population is known as ACORN. This is **A C**lassification **O**f **R**esidential **N**eighbourhoods and is derived from a composite of census data. ACORN provides a socio-demographic index. The data is available for units of population of 300. This scale of data is useful to the PHC team, particularly if the community assessment is focused upon a general practice population. ACORN data is usually available from marketing companies and the best place to obtain this information is the local public health department or from an academic department of general practice.

Planning for the provision of services usually splits needs and the responsibility for meeting them into health authority responsibility and social services or local authority responsibility. The Community Care Act (1990) clearly delineates responsibility for health and social care into social service provision and health care provision and demands that there is joint planning between the health authority and social services departments so that artificial administrative delineation between the two organisations does not damage adequate holistic planning.

Bradshaw's (1972) taxonomy of need defines need in four categories (Box 9.5).

Box 9.5   Bradshaw's taxonomy of need (1972)

- Normative need: need defined by a professional
- Comparative need: one group of people are compared with another
- Felt need: needs which clients express, but which may not result in action being taken
- Expressed need: a felt need translated into action

For some people, need is related to the ability to benefit from a healthcare intervention, which in turn depends upon morbidity and the effectiveness of any intervention offered. Another type of need might be considered as demand, what people asking for health care actually want. The relationship between need and demand must be analysed, in terms of community needs and shaping services accordingly, with the concept of supply, that is, the health care service which it is possible to provide. In terms of shaping services based on community needs assessment, it is rational to provide those services from which there can be a maximum health gain. The ability of the population to benefit from health care depends upon two factors (Mathew 1971):

- The number of individuals affected, i.e. the incidence and prevalence of the condition under scrutiny
- The effectiveness of services which are designated to meet the needs identified.

TYPES OF COMMUNITY ASSESSMENT

Health profiles

A health profile is a multi-faceted tool which can be used in a variety of ways. It is:

- A means for analysing the social, demographic, economic and epidemiological characteristics in relation to an agreed population
- A tool in which need is identified and communicated throughout healthcare structures in policy and planning
- A means through which the CHCN and other members of the PHC team can become familiar with the needs of the client population
- Practice-based
- A means to allow the full skill mix of the PHC team to be deployed
- A means to allow appropriate and best use of available resources
- A means to address inequity
- A means through which gaps in services can be identified
- An essential adjunct to strategic planning.

Twinn et al (1990) identified two components of compiling and interpreting a community health profile: the systematic collection of data; and data analysis to assess priority needs, and to compile a care strategy.

Compiling a health profile

1. Define the community. This involves developing a brief history and understanding of the community and the area it occupies, its boundaries and the size and density of the population. Factors such as traffic patterns, environmental considerations and industry and leisure facilities are also important.

2. Collect the data. Data should be collected to describe the population by age, sex, culture, ethnicity, income, social class and unemployment/employment patterns. Also, patterns of consultation and reasons for consulting members of the PHC team should be analysed.

3. Analyse the data. This process involves summarising the information, emphasising any particular problems, and highlighting priorities for targeting services.

4. Compile the profile. This must be a collaborative process, involving all members of the PHC team. Priorities must be set and objectives established, so that service provision can be formulated. Resources required to meet any needs which have been identified must be assessed.

Local health profiles should feed into the wider, district profile as practices and PHC teams are encouraged to share data, although it may be difficult to encourage this in small businesses such as general practices. Regional and national profiles can be compiled to contribute to health service strategic planning.

Caseload review

A caseload is a population for which the CHCN has designated responsibility (ENB 1991). Workload constitutes activities which the CHCN is responsible for undertaking to meet the needs of the caseload (ENB 1991). The CHCN should:

- Monitor levels of appropriateness of nursing intervention
- Identify the CHC nursing response to local needs and improving services
- Identify client health need in relation to community health needs and balance these in order to offer appropriate proactive care
- Set priorities for practice and contribute to local community health profiles.

In thinking about caseload activity the CHCN should ask certain questions:

- What should be happening?
- What is happening?
- What changes are required?
- How can changes best be achieved?

Data generated by profiling activities provides essential information to managers and policy makers (Drennan 1990) and gives information which informs health promotion strategies and quality initiatives (David 1991).

A caseload review should be systematic and ongoing, ideally carried out at 3 to 6 monthly intervals. It should show:

- Total number of clients and variations in client patterns over time
- Client characteristics
- Gender and ethnicity characteristics
- Client dependency levels.

The general practice population profile

The practice population profile is a profiling tool to enable decisions to be made for health gain with regard to prioritising of service need, purchasing, resource allocation and targeting. A profile generates information which determines priorities for proactive and reactive health care. General practice is the focus of primary health care provision and a practice population profile should contain elements from a range of areas of activity:

- Multidisciplinary health needs assessment
- Neighbourhood study
- Community profile
- Nursing workload analysis
- Medical consultation and workload analysis.

General practice profiling, in common with all community profiling, must be a multidisciplinary undertaking. It should also include the perspective of clients and users of the service. Profiling should identify:

- The health needs of the practice population
- The social needs of the practice population
- Current service provision

- Gaps in service
- Future strategic plans for developing services
- The skills and expertise required to best meet identified needs.

The practice profile should include details on a range of aspects relating to the population's health (Box 9.6).

Box 9.8 contains suggestions for CHCNs of sources of data relevant to compiling the profile.

Assessing the community perspective

Most assessment of need considers normative, comparative and expressed need. In order to gain an holistic perspective, the felt need of the population is critical. There are several ways in which the views of the population can be obtained.

Informal discussion. To obtain information the PHC team can identify key members of the community and make links with them through the establishment of informal networks. People such as community leaders, teachers, youth workers, patient groups, and special interest groups are useful sources of information about what is important to the community. Informal contact can be made in a non-systematic way initially, and if it proves useful to both groups, then informal meetings could become a more formal part of the process of needs assessment and lead to continued working with the community and developing a community agenda for action.

Formal discussion. In some situations it is important to gain a formal viewpoint from the community and this requires a structured approach. There are several ways to conduct formal discussion or consultation, including:

- Advertising an issue and inviting people to participate
- Contacting existing groups known to have an interest or influence regarding the topic
- Selecting people and inviting them to join in.

Whichever means is selected, the views of some sections will inevitably be missed. To overcome

Box 9.6 Information to include in a profile

Age/sex characteristics of the client group. People of different ages have different health needs and, therefore, require different service provision. The health needs of men and women also differ and should be taken into account. The health authority, formerly the family health services authority (FHSA), maintains a register of all people on the registered list of GPs in an area. The data helps the authority calculate payments for the GP. The information includes age, sex, address and date of birth. The data is used to provide information on the age, sex and geographical spread of clients and is also used to operate call and recall systems for services such as breast screening and cervical cytology. In using data which only applies to registered patients, it should be remembered that some of the most disadvantaged people in society may not register with a GP. In some inner city areas this may be as many as 1 in 7 of the population. Figures for rates of morbidity and mortality should also be included.

The ethnic and cultural mix of the population. Some minority groups may be disadvantaged, e.g. non-English speakers, and require additional services, such as advocacy services, in the practice. Some healthcare practice may be unacceptable to certain cultures or religions. This must be taken into account when designing service provision and compiling staffing profiles.

Family patterns. How many single parents are there in the area? How many couples with children? How many elderly clients live alone? What is known about kinship patterns and extended family networks locally? How many clients act as carers? What are the birth and death rates?

Social class, income and occupation. This is important because the patterns of mortality and morbidity differ between social classes and occupational groups. Some occupational groups are prone to particular disease patterns.

The numbers of vulnerable people in the population. These people will include travelling families, those in temporary accommodation and the homeless. Some of these vulnerable groups may not be covered by the practice list. In a full profile, their needs should be considered so that strategies are developed to meet their needs outside the main pattern of service provision, if that is what they require and wish.

Patterns of consultation with members of the PHC team. Why do clients seek consultations? What are the disease patterns, prescribing patterns, etc? The health authority collects data from the GP relating to items of service procedures which are part of the GP's contract with the authority and which attract a payment. The data includes information on immunisation, contraceptive services, maternity care, child health surveillance, night calls and health promotion activity. Some of this activity is carried out by the doctor and some is carried out by the practice nurses or attached community nursing staff within the PHC team. Other activity, such as screening elderly people, is carried out in general practice and does not carry a specific payment. This data is also obtainable through the health authority. Health promotion activity is also measurable either through figures held at the practice or through the health authority. In the previous banding system, the practice was obliged to collect data to support activity. This is no longer compulsory, but many health authorities encourage general practices and PHC teams to continue to collect the data because of its relevance to community profiling. Data is also available in relation to prescribing and derives from the Prescription Pricing Authority (PPA) which launched a scheme in 1988 to show prescribing data. This is known as prescribing analysis and cost (PACT) data, and is obtained from reviewing prescription forms (FP10s) signed by the GP. PACT data may be replaced in future with a similar format.

---

this problem and to make the consultation process as fair and as open as possible, it is useful to have several stages in the formal consultation process. It should be emphasised that the process is lengthy and time-consuming and can be costly, but is worthwhile ultimately. Without open consultation any decisions taken and services implemented as a result may not have community acceptance. The stages involved in developing formal discussion groups are as follows.

1. Advertise the issue locally to raise public awareness and stimulate thought.

2. Hold initial discussion around the issue with representative groups selected through the advertisements.

3. Summarise the views raised so far and any ideas for a way forward.

4. Hold an open forum discussion, well advertised and at an accessible time; perhaps hold more than one at various times. Put the initial ideas to the public and take views and comments.

5. The initial group considers the comments and tries to incorporate them into planning, producing a draft report.

Box 9.7 Factors to include in a community assessment

- Economics
- Recreation
- The physical environment
- Education
- Safety and transportation
- Politics and governmental factors
- Health services
- Social services
- Communication networks

Box 9.8 Sources of data for profiling (NHSME 1992)

- Office for National Statistics (formerly the Office of Population Census and Survey) which can supply figures from the household survey, the Director of Public Health Report.
- Social service/health authority community care plans.
- Census information by ward or postcode, available from the town hall or libraries.
- General practice age/sex register and/or computer data linking this to disease patterns, e.g. the number of hypertensive men over 40. Practice mortality and morbidity can also be obtained in this way.
- Community health care nursing record systems.
- GP patient/client records.

---

6. A further open meeting is held to discuss the draft report.
7. Consensus is reached and action planned in a final report and taken.
8. The process is reviewed regularly to assess effectiveness.

Issues in population surveys

Using a survey methodology is a useful way to assess the population's viewpoint. A survey can be large or small scale. Surveys carried out amongst users of health services tend to reflect similar issues (Yorkshire RHA et al 1994).

Accessibility. People want to see the health professional of their choice as soon as they need to and at a time convenient to them. This includes attendance at surgery and home visiting.

Telephones. These should be answered quickly and courteously.

Consultations. Clients want enough time to explain their concerns to the health professional. They want a sympathetic hearing and an explanation of the issues, including medication, treatment, prognosis, and so on. In particular, clients referred to hospital want to know what to expect.

Consumer satisfaction. In general, clients are satisfied with the PHC team. Usually satisfaction is higher in relation to CHCNs than with doctors. People who are not happy with the service they have received may find it difficult to express this to the team.

Waiting times. Length of waiting time is very important to clients. A wait of more than 20 minutes is generally unacceptable to most people unless they are given a valid reason for the delay. Waiting room environments, although important to the primary care team staff, tend not to be so critical to clients.

Health issues. The issue raised by the largest number of people is back pain. All other issues, although important, are considered so by small numbers of the population in comparison. Issues which health professionals consider important, such as giving up smoking, are not so important to the population.

FRAMEWORK FOR HEALTH NEEDS ASSESSMENT

For the purpose of assessing health needs, the population should be divided into meaningful groups, such as client groups or disease groups. There are, however, problems with this approach. These are:

- Overlapping groups
- Some of the population is excluded
- Focus is on users of the services and not those outside the mainstream who are often vulnerable and may be left out.
- It tends to be problem oriented rather than health oriented and holistic.

It should also be remembered that examination of health need has tended to look at the services that exist rather than what is the need and how, ideally, that need should be met.

An approach to needs assessment which avoids some of these problems was devised by Picken & St Ledger (1993) and examines the different requirements people have at various stages of the life cycle. This is known as the life cycle approach (Box 9.9).

There are several benefits to using the life cycle approach. It allows the whole population to be looked at coherently but also allows specific groups within the population to be investigated. The information required can be collected without necessarily looking at which services are already being offered and the information can be linked between groups. Using this approach means that healthy influences can be related to proposed or current service provision. Finally, the life cycle approach tries to explain the health of the population rather than just describe it and can accommodate changes in knowledge of the determinants of health.

The checklist in Box 9.10 is developed from the original in Yorkshire RHA et al (1994) and is a useful tool to enable a PHC team to begin the process of profiling/community needs assessment. It provides a starting point and suggests what to consider, but is not intended to be prescriptive. Each practice population and community is unique, therefore the framework should be adapted to suit the circumstances of particular practices.

How profiling can shape services

If used proactively and integrated into planning and service delivery, profiling can determine the nature of services to be offered, particularly if the profile is linked to primary health care-led commissioning. It is worth considering at this point how profiling can influence service provision. This account is based on an RCN paper (1993), the GP practice population profile.

Profile finding. There is a high rate of pregnancies amongst teenage girls between the ages of 14 and 16 years leading to abortion. Following this the girls generally attend surgery more frequently than before the event and many develop eating disorders.

Action. The PHC team selects the above finding as a priority issue for action.

The team sets goals recognising that the problem is larger than simply a health service remit. The goals are to:

- Develop stronger networks with the school nursing service, schools and community youth groups
- Establish a link with the local authority social services youth project
- Link with the local pregnancy advisory service

Box 9.9 Stages in the life cycle approach to needs assessment (Picken & St Ledger 1993) (Reproduced with kind permission from Open University Press.)

- **Late pregnancy to 1 week after birth.** The suggested parameters to explore are the quality of the pregnancy, delivery, birth, early life, the mother's health and social support.
- **1 week of age to 1 year old.** The parameters to explore are the quality of the external environment, the home circumstances, immunisation uptake, developmental surveillance, and the patterns of family life.
- **1 year to 4 years old.** The parameters considered important are immunisation patterns, accidents, the environment, special needs, and the family.
- **5 years old to 14 years old.** Important factors for this age group are accidents, malignancies, education, how healthy the lifestyle is, and the influence of peer groups.
- **15 years to 24 years old** This age group should be assessed in relation to sexual activity, lifestyle, alcohol, drug use, family planning and social stresses such as unemployment and homelessness.
- **25 years of age to 44 years.** This group should be assessed in relation to child bearing and child rearing, accidents, malignancies, mental health issues and continuing autonomy in lifestyle and health choices.
- **45 to 64 years.** Consideration should be given to acute and chronic illness, mobility and preparation for retirement.
- **65 to 74 years.** Important factors to assess include looking at patterns of social support, potential isolation, depression and limited mobility problems.
- **75 plus.** This group may experience multiple morbidity, dementia, loss of independent living and carers.

Box 9.10   Health profile check list

Causes of substantial mortality
- Coronary heart disease
- Stroke
- Cancers

Causes of substantial ill health
- Smoking
- Respiratory tract infections
- Asthma
- Ischaemic heart disease
- Hypertension
- Musculoskeletal pain, especially back pain
- Skin disease
- Mental illness and neuroses
- Indigestion
- Gastroenteritis
- Diabetes

Areas Of concern
- Socio-economic problems/deprivation indices
- Access to healthcare workers
- High rates of hospitalisation
- Parental skills
- Teenage pregnancy
- Dental health
- Diet
- Exercise
- Sexually transmitted disease
- Health needs of 15–24-year-olds
- Accidents
- Maternity services
- Child welfare
- Rehabilitation post-operatively, following trauma or illness
- Dignity and comfort for the terminally ill and their carers
- Drug and alcohol misuse
- Crime
- Housing
- The environment

Other considerations
- The primary health care team philosophy
- The Patients' Charter
- The GP contract
- Pattern of employment/attachment of CHCNs; are the nurses integrated?
- Health promotion priorities
- The Health of the Nation targets
- Is the practice fundholding or non-fundholding?
- Links with other agencies, social services, housing, education, community groups, the voluntary sector, pressure groups, etc.

- Link with relevant voluntary agencies
- Liaise with the community, parents and young people to ascertain what they perceive as a necessary issue.

The PHC team identifies members of the team with an interest and skill in counselling and working with young people. The brief of the staff selected is to work with the community and other interested agencies to establish a drop-in centre for young people. Funding for 1 year is obtained from the health authority development budget. The GPs, who are fundholders, add funds to the budget and the community trust supports nurse involvement.

Following close consultation with the community and the young people concerned, the drop-in centre is established in a venue acceptable to the young people, away from the school and surgery. It is open at times convenient to the young people. Advertising of the centre and range of services offered is arranged and leaflets and posters are distributed to schools, youth groups, churches, libraries, shopping centres and so on. The local radio station carries a feature about the service on its teenage slot.

The centre runs for 1 year and is evaluated at 6 months and 12 months. The project is deemed successful and the results are used to influence future purchasing.

PRIMARY HEALTH CARE-LED PURCHASING (PCLP)

Primary health care-led purchasing, in tandem with the primary health care-led NHS, is now the dominant model of healthcare commissioning within the NHS and the success of commissioning of services will be measured through the application of the Patients' Charter (Department of Health 1993). This has arisen as a result of the NHS reforms, principally devolved fundholding and purchasing in general practice. In the early stages of the NHS reforms, the GP fundholder was charged with purchasing elements of secondary care for clients registered with the practice. This has progressed in some areas so that the budget holder is charged with purchasing total care, primary care as well as secondary care, for the practice population, including nursing care. The aim of purchasing health care is to maximise health gain. Services for non-fundholder GPs are purchased through the health authority, although the tendency is towards devolved budget holding.

There are two themes within PCLP. These are:

- Purchasing by primary care
- Purchasing decisions advised by primary care.

Within the new structure of the NHS there are clear regulations regarding fundholding and the operation of funds which are undertaken nationally to the same standards. With respect to PCLP, no framework exists and there are vast differences in how purchasing is operated. PCLP is critical in shaping the health services of the future and should be regulated. McCall (1995) suggests certain criteria for the national regulation of PCLP.

- The overall aim of the NHS must be protected; that is, to deliver high quality health care, irrespective of age, race, means or creed, free at the point of delivery.
- Regulated PCLP should ensure national equity of healthcare delivery.
- Regulated PCLP must not be prescriptive in how healthcare services should be delivered, but build upon the strengths of current service and develop the concept of flexibility.
- Regulated PCLP must be enabling to the process of change.
- Regulated PCLP must assist the principles of a managed health service.

Health gain. In simple terms, health gain can be defined as the benefit derived when care or intervention is applied in a given circumstance to an individual or community. The dilemma is to assess which intervention, of the many available possible choices, gives the most benefit to the most people. Health gain measurement is inevitably linked to decisions about healthcare priorities, 'prioritisation' or 'rationing' of services. Rationing is an unpopular concept but is, and always has been, a necessity in health care. The difference now is that the decisions are more explicit and the topic is debated in the public domain. Ways in which interventions are deemed to be successful and yield a positive or negative health gain are through:

- Evidence-based practice

- Audit, quality and evaluation
- Consultation and partnership with the community concerned.

Purchasing health care to meet population healthcare needs linked to measurable and achievable health gain, is a relatively new concept within the NHS. In the past healthcare delivery was provider-led. The emphasis is now on purchasers to identify and define local needs and purchase services to meet them. The health service, whilst it should have basic core services which are the same throughout the UK, will have local differences of emphasis in how the services are provided. When purchasing by GP fundholders began there was a move to replicate existing service patterns. However, the analysis of community health needs has developed since then and there are now more complex packages of purchasing led by primary health care. Health analysts have recognised that the more complex the healthcare requirements, based on needs assessment, the greater the multidisciplinary input from all members of the PHC team required.

The main functions of a purchasing authority, whether that be a GP fundholder, GP consortia or health authority, have been defined by Dearden (1991) as:

- Vision
- Analysis
- Creative specification
- Total quality management
- Financial management
- Negotiation.

In May 1993 the Audit Commission produced a document entitled 'Their health, your business: the new role of the DHA'. In this, the Commission identified the skills required of purchasers of health care, which must be developed through the allocation of appropriate resources of time and money, to fulfil their remit appropriately. These are the:

- Needs assessment of local community needs, based on the collection of data
- Identification of appropriate services to meet the needs identified

- Ability to negotiate and achieve a contract with providers.

The extension of the remit of GP fundholders in relation to the purchasing of services for the practice population, to include community nursing services, has benefits, outlined by Martin & Eveleigh (1994):

- Improved communications between professional groups
- Definition of shared goals and objectives
- Better understanding of the respective contributions to patient care of GPs, practice nurses and other contracted groups, including health visitors and district nurses
- Agreement over the attachment of CHCNs to PHC teams
- Multidisciplinary training and team development and closer integration of primary and secondary health care provision
- PHC teams can plan more effectively for patients and improve the quality of care.

In 1993, McCall stated that 'Primary care-led purchasing represents the currently best available means of assessing and delivering the [health-care] needs of the population' (McCall 1995). McCall's assertion was criticised subsequently but he defended his claim in 1995 (McCall 1995) and cited a range of reasons as to why PCLP was the most appropriate arrangement. He drew on evidence of existing models of primary care-led purchasing to maintain that, from the patients' perspective, the PHC team is the most accessible part of the NHS, a powerful public relations position, and that teams have at their disposal considerable data to assist in the assessment of patients' wants and needs. With the relevant support and education, the PHC team can use the data to plan the most cost-effective patient-centred means of health care delivery. Finally, he pointed out that members of the PHC team also act as the agent of the patient, liaising between patient and provider, and as influential change agents within the NHS.

If PCLP is to be successful, three main areas must be taken into consideration.

The effect of purchasing on the PHC team. PHC team members must be trained in the skills required to gather and interpret data, and to commission the necessary services to meet needs. However, initially, the management capabilities of team members must be assessed to allow an appropriate management structure for PCLP to be developed within the PHC team. Existing service provision will be affected by decisions taken as a result of PCLP processes: which services will be retained, which will be lost, and what new services will be required? Consideration of these factors will influence PCLP decisions. The PHC team will need somewhere to operate PCLP from, so the question of premises and other logistical issues should be considered.

The effect of PCLP on health commissioning. Under a PCLP system, the workload of the health commission might be increased, particularly if there is no agreed formula for PCLP and the commission has to process and negotiate several variants. The health commission might also need to employ specialist managers with the appropriate skills to undertake the work required by PCLP.

The effect of PCLP on providers of health care. The patterns of workload generated by PCLP for providers of health care must be assessed: for example, an imbalance in some services could be detected requiring a change in the types of service providers are required to give, and minority specialties in secondary care might become redundant in certain areas. As with the other two areas, an appropriate management structure will be required to deal with, for example, alterations in the profile of the workforce, the size the workforce and the skills required by the workforce.

Summary

Community health needs assessment based around a general practice population is a powerful adjunct to planning and shaping health services through primary health care-led purchasing. Community health care nurses can make a significant contribution to multidisciplinary health needs assessment, and in so doing influence healthcare purchasing through linking with general practice fundholders and other local budget holders. However, to manage this effectively, community health care nurses must be active participants in the process. They must possess the appropriate knowledge and have at their disposal a variety of tools, to enable them to collect the information required to inform the assessment and review of the nursing needs of the community.

REFERENCES

American Nurses Association Executive Committee and Standards Committee. Division On Community Health Nursing Practice 1974 Standards of community health nursing practice. In: Higgs Z, Gustafson D (eds) 1985 Community as a client: assessment and diagnosis. F A Davis, USA

Audit Commission 1993 Their health, your business: the new role of the DHA. HMSO, London

Bradshaw J 1972 The concept of need. New Society 30: 640–643

Community Care Act 1990 HMSO, London

Connor D M 1969 Understanding your community, 2nd edn. Development Press, Canada

David 1991 Whose definition of quality? Queens Nursing Association, Quality Conference, London

Dearden B 1991 Purchasing with vision. Health Services Management 171–173

Department of Health 1992 The health of the nation. HMSO, London

Department of Health 1993 Press release, H93/782, 3 June. HMSO, London

Drennan 1990 Gathering information from the field. Nursing Times 86(39):46–49

English National Board for Nursing, Midwifery and Health Visiting 1991 Circular 1991/05/MB. ENB, London

Higgs Z, Gustafson D 1985 Community as a client: assessment and diagnosis. Davis, New York.

Hilleboe H, Larimore G 1966 Preventive medicine. Saunders, Philadelphia

McCall C 1995 Primary care led purchasing: plugging the gaps. Primary Care Management 5:7–11

Martin C, Eveleigh M 1994 Buying in better standards of care. Primary Health Care 4(6):12–15

Mathew G K 1971 Measuring need and evaluating services. In: Stevens A, Gabbay J (eds) 1991 Needs assessment needs assessment. Health Trends 23(1):20–23

NHS Management Executive 1992 Document EL (92) 48. HMSO, London

Picken C, St Ledger S 1993 Assessing health need using the life cycle framework. Open University Press, Buckingham

Royal College of Nursing 1993 The GP practice population profile: a framework for every member of the primary health care team. RCN, London

Royal College of Nursing 1995 The role of nurses in purchasing for health gain, Information Sheet 00292. RCN, London

Stevens A, Gabbay J (eds) 1991 Needs assessment needs assessment. Health Trends 23(1):20–23

Townsend P 1988 Health and deprivation: inequality and the north. Routledge, London

Townsend P, Davidson N (eds) 1988 The Black report – inequalities in health. Pelican, Harmondsworth

Twinn S et al 1990 The process of health profiling. Health Visitors' Association, London

World Health Organization 1985 Health for all. WHO Regional Office For Europe, Copenhagen

Yorkshire RHA, North West Region, South Thames Region (West), NHS in Scotland, NHS in Wales, NHS Training Division 1994 Using information in practice management. Health needs assessment and health gain. Greenhalgh [Crown Copyright], London

10

Health promotion

Susan M. McKnight
Marilyn Edwards

Health promotion is an essential component
of the community health care nurse's work.
Health and health promotion are complex
concepts for which there are no clear,
single definitions, nor any universal
agreement on the model or approach to guide
best practice. Many of the health promotion
activities which community health care
nurses concentrate on derive from
epidemiological data and relate to
government strategies. The example focused
on in this chapter relates to school nursing,
but the principles applied can be transferred
to other health care settings. To carry out the
health promotion component of the role, the
community health care nurse should be aware
that:

- There are three main areas of knowledge
  which are important for health promotion in
  practice
- The first two are models which fall into one
  of the theoretical categories: descriptive or
  prescriptive
- The boundary between these two types of
  health promotion model is not inflexible and
  aspects from both can be employed at the
  same time
- The third area is knowledge of a process
  approach which draws on teaching and
  learning theory to put health promotion into
  practice
- Health promotion is subject to conceptual
  and ethical problems which must be

considered by the nurse in relation to individual clients.

INTRODUCTION

Health promotion is an essential component of community health care nurses' (CHCNs') work. This chapter aims to outline the meaning of health, and relates health to theoretical concepts and models of health promotion.

Health and health promotion are complex concepts and the authors emphasise that no single model or approach to health promotion provides the CHCN with a total guide for practice. The temptation is to regard the multiplicity of models as academic hot air and therefore of little practical value, but when used judiciously, these models can enhance the CHCN's understanding of the nature of practice.

There are three main areas:

1. Descriptive theoretical models
2. Prescriptive theoretical models
3. A process approach, which draws on teaching and learning theory to put health promotion into practice.

The boundary between the first two is not a hard and fast one.

Descriptive theoretical models

These models describe the different activities included within health promotion, illuminating the relationship between these different activities and classifying the nature of health promotion activities in terms of both the institutions involved and the power relationship embodied in these types of activity. The model outlined by Downie et al (1991) clearly defines the types of activity included in health care and how they overlap. The Beattie model (1991) provides a comprehensive 'definition' of health promotion, and makes us aware of the nature of health promotion activities.

The descriptive models are often overlooked but they do have a direct relevance to the CHCN. Awareness of the many different aspects of health promotion helps to broaden health promotion strategies and enables us to be more aware of the wider structural inequalities that can limit individuals' potential for health. At a more complex level, the different activities that make up health promotion put into sharp relief questions of ethics and politics. Ultimately, the discovery that the nature of your activity is to attempt to disempower individuals may shed light on why so much 'good advice' goes unheeded. The descriptive models make it clear just how all-inclusive health promotion can be as an activity. It is essential to be aware that health promotion is not just an objective professional activity as it cannot be divorced from wider social and political questions. The dichotomy between different aspects of health promotion is vast, and just a simple contrast makes the point that this activity cannot be seen as a matter of objective professional opinion. Some health promoters put the focus on the individual changing and being responsible for their actions, and therefore potentially blameable. In contrast, others venture into broad political areas, such as a focus on unemployment being detrimental to health.

Prescriptive theoretical models

The prescriptive models provide guidance on approaching health promotion to enable individuals to change their behaviour and have immediate practical relevance to the health promoter. These models are grounded in social psychology and recognise the complex interplay between beliefs, attitudes, values and perceived social norms in changing behaviour. There is more widespread awareness of these models and, for this reason, they are not explored specifically in this chapter.

Many of the health promotion activities on which CHCNs concentrate are epidemiologically derived and relate to governmental strategies, such as the Health of the Nation document (DoH 1992). In this chapter, examples of health promotion in action relate to the primary health care setting of school nursing, but can be transferred to any other health care setting. The reader is invited to undertake further reading of key texts to expand specific areas. Activities to apply theory to practice are included throughout the chapter.

THE CONTEXT OF HEALTH PROMOTION AND HEALTH EDUCATION

WHAT IS HEALTH?

Look to your health, and if you have it praise God, and value it next to a good conscience, for health is the second blessing that we mortals are capable of; a blessing that money cannot buy
                    Izaak Walton 1593–1683, *The Complete Angler*

The meaning of the term 'health' has profound implications for the health promoter, and differing definitions of what is meant by health can be used to justify a very narrow approach to health promotion, or such a wide approach that virtually all decisions can be cast in terms relating to health. There have been numerous attempts to produce both definitions of health and 'models of health' to enable healthcare professionals to make sense of what they are both promoting and providing. Given the implications of how health is defined, it is not surprising that this is an area of great dispute, but CHCNs ignore this debate at their peril, as it will define the parameters within which they as health promoters operate.

Definitions

Health has its semantic origins in the old English word 'hal' meaning whole. Health was seen to be good and valuable, health and happiness being closely allied. The term clearly meant more than 'not being ill', but the problem is what is meant by 'whole'? If to be healthy means being 'complete' with no parts missing, what are the 'parts' that make up this thing called health?

A useful starting point in attempting to define health is the commonly quoted definition outlined by the World Health Organization (WHO) in 1946, which attempted to identify the parts which make up health, describing it as 'A state of complete physical, mental and social well-being and not just merely the absence of disease or infirmity'.

This definition has been widely criticised (Seedhouse 1986, Noack 1987), in part because this concept of health is so broad that what might be seen to be 'ideal' health is unattainable, and that no healthcare professional could ever completely promote it. Indeed, if everybody can in some way be regarded as 'unhealthy', or 'not healthy enough' the health promoter's task becomes endless. The WHO definition's breadth enables social and political issues to be transformed into health issues, potentially expanding the role of healthcare professionals into one affecting virtually all decisions. The WHO's definition of health, by focusing on well-being, also questions the traditional view of health care being dominated by reacting to ailments. Despite the breadth of the definition, it was revised further in 1984:

The extent to which an individual or group is able, on the one hand, to realise aspirations and satisfy needs; and, on the other hand, to change or cope with the environment. Health is, therefore, seen as a resource for everyday living, not an object of living; it is a positive concept emphasising social and personal resources, as well as physical capacities.

The 1984 WHO definition clearly includes what may be labelled as 'positive health' in that it attempts to define health to mean more than the absence of illness – which can be labelled 'negative health'. It has been widely recognised that not only is the definition of health in negative terms too limited a way of defining whether one is healthy, but it also underpins the traditional medical model in which health care consists of responding to illness. It has become fashionable to see health in positive terms of enhancing well-being, but it is important to realise that positive health as a concept has implications for the boundaries of health promotion which some, understandably, find disturbing.

A definition of health which is positive will mean different things to different people. Different countries, societies, cultures and religions have varying political beliefs and economic circumstances which may influence health. Health is a value laden concept and, although it is frequently stated that health promoters should not impose value judgements on the people whose health they are trying to promote, they are clearly working with the assumption that there is a more desirable state of affairs that they are attempting to bring about.

There is little logical difference between regarding someone who smokes as engaging in an unhealthy, therefore undesirable, activity, and regarding involvement in political dissent as a manifestation of mental illness, therefore unhealthy or undesirable. It is important to appreciate the variety of 'health promoting' activities that could be justified within a broad positive definition of health.

Despite the dangers of a broad definition of health, it is clearly undesirable to espouse a definition rooted in a concept of negative health. Definitions like the WHO's enable health to be seen as a state of dynamic balance and interdependence. For example, it is not uncommon for a person who is physically unwell also to feel depressed, or a person who is having social difficulties to become mentally and physically unwell, complexities which are ill-handled if health is defined in terms of negatives. Larger social issues, such as health inequality in relation to income (Blaxter 1990) are clearly relevant to health, and indeed by ignoring them the health promoter is liable to be treating the symptoms of problems rather than the cause, but these would not be accommodated in a narrow definition of health.

An accessible example of a broad model of health is that suggested by Downie et al (1991) (Fig. 10.1). This concept of health underpins the Tannahill model of health promotion (Fig. 10.2 p. 183). Downie et al's model brings together the positive and negative aspects of health, attempting to synthesise a picture of the many components of health and their interrelationships. Health is not seen as an absolute utopian concept but as a relative concept, enabling someone who is disabled or who has diabetes to achieve his overall 'quantity' of health; health is not simply the absence of disease. Downie et al's definition of health leads to health promotion aiming to achieve better health, rather than seeking to attain a specified level of health. The broad definition of health that Downie et al advocate inevitably leads to health promotion being seen as a wide ranging activity, and states:

The overall goal of health promotion is the balanced enhancement of physical, mental and social facets of positive health, coupled with the prevention of physical, mental and social ill-health.

Downie 1991

This definition is not without its problems. It clearly represents a very broad definition of health. There is a danger that, in practice, this

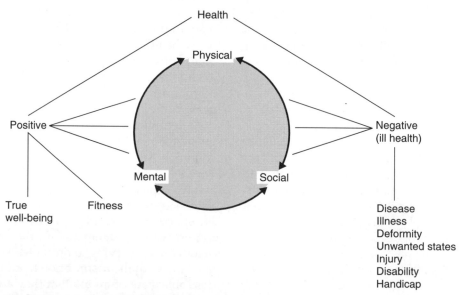

Figure 10.1 A model of health (Downie et al 1991). (Reproduced by kind permission of Oxford University Press.)

concept of health will not be adhered to. The positive aspects of health are hard to measure, in contrast to the negative dimensions of health; in particular physical preventive dimensions, such as screening, are likely to take precedence over the positive aspects of fitness and well-being.

CONCEPTS OF HEALTH PROMOTION AND HEALTH EDUCATION

Health promotion first appeared as a term and concept in 1974, in a publication by Lalonde, the Canadian Minister of National Health and Welfare, entitled 'A new perspective on the health of Canadians'. This document altered the emphasis of the Canadian government's public health policy, resulting in a move away from treatment to prevention, and ultimately to the promotion of health. This paper suggested that all causes of death and disease could be attributed to four factors:

1. Inadequacies in current health care provision
2. Lifestyle or behavioural factors
3. Environmental pollution
4. Biophysical characteristics.

It is important to note that factors 1 and 3, and arguably 2, fell outside the traditional sphere of activity for healthcare professionals at that time.

The report prompted a series of WHO initiatives, commencing with the Alma Alta declaration (WHO 1978) which directly influenced the formulation of government health policies in the western world. They have been instrumental in the evolution of what has been termed the 'new public health movement' (Bunton & McDonald 1992). Despite formally acknowledging this approach, and the targets that the WHO has advocated, the UK has trailed behind countries such as the US, Sweden, Norway, Canada and New Zealand in implementing policies.

Differences between health promotion and health education

A multitude of books and journal articles use the terms 'health education' and 'health promotion'. Sometimes the terms appear to be interchange-able, at other times there is lengthy debate on their very different meanings, and occasionally they are seen as antagonistic. To add to the confusion, descriptive models have been produced over the last few years which purport to explain the distinctions between, and nature of, health promotion and education. The distinction between the terms appears contentious and confused; the inevitable product of health promotion being a revolution in thinking and in knowledge. In the UK, the term 'health education' was used until the late 1980s, when the term 'health promotion' was introduced.

The problem of differentiating health education from health promotion can be partly traced back to the way the parameters of health education were extended in the 1970s. Prior to the advent of health promotion as a term of importance, and as part of the evolution of the concept of health, health educationalists were starting to include consideration of broader structural features within society and advocating social reform.

Green & Johnson (1984) attempt to make a clear distinction between the two terms. Health education is 'Any combination of learning experiences designed to facilitate voluntary adaptations of behaviour conducive to health in individuals, groups, or communities'. Health promotion in contrast is 'Any combination of educational, organisational, economic, and environmental supports for behaviour conducive to health'.

These definitions have common features. They acknowledge a combination of strategies as being more successful than a single approach. They also suggest a planned structure designed to help or support positive health behaviour. Where they differ is in the absence of the word 'voluntary' from the health promotion definition. 'Voluntary' suggests that choice is built in to the process. Absence of this word suggests that the process is less inherently consensual. Indeed the approach of health promotion has been seen to be more coercive and more of an 'aggressive hard sell' which might force people to be healthy. If central government passed legislation banning smoking in all public places, launched an aggressive TV advertising campaign against smokers as dirty and antisocial and refused to supply smokers with certain NHS treatments, this could be seen as a very coercive approach to persuading people not to smoke.

The WHO definition of health promotion (1984), which links closely to the earlier definition of health and attempts to overcome some of the above problems by recognising the need for personal choice, is 'Health promotion has come to represent a unifying concept for those who recognise the need for change in the ways and conditions of living in order to promote health. Health promotion represents a mediating

---

Box 10.1 Approaches to health promotion (Naidoo & Wills 1994)

1. Medical approach
Aim: to reduce premature mortality and morbidity. Uses scientific objective methods, for example epidemiology, to target high risk groups or whole populations.
Methods: preventive programmes involving specific screening procedures such as immunisation, cervical and breast screening or scientific methods of assessment, for example cholesterol levels, body mass index.
Worker/client relationship: Expert-led. Client conforming/passive.
Evaluation: two key ways.
(i) Long-term research into the effectiveness of preventive procedures such as cervical screening
(ii) Short-term measurement of uptake of a procedure by the target population, for example percentage of individuals immunised.

2. Behaviour change approach
Aim: Encourages individuals to improve their health by adopting healthy behaviour. Relies on individual being motivated to take action. Is the bedrock for many of the targets in the Health of the Nation strategy (Department of Health 1992).
Methods: Many campaigns undertaken by the Health Education Authority (HEA) use this approach, such as the 'Look after your Heart' campaign (Naidoo & Wills 1994). Through one-to-one information and counselling individuals may be persuaded to change their behaviour. If they do not, it could be seen that any resultant ill-health is their fault. Groups may also be targeted by use of the media.
Worker/client relationship: Expert-led, dependent client. Can result in 'victim blaming' ideology.
Evaluation: Can be problematic as may not be possible to measure objectively.

3. Educational approach
Aim: To provide knowledge and enable clients to develop the appropriate skills to make informed choices about their own health behaviours.
Methods: Linked to psychological theories of learning. Recognition of three main foci for learning:
(i) Cognitive – information and understanding
(ii) Affective – attitudes and feelings
(iii) Behavioural – skills activity.
Usually teacher/facilitator led but focus for discussion may be determined by client. Role play may be used

to explore attitudes, one-to-one counselling or group discussion.
Worker/client relationship: Can be expert-led but should have negotiation with client.
Evaluation: Increases in knowledge can be measured. This is not enough, however, to change behaviour.

4. Empowerment approach
Aim: Helps people identify their own concerns/health issues and gives them the skills and confidence to deal with them. Focuses on two main areas:
(i) Self-empowerment: based on non-directive client centred counselling approach
(ii) Community empowerment: way of working with communities which enables them to challenge and change aspects of their environment. Linked to community development.
Methods: Health promoter works with client or community to identify perceived health needs. Advocacy, negotiation and networking are key methods used. May involve facilitation of client self-help groups.
Worker/client relationship: Health promoter acts as a facilitator/advocate enabling client to become empowered.
Evaluation: Is difficult as many of methods used may take a long time to produce results. Evaluation of the process; for example has self-help group worked or client been empowered.

5. Social change
Aim: Emphasises the importance of socio-economic factors such as class, race, culture, gender and geography in determining health. Focus is on structural issues such as policies and the environment which can cause inequalities in health. Tries to make healthy choices easier choices by looking at availability, accessibility and cost as factors which may limit choices.
Methods: Focuses on government and institutional policies, legislation and fiscal controls. Involves activities such as lobbying, which are essentially seen as political in nature.
Worker/client relationship: Top down approach. Involves social regulation.
Evaluation: Successful if focus of social change occurs, for example the implementation of policies, legislation.

strategy between people and their environments, synthesizing personal choice and social responsibility in health to create a healthier future'.

Although the WHO makes a distinction between prevention and health promotion, health education and prevention are seen as being integral components of health promotion.

If one considers the practical application of the approaches to health promotion practice (Box 10.1), it becomes clear that professionals are likely to employ several of these approaches with a client or group. It is important for health promoters to have a conceptual framework which enables them to reflect on what must be the important components of their health promotion practice.

A plethora of health promotion models have been developed in an attempt to provide a theoretical framework for practice. Many have developed in response to a growing disenchantment with the traditional and dominant medical model, which placed the focus on improving health largely on the activity of curing and preventing disease. In simple terms there are two main categories of model:

- Descriptive – these describe different activities within health promotion. They highlight the relationship between differing activities, and classify the nature of health promotion in terms of both the institutions involved and the power relationships. The models of Tannahill and Beattie (Figs 10.2, 10.3) fall into this category. Tannahill's model has been selected as a pure descriptive model. In contrast, Beattie's model is not purely descriptive but has elements of practical application. It acknowledges the complexity of human behaviour and suggests different ways of working for health.
- Prescriptive – for example, Becker's health belief model (Naidoo & Wills 1994) and Prochaska & Diclemente's stages of change model (Naidoo & Wills 1994). These provide guidance as to how health promotion should be approached to enable individuals to change their behaviour. These models recognise the fact that changing behaviour is a

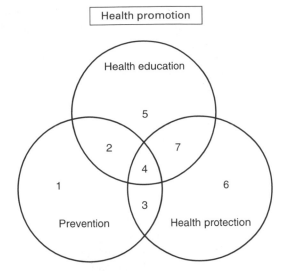

Figure 10.2 Tannahill's model of health promotion (Downie et al 1991). (Reproduced by kind permission of Oxford University Press.)

1 Preventive services, for example immunisation, cervical screening, hypertension case finding, developmental surveillance, use of nicotine chewing gum to aid smoking cessation.
2 Preventive health education, for example smoking cessation advice and information.
3 Preventive health protection, for example fluoridation of water.
4 Health education for preventive health protection, for example lobbying for seat belt legislation.
5 Positive health education, for example lifeskills work with young people.
6 Positive health protection, for example workplace smoking policy.
7 Health education aimed at positive health protection, for example lobbying for a ban on tobacco advertising.

complex process and may involve examining individuals' beliefs, attitudes, values and perceived social norms. It has been suggested that there are large areas of overlap in the many models which have been developed but little consensus on terminology or underlying criteria (Naidoo & Wills 1994).

The following descriptive models of health promotion demonstrate the overlap suggested by Naidoo & Wills (1994).

Tannahill (Downie et al 1991) considers health promotion to be an umbrella concept with health education, prevention and health protection forming part of health promotion. Health is seen to comprise positive and negative aspects (see Fig. 10.1). Figure 10.2 depicts the three areas of health promotion as overlapping spheres; additional activity is identified where spheres overlap. This highlights the complexity of interaction between the three main parts of health promotion. Health promotion is seen not as a unique activity in itself, but as a method of enhancing positive health and preventing ill-health through the overlapping spheres of health education, health protection and health prevention.

Health education (Downie et al 1991) refers to the 'communication activity aimed at enhancing positive health and preventing, or diminishing, ill health in individuals and groups, through influencing the beliefs, attitudes and behaviour of those in power and the community at large'. Health protection (Downie et al 1991) 'comprises legal or fiscal controls, other regulations and policies, and voluntary codes of practice, aimed at the enhancement of positive health and the prevention of ill health'.

Health prevention is described as focusing on four areas (Downie et al 1991), which are:

- Prevention of the onset or first manifestation of a disease process or some other first occurrence, through risk reduction
- Prevention of the progression of a disease process or other unwanted state, through early detection when this favourably affects outcomes
- Prevention of avoidable complications of an irreversible, manifest disease or other unwanted state
- Prevention of the recurrence of an illness or other unwanted phenomenon.

Although similar, these four areas challenge the traditional definitions of primary, secondary and tertiary prevention described by Naidoo & Wills (1994). These are as follows.

- Primary prevention is the prevention of the occurrence of a disease or ill-health. This may be through the provision of child immunisation, or through activities aimed at maximising bone mass in girls to prevent osteoporosis.

- Secondary prevention prevents ill-health becoming chronic and restores people to their previous level of health. Health promotion on smoking cessation for patients with respiratory conditions meets this criteria. Another example is cancer screening.
- Tertiary prevention refers to assisting people with chronic or irreversible ill-health to cope with their condition and maximise their health potential. Diabetes is a chronic condition which is an example of this level of prevention.

The Tannahill model describes seven areas of potential health promotion activity. The overlapping areas can become confusing if not followed carefully and for some health promotion initiatives it may not be appropriate to use all sections. The practical value of this model for the CHCN is that it demonstrates the interplay between the three key components of health promotion and highlights some of the broader social and political activities (for example numbers 6 and 7) in which the CHCN may need to become active.

Beattie (1991) draws on sociological theory and attempts to combine models of health and models of education. Two intersecting axes are seen to be the fundamental dimensions of health education and they create a structural map of possible health promotion strategies or approaches (Fig. 10.3). Beattie suggests that the authoritative/ negotiated (vertical) dimension on the map can serve to draw a parallel with debates about paternalistic, prescriptive, or top-down forms of social intervention, versus negotiated, participative client-centred, or bottom-up forms. The individual/collective (horizontal) dimension stands in its own right as a stable axis of conflict in social theory and social policy.

The Beattie model is a useful way of looking at some of the key features of the strategies used in health promotion. It can focus the CHCN's attention on how she interacts with clients and in particular, the power and control she may use as a so-called professional 'expert'. Health persuasion techniques (quadrant A) are seen as a cluster of interventions which might be employed by health professionals who may be seen to be

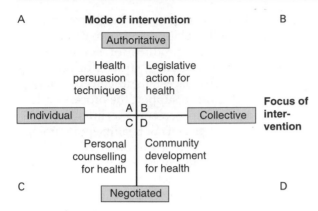

Figure 10.3 Strategies of health promotion (Beattie 1991). (Reproduced with kind permission from Routledge.)

expert by the client (doctors, health educators, health visitors, nurses) to redirect the behaviour of individuals in top-down, prescriptive ways. This may be on a one-to-one basis or via media campaigns. Historically, this strategy has been very popular, particularly the use of the media. It entails selecting specific messages from current medical knowledge about the risks involved with a particular behaviour. These messages are then presented to the public via a convenient medium. Beattie (1991) explains how socio-psychological theories, such as Becker's (1974) health belief model, have been used in campaigns directed at lifestyles. Unfortunately mass media campaigns alone have had little effect.

Legislative action for health (quadrant B) is the term used to describe interventions which use the expertise of health professionals to change civic policies and thus improve health. Action is directed principally at ecological, fiscal, legal and political modes of change. The case for this form of intervention has been argued forcefully during the 1980s and is linked to social and geographical determinants of health. This quadrant thrusts health promoters into an area which they may not have seen as part of their role – the political arena.

Personal counselling for health (quadrant C) invites individual clients to engage in active reflection and review of personal lifestyle, and to assess their scope for change. Counselling is provided either on a one-to-one basis or through processes within a group of peers. This is often

supplemented by printed self-study material. Beattie (1991) outlines a number of studies that have reported the benefits of this approach and cites examples of major health promotion agencies who, throughout the 1980s, have adopted this approach, e.g. the Family Planning Association, MIND and RELATE.

Community development for health (quadrant D) is characterised by groups of people who have similar health concerns or similar circumstances coming together to take joint action to improve health prospects; for example obsessive eating groups, ASH. It has been seen as one way of altering the balance of power and control between medical and collaborative social approaches focusing on positive health.

The Beattie model focuses attention on the nature of the differing modes of intervention. The bottom half of the diagram refers to both individual and collective approaches which ought to empower the client. The top half of the diagram makes CHCNs aware of more expert controlled, authoritative aspects of health promotion which might be used to control the individual. Health promotion will not be static in one quadrant and the CHCN should expect to move between quadrants in order to carry out effective health promotion. It is likely, however, that if the percentage of time spent with a client in each quadrant was analysed, most of the time would be spent in quadrants A and C.

EPIDEMIOLOGY AND HEALTH

Epidemiology is an important aspect of health promotion, seen by many to be the primary feeder discipline which helps assess health needs of individuals and communities and thereby underpins health promotion activity. It provides the scientific, objective foundation for one of the commonly used approaches, namely the medical approach. In relation to Beattie's (1991) model (Fig. 10.3), it is a major driving force for activities in quadrants A and B.

Barker & Rose (1984) define epidemiology as 'the study of the distribution and determinants of disease in human populations'. Distribution of disease, or so-called descriptive epidemiology, describes aspects of the burden of disease in communities. Routine data collection identifies the amount of disease by collecting mortality and incidence figures linked to morbidity. Determinants of disease in descriptive epidemiology may help identify some of the supposed causes of disease. These causes must be researched further to ensure risk factors or risk behaviour can be scientifically validated.

Tannahill has identified some of the problems linked to the application of epidemiology to health promotion (Bunton & McDonald 1992). He has suggested that a broader new approach to epidemiology, emphasising positive as well as negative aspects of health, is needed. Categories of ill-health and risk factors identified through quantifying causes of morbidity and mortality can be directly translated into health promotion programmes. However, this may result in health promotion in action being a very narrow activity unlinked to the concepts and models described previously. Identified problems are:

• Unsound programme planning: programmes may be devised which focus on disease or risk factor but take no account of areas of overlap between programmes, or neglect socio-economic factors, locus of power and control and peer pressure. Examples include a smoking programme, a coronary heart disease programme and a cervical cancer programme. There may be duplication of health promotion messages with resultant waste of money, human resources and public confusion.

• A neglect of methodological issues: a programme based on diseases and risk factors ends up focusing in reality on targets for achievement with an emphasis on giving information and advice, either individually or via campaigns, at the expense of modes of action which empower and develop individuals.

• An over-emphasis on individual behaviour: health promotion which is driven by epidemiology can focus blame for health-related behaviour on the individual in the community with the resultant 'victim blaming' approach. It may fail to take into account the social context of health and the need to develop public health policy.

• A narrow view of outcomes: the outcomes in

an epidemiologically driven health promotion programme will relate to objective statistical measurement of the product, for example effect on disease incidence rates, uptake of screening services. This approach fails to consider important human factors to support the process such as psychological fear of screening techniques.

• An incomplete view of health: epidemiology as previously defined focuses on disease. It therefore fails to include positive and often motivational aspects of health which were clearly evident in the model of health given in Figure 10.1 (p. 180) and the concepts of and models of health promotion. This can result in health promotion in practice failing to match stated aims.

Tannahill suggests that what is needed to overcome the above problems, and to enable epidemiology to support the values identified in his model of health promotion, is epidemiology which focuses on the distribution and determinants of good health, which has positive and negative components, rather than just disease. This will include not just objective determinants, but also subjective determinants. The Nottingham health profile (Hunt et al 1986) is just one example of a broader subjective epidemiology of health on which to base health promotion activities. This profile was devised from research which asked ordinary people what they thought were important aspects of health. From this research, a six dimension profile (physical mobility, pain, sleep, social isolation, emotional reactions, energy level) was devised. Each of the dimensions is scored independently on a questionnaire and provides a subjective assessment of a person's health status with equal value being placed on mental and social aspects of health.

It has been claimed that this profile is a better predictor of subsequent health outcome than objective measures of health status (Hunt et al 1986). Health profiles of entire areas can be developed if the Nottingham profile is used in conjunction with other socio-environmental measures.

Epidemiology and public health

Epidemiology is considered to be the basic science of public health because it describes relationships between health and disease and other factors in human populations (Detels 1991). The Royal College of Nursing (RCN 1994) defines it as:

a collective view of the health needs and health care of a population rather than an emphasis on an individual perspective. A central component of this collective approach is partnership at all stages and levels of the public health process. This means partnership with communities, and clients within them, as well as partnerships across professional groups. Teamwork is an essential prerequisite to effective public health work.

Components of public health are:

- Mortality and morbidity statistics and their associated factors
- Socio-structural and environmental factors known to impact upon health
- Service provision, including non-NHS services such as clean water
- The knowledge, beliefs and perceptions about health and health care held by the general public ('lay beliefs')
- Specific client groups, particularly vulnerable groups such as the homeless and those living in poverty
- Social policy measures, especially legal and fiscal measures
- A particular method of working using community development or community participation approaches.

There are clearly areas of similarity and overlap between these components and those identified earlier as being part of health promotion. This is not surprising as health promotion has not developed in isolation. The term and theoretical framework for health promotion preceded what is now termed the 'new' public health movement. Bunton & McDonald (1992) suggest that health promotion will contribute to, and form part of the new public health movement, contributing to the concepts used in public health and healthy public policy.

One example of a national strategy which has influenced public health is the Health of the Nation document (Department of Health 1992). Its aim is to improve the overall state of health in

England and it responds to Targets for health for all by the year 2000 (WHO 1985). The Health of the Nation document emphasises disease prevention and health promotion as ways in which even greater improvements in health can be secured, while acknowledging that further improvement in treatment, care and rehabilitation remains essential.

The five key areas, selected partially from epidemiological data, are:

- Coronary heart disease and stroke
- Cancers
- Mental illness
- Accidents
- HIV/AIDS and sexual health.

The chosen areas are seen as being major causes of premature death and preventable serious illness which offer scope for effective action. Each key area has a national target with action plan for achievement by the year 2000 and beyond.

In order for the strategy to work, it is suggested that there should be not only commitment at government level, but also commitment from the NHS and health professions, statutory and other authorities, the health authority, voluntary bodies, employers and employees and the media. This has been implemented through health promotion incentives in general practice. The term 'healthy alliances' is used to describe the partnerships which must occur between the many organisations and individuals involved in order for the strategy to work. This strategy therefore draws, at least in part, upon the WHO's identification of a need for commitment to community participation and intersectoral action.

The Health of the Nation document (Department of Health 1992) has been heavily criticised for several reasons.

- It has a very narrow focus (HVA 1991a), mostly on medical intervention and secondary prevention, rather than the broader aspects outlined in the health promotion models.
- It neglects important issues of equity, access and partnership (HVA 1991a, RCN 1991).
- There is an overemphasis on individual lifestyles and behaviour change with no

recognition of the important structural influences on health, and social, economic and environmental issues (HVA 1991a, RCN 1991).

Healthy alliances

Central to the concepts of health promotion and the new public health is a collective approach. This can only be achieved by people in a wide range of agencies and organisations working in partnership to promote health. Naidoo & Wills (1994) emphasise that there are different ways of developing healthy alliances for health promotion and provide useful definitions of the different ways of working.

* Multi-agency refers to organisations belonging to the same sector; for example health, social services, education are all statutory providers of public services.
* Intersectoral refers to working with other sectors, for example voluntary groups or private enterprise.
* Inter- or multidisciplinary working describes joint working of people with different roles or functions within the same organisation or across sectors.
* Joint planning occurs when organisations (within or across) agree objectives and have regular meetings to develop and implement a joint plan.
* Teams usually have a common task and consist of people with relevant expertise. They may be multidisciplinary or interagency.

There are both advantages and disadvantages to working together to create healthy alliances. One of the key advantages of collaborative planning is that it enables a clearer picture of local health care needs to be established and reduces duplication of activity, resulting in better use of resources. However, difficulties arise when partnerships fall apart due to lack of commitment, professional rivalry, lack of skills and differences of opinion.

An alliance can be as simple or as complicated as the participating groups wish. The size and range of the working group will depend upon the

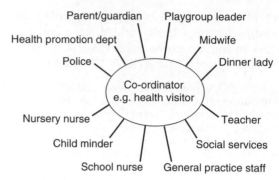

Figure 10.4 Health promotion initiative: a community approach to reduce the number of accidents in children aged 0–5 years.

planned health promotion initiative designed to meet an identified need. A co-ordinator is required to initiate, and invite members to contribute to, the alliance. Each member will have a specified role, to maximise expertise and resources. Feedback and evaluation are integral to the alliance. It is inevitable that not all proposed members will share the enthusiasm and commitment of the co-ordinator; this will be compensated for by the commitment of the remaining members.

Figure 10.4 demonstrates the range of agencies which may be invited to join a healthy alliance.

The Health of the Nation strategy proposes a variety of settings in which healthy alliances may be developed, including:

* Healthy cities
* Healthy schools
* Healthy hospitals
* Healthy workplaces
* Healthy prisons
* Healthy environments.

These settings target people in particular social organisations, for example students in schools, patients in hospitals and workers in the workplace. Whichever setting health promoters target, there will be sections of society who will be missed, for example the unemployed and travellers. Another way of targeting people is through community development initiatives. Practical application can be transferred to all other settings.

COMMUNITY EMPOWERMENT AND DEVELOPMENT

The role of health education and health promotion

Ross (1995) has defined community development as:

A process by which a community identifies its needs or objectives, orders (or ranks) these needs or objectives, develops the confidence and will to work at these needs or objectives, finds the resources (internal and/or external) to deal with these needs or objectives, takes action in respect to them, and in so doing extends and develops cooperative and collaborative attitudes and practices in the community.

Community development features as one of the quadrants of Beattie's model in Figure 10.3.

Green & Raeburn (1990) claim that community development is the central defining strategy for health promotion and that the essence of health promotion is empowering the community. Community development is user-led and demands different ways of working with individuals or groups to approaches such as the medical or behaviour change models. It has been viewed as being a highly political activity which can challenge power structures in society, for example medical dominance. The women's health movement of the 1960s and 1970s used elements of this approach to enable women to gain knowledge about their bodies and share personal experiences in group settings.

The role of the CHCN

Historically, strategies for promoting health have been derived from psychological theory, the main thrust of action being directed at changing an individual's behaviour or lifestyle. It is important that the CHCN involved in health promotion does not focus solely on the individual approach at the expense of the broader structural issues which can limit an individual's ability to make 'the healthy choice the easier choice'. The descriptive category of health promotion clearly directs the CHCN to the main components of health promotion.

In addition, McBride (1995) puts forward three main areas which can be the practical focus of health promotion:

- Changing attitudes
- Changing behaviour
- Changing environments.

Attitudes towards certain behaviours are directly influenced by two interlinked key factors, beliefs and motivation. To address the first two areas, the health promoter will need to provide clients with information which challenges their beliefs, allows them to explore their feelings about a certain behaviour and enables them to develop skills to cope with a change in behaviour. The third area will require action at the level of healthy public policies.

In order for the CHCN to work with individuals or groups, a systematic process needs to be employed. The nursing process approach, familiar to CHCNs, is a practical way of successfully organising health promotion activity by:

- Assessing health needs – individual and societal (discussed in Ch. 9)
- Planning health promotion activity
- Implementing health promotion interventions
- Evaluating health promotion.

The CHCN will also need skills in specific areas to successfully work with clients. These include an up-to-date knowledge base in specific areas of health promotion activity, and good communication skills. The CHCN will need to be competent in preventive skills such as cervical cytology or immunisation, or be able to refer the client to the appropriate person to undertake these tasks. Good communication skills do not only include eliciting information from the client during assessment in a way that respects the client, but also include elements of educational psychology relating to teaching and learning (Box 10.2).

The importance of skilful communication has been highlighted in research into helping clients stop smoking (McCleod-Clark et al 1990). In this research, there appeared to be a relationship between the use of open questions, listening and positive response to cues and successful outcome in terms of smoking cessation. Health promotion

---

Box 10.2 Practical elements of communication (McBride 1995)

- Check existing understanding and attitudes towards issue
- Motivate the client
- Give information and advice early in discussion, when it is more easily remembered
- Structure information in categories. Use short sentences and words that are easily understood. Do not use jargon
- Tackle one issue at a time. Do not expect too much
- Reinforce by repeating information and advice if necessary
- Offer written, visual or audio sources to take away. These should be sensitive to cultural issues and the client's learning ability
- Check the client's understanding of the information given
- Record in the notes what you have covered.

---

activity in relation to smoking also seemed to be more successful if the client was directly involved with planning. There appeared to be a direct link between full participation of the client and success, indicating that client-centred approaches (personal counselling for health, quadrant C in Beattie's map, p. 185) seemed to be more successful than top-down prescriptive approaches. Good communication skills are also essential for liaising with other agencies, including the media, which has the advantage of sharing the health promotion message with a very wide audience.

The CHCN will have to develop skills at using a variety of teaching methods. These include large group work, small group work and one-to-one interventions. There are many examples of prepared teaching material for use in a variety of health promotion topics. These resources can usually be obtained from local health promotion departments.

Community development approaches, as defined by Ross (1995), are increasingly becoming a part of the public health nursing role. Gilbert & Brett (1996) explain this approach in relation to the setting up of a project on a council estate, and outline a framework which seeks to reconcile the demands for community action with the development of mainstream services. The challenges of working in this way compared to the tradi-

tional primary health care team are considered along with the implications for all areas of nursing practice.

HEALTH PROMOTION IN ACTION – ETHICAL DILEMMAS FOR PRACTICE

Health is a value-laden concept. It is important for professionals involved in health promotion to be aware of, and base their practice on, clients' beliefs and values. It is clear from the health promotion models and approaches described that each is based on different ways of working with and valuing people. Health promotion must also be considered in relation to the principles of autonomy, beneficence, non-maleficence and justice discussed in Chapter 13, and shown in practical terms in Case study 10.1 (McKnight 1994).

HEALTH PROMOTION IN PRIMARY CARE

The WHO sees primary health care as a key setting for national and international health promotion policies.

The principles of health promotion in primary care can be applied to any health care setting. Models of health promotion should be used to guide the health promoter, and it may be appropriate to use a combination of models and approaches in an initiative. A locality health needs assessment identifies specific areas of need, to which health promotion should then be directed. New health promotion guidelines for GPs were issued in 1996 (NHSE 1996) and replaced the banding system for health promotion activity previously used. Payment for health promotion activities is dependent upon written approval from health promotion committees. Written proposals should include consideration of four criteria:

- Modern authoritative medical opinion
- The Health of the Nation strategy (Department of Health 1992) or regional equivalent
- The needs of the practice population
- Local priorities presented in the health authority's annual report.

Case study 10.1

Mr A is a 30-year-old man who enrols as a new patient at a general practice. At registration the receptionist offers him the opportunity to come for a well-person check, a facility which is offered to all newly registered patients. During the interview the practice nurse identifies that as a result of gross obesity the man becomes breathless on exertion and also has a raised blood pressure. The nurse uses Beattie's (1991) model (Fig. 10.3) to plan an approach to Mr A's care.

Approach 1
The nurse begins the interview in quadrant C of the health promotion map. She asks Mr A about his health and encourages him to express his perceptions relating to excess weight and consequential ill-health. During the interview, she moves into quadrant A and gives Mr A information, including up-to-date research about the consequences of obesity for his long-term health, and strategies to lose weight. Drawing on information she obtains from the man in relation to his way of life and preferences, she formulates a jointly agreed action plan with review meetings. She also moves into quadrant D and gives Mr A the address of a self-help group for overweight people. The well-person check takes 1 hour.

Approach 2
The nurse begins in quadrant A and tells Mr A that he is grossly overweight and informs him of the possible health consequences. She points out that if he does not lose weight within the next 6 months the GP will ask him to leave the practice. She also points out that if he requires any form of routine surgery it is likely to be refused until he loses weight. The nurse then outlines an action plan Mr A should follow to lose weight, and gives him details of a self-help group. The well-person check takes 15 minutes.

Both these approaches are examples of health education. The first appears to be giving the client choice. The second approach is more coercive in its approach and includes the explicit threat of the sanction of withdrawal of medical services.

GPs must send a report of their health promotion activities to their local health authority each year (Department of Health 1996). GPs are envisaged to have a key role in health promotion (Bridgewood et al 1996), although the RCN suggests that CHCNs, and in particular health visitors, are the key professional group who promote health and prevent disease in communities (RCN 1995).

The strategy encourages the PHC team to identify people at risk of certain preventable diseases, and promote a healthier lifestyle to reduce these risk factors. Many people do wish to modify their lifestyles and turn to the health promoter for guidance and support.

Two-thirds of adults in the UK have cardiovascular disease (CVD) risk factors and it is suggested that resources must be focused on those at greatest risk (Working Group of the Coronary Prevention Group 1991). How do we identify those people? One method of identifying people at risk is through screening, which may be regarded as a form of secondary health prevention.

Screening

Screening can be defined as the active early identification of disease or the identification of risk factors for disease in asymptomatic individuals. Screening tests are not diagnostic but are the means of selecting individuals for further examination. A condition or disease is subject to specified criteria for screening to be effective. These include:

- A long preclinical phase which allows screening to identify asymptomatic disease
- Proven data that earlier treatment improves outcomes. This is controversial in some conditions, for example screening for prostate cancer (Edwards 1996)
- A test which is acceptable, easy to perform and safe
- A test which correctly identifies all those persons with the condition (sensitive), and none of those without (specific). Cervical screening and breast mammography are examples of tests which may identify false positive results
- A cost effective programme. The number of cases screened identify a number of positive cases.

Screening of populations may be conducted in several ways. Mass screening, which includes the national programmes for breast and cervical cancer, offers individuals the service and they participate on a voluntary basis. Routine screening, including checking the newborn baby for congenital abnormalities and schoolgirls for scoliosis, follows defined programmes and protocols, whereas opportunistic screening involves a person presenting with one condition and being screened for another. For example, it is appropriate to check the rubella status of a young woman who presents for travel advice and who is planning a family in the near future.

Selective screening can be directed towards high-risk groups, for example checking the blood cholesterol levels of all diabetic patients, and multi-phasic screening involves tests for numerous diseases and/or risk factors at one time. This may become a common practice, as GPs face rising numbers of litigation actions.

The advantages of screening include:

- Disease is identified at an early stage
- Reduction in morbidity and premature mortality
- Early diagnosis may lead to non-pharmacological management, for example reducing plasma cholesterol through diet and lifestyle modification.

Screening does, however, have disadvantages:

- Negative psychological effects and behavioural outcomes from labelling patient as 'hypertensive', or having abnormal cervical cells
- Reinforcement of unhealthy lifestyles when a health check identifies no disease, for example patient continues to smoke.

An audit in general practice demonstrated the advantages of health checks as a method of screening asymptomatic patients for a variety of conditions (Edwards 1994). Edwards (1996) also reviewed the literature and explored the advantages and disadvantages of screening for prostate cancer. She concluded that the patient should be given sufficient appropriate information to be able to make an informed decision whether or not to be screened for a condition. Participation by individuals in screening procedures should be voluntary. There is a legal requirement to informed consent; the nurse may be required to act as the patient's advocate to ensure this occurs (discussed in greater detail in Ch. 13).

Delivering the message

Health promotion and health education can be delivered by a variety of methods. These include:

- Posters and displays in public places, for example library or sports centre
- Targeted displays within general practice, for example safety with fireworks prior to November 5th
- Group education at antenatal or postnatal classes
- Through the post, for example breast mammography invitation including breast self-awareness leaflet
- One-to-one, for example personal lifestyle advice
- Group session, for example slimming club
- Regional or national campaigns through the media, including local free newspapers, the press and radio, for example during national continence week, or the measles/rubella campaign of 1992
- Use of theatre groups. These multi-agency projects use drama to reach groups in a variety of settings. One project targeted women in Yorkshire (Crawley 1996).

There are advantages and disadvantages with each of the suggested methods. Home mailing may offend some people, while community awareness displays will attract a limited audience. Some clients participate well in group sessions. Some prefer one-to-one contact, such as for menopausal clinics. Some women are embarrassed to talk about personal problems in public, while others benefit by sharing experiences.

There is no one method which is appropriate to meet the needs of all prospective health advice recipients. Health promotion must be delivered to suit each situation and each individual. This may include the need for an interpreter.

Health includes all health issues, not merely Health of the Nation targets. The following example of the folic acid campaign demonstrates the potential diversity of health promotion initiatives.

A campaign in action – folic acid

In 1996 the Department of Health began funding a $2\frac{1}{2}$-year campaign to increase public and health professional awareness of the benefits of folic acid (HEA 1996). This follows research which suggests that women who take extra folic acid before conception and in the early stages of pregnancy reduce their risk of having a baby with neural tube defects (spina bifida or anacephalus) (HEA 1996). The HEA circulated guidelines which suggest how local action can be effectively organised in a variety of settings, including pharmacies, general practices and gynaecological outpatient clinics. This campaign meets the NHSE criteria because:

- The health promotion is based on activities of proven benefit
- It is aimed at all pre-conceptual or pregnant women, hence meets the needs of a practice population.

This campaign, using primary health prevention, demonstrates the value of health promotion for conditions other than those cited in the Health of the Nation document (Department of Health 1992). It involves minimal expense for maximum benefit. National campaigns may reduce some of the regional inequalities in health by standardising health promotion activities.

Cost–benefits of health promotion

Cost–benefits may be difficult to assess in long-term health promotion strategies (Tolley 1995) for a variety of reasons.

- Resources spent in improving the health of young people through health education and school health policies (including the re-introduction of free school milk and regular physical exercise) will be recouped by savings in treatment for osteoporosis in later years and so cannot be accurately assessed now.
- Resources necessary for devising, printing and distributing leaflets and posters versus the cost of long-term care and medical treatment for a child born with a neural tube defect cannot be assessed. Family costs must not be ignored

either. These include the stress of coping with a handicapped child, the effect on siblings, and bereavement, and are almost impossible to quantify.

Evaluation

It is essential to evaluate the health promotion programme to ensure that the aims are being met. This is usually an ongoing process, allowing changes to be made to the activity to address any shortcomings in the programme.

Process evaluation measures the current activity and the quality of the programme. It will highlight any deficiencies, such as training needs of alliance members, or lack of resources such as publicity leaflets. Impact evaluation measures the immediate effect of the strategy, and this may include numbers recruited for smoking cessation clinics. Outcome evaluation measures the long-term effect. In the example of smoking cessation, this may be the number of quitters in 1 year.

HEALTHY SCHOOLS

Schools are key settings for health promotion for several reasons, chiefly because they provide a captive audience and some health education is usually included throughout the educational curriculum.

There is evidence that risk factors for diseases in adulthood can often be linked to unhealthy lifestyles in early life (Townsend et al 1992). The health education offered as part of the ongoing spiral curriculum includes a cross curriculum theme which builds on the Health of the Nation target areas, for example accident prevention and reduction of obesity. It is important, however, to appreciate that education given through school may not be reinforced in the home environment.

From a broader holistic health promotion perspective, schools can provide appropriate preventive measures including some immunisation and dental care, by forging links with relevant professional groups. Health protection measures should include not just statutory health and safety policies, but the implementation of healthy school policies, for example no-smoking policies, healthy food options in the school canteen, stress management.

The national curriculum is quite specific in the content of programmes of study schools must offer. Health education is included in the National Curriculum Council (1990) Guidance Document 5 which provides an overview of a health education programme for children aged 5 to 16. The Education Act 1993 provides additional arrangements for sex education with a stronger emphasis on family values and a moral framework. The provision of sex education in primary schools is discretionary, but it is compulsory in secondary schools. HIV education was included in the Statutory National Curriculum for Science in 1991, but was withdrawn in 1994 (except for biological aspects) due to intense reactions from various religious groups. The level of education will, however, depend upon approval of the school governors. Parents have the right to withdraw their children from sex education sessions, but these are probably the ones who would benefit most from the lessons. The quality and depth of education will vary between, and within, schools, both regionally and nationally.

In 1991 the Health Visitors' Association highlighted the potential for the role development of school nurses (HVA 1991b). This has resulted in many community trusts reviewing their school health services and developing the skill mix (Bagnall 1993). Screening is now carried out by school nurses based on guidance issued in the Hall (1991) report.

Additional training in key areas such as health promotion skills has been offered by many trusts to develop the skills of their existing school nurses. Some exciting intiatives have been undertaken in response to the Health of the Nation target for sexual health – to reduce by at least half the rate of conceptions amongst the under 16s by the year 2000. It is recognised that there is a reluctance by young people to consult their GP for formal contraceptive advice (Hudson & Ineichen 1991, Hadley 1992). Analysis of this author's (Edwards's) local family planning clinic data reveals that young people do not use this facility. This begs the question, where do the young peo-

---

Case study 10.2   Health promotion in schools

Topic: sexual health
Health promoters: school nurse, family planning nurse, health visitor community midwife, practice nurse (liaise with school teachers to meet curriculum guidelines)

Venue: school, community clinic, youth club

Role of health promoter:

- School nurse – known by target population, friendly face, continuity
- Family planning nurse – expert in subject, resource
- Health visitor – often has family planning training, may be contact for the future
- Community midwife – specialist knowledge of conception
- Practice nurse – link with general practitioner and other professionals

Material resources: include the use and availability of all visual aids on contraception, workshops on how to say 'no', leaflets, details of local family planning clinics and genitourinary clinics.

Methods: may have a roadshow at school, community clinic or youth club

Outcome: health promotion which meets criteria within school curriculum which includes relationships, safer sex and consequences of unprotected intercourse. This is delivered through a health alliance which draws on the expertise of the CHCNs.

---

ple in this area receive their sexual health advice when there are no special young people's contraceptive clinics such as Brook Advisory?

The scenario in Case study 10.2 demonstrates how CHCNs and the PHC team can address the Health of the Nation target to reduce conceptions in the under 16s.

Having identified a need for accessible health promotion for young people in a rural area, a CHAT clinic (confidential health advice for teenagers) was initiated in April 1996 at a local health clinic. A family planning nurse and school nurse run the session during the school lunch period. Young people (boys and girls) have maximum opportunity to access the facilities, where they are encouraged to discuss all aspects of health, receive counselling and support, and collect condoms. Girls who require emergency contraception are referred to a sympathetic GP or family planning clinic, where future contraceptive needs can be assessed. It is not a requisite to be on the GP's list to be registered for contraception. This is particularly important in an area where children are bussed to school and require support during school hours, without parental knowledge. Advantages of this service include the opportunity for young people to access a confidential sexual health advice service.

CHCNs who disapprove of premarital sexual relations may consider any initiative to promote safer sex as unethical. However, any initiative which reduces unplanned conceptions should be encouraged.

Another example of good practice is in Forest Health Care Trust, London (Pavitt & Clark 1992). They have targeted school nurses for family planning training. This enables the school nurses to provide contraceptive and sexual health advice sessions in clinics located close to the schools for which they are responsible. This provides both continuity and accessibility to a confidential service.

Community psychiatric nurses (CPNs) also have an important role in school health, although their role often goes unrecognised.

A healthy school involves the collaboration of educational and health professionals. Health promotion is an integral part of current higher education for health visitors, practice nurses, midwives, school nurses and district nurses. Much of this knowledge may not be directed towards schools, but as previously demonstrated, there is a wealth of expertise to share. CHCNs must maximise their opportunities to promote healthy schools and to reduce future morbidity and premature mortality.

WHO LISTENS TO HEALTH PROMOTION MESSAGES?

Many of the Health of the Nation targets (Department of Health 1992) aim for improvements in mortality and morbidity figures, which can only be measured in the long term. The Health Education Monitoring Survey (HEMS) was established as a way of monitoring intermediate progress towards these targets.

In one survey, 91% of respondents said they led 'very healthy' or 'fairly healthy' lifestyles (Bridgewood et al 1996). These figures suggest an individual's perception of a healthy lifestyle is subjective, as epidemiological data does not support these figures. Also, 65% of respondents had talked to a doctor at the surgery in the previous year, while an additional 4% had spoken to another health professional, for example a nurse or health visitor. If these figures are replicated nationally, health promotion in primary care would target nearly 70% of the population.

The confusion created by changing recommendations may lead people to ignore future advice on healthy eating. In the survey (Bridgewood et al 1996), 70% of respondents stated that 'experts never agree about what foods are good for you'. This lack of consensus may have repercussions on the long-term health of the nation as shoppers ignore the healthy eating messages.

Summary

Although the focus of government strategies currently relates to the Health of the Nation, it is essential that health promotion resources and activities are directed to ALL areas of health where levels of morbidity and premature mortality can be reduced. The HEMS survey results suggest that the health promotion message has been heard by the majority of the population. This should encourage health promoters, although it does not follow that knowing the benefits of a healthy lifestyle will necessarily lead to application of these benefits. Health promotion sows the seeds of the benefits of lifestyle modification to achieve optimum health. Although these seeds may not reach maturity for several months (or years), the benefits may still be reaped through a reduction in morbidity. Health promotion enables the individual to make an informed choice of lifestyle, within the limitations of the social and economic environment.

However, as health promoters, nurses may promote longevity by preventing for example coronary heart disease, but may offer an individual increased dependence through alternative morbidity and the ageing process. Nurses must recognise that the benefits of some health promotion may never be measurable.

REFERENCES

Bagnall P 1993 Health promotion, school nursing and the school age child. In: Dimes A, Cribb A (eds) Health promotion: concepts and practice. Blackwell, Oxford

Barker D J P, Rose G 1984 Epidemiology in medical practice, 3rd edn. Churchill Livingstone, Edinburgh

Beattie A 1991 Knowledge and control in health promotion: a test case for social policy and social theory. In: Gabe J, Calnan M, Bury M (eds) The sociology of the health service. Routledge, London

Becker M H (ed) 1974 The health belief model and personal health behaviour. Slack, New Jersey

Blaxter M 1990 Health and lifestyles. Routledge, London

Bridgewood A, Malbon G, Lader D, Matheson J for the Office for National Statistics and Health Education Authority 1996 Health in England 1995. What people know, what people think, what people do. HMSO, London

Bunton R, McDonald G (eds) 1992 Health promotion: disciplines and diversity. Routledge, London

Crawley M 1996 Don't lose heart. Nursing Times 92(40):50–52

Department of Health 1992 The health of the nation. A strategy for health in England. HMSO, London

Department of Health 1996 Statement of fees and allowances. Paragraph 30. HMSO, London

Detels R 1991 Epidemiology: the foundation of public health. In: Holland W W, Detels R, Knox G (eds) Oxford textbook of public health, vol 2, Methods of public health. Oxford University Press, Oxford

Downie R S, Fyfe C, Tannahill A 1991 Health promotion. Models and values. Oxford Univeristy Press, Oxford

Education Act 1993 HMSO, London

Edwards M 1994 Health checks: a positive approach. Practice Nursing 5(20):32–33

Edwards M 1996 Prostate cancer: to screen or not? Practice Nursing 7(3):40–42

Gilbert A, Brett S 1996 A public health nursing post: the tools for getting started. Nursing Times 92(16):33–35

Green L W, Johnson K W 1984 Health education and health promotion. In: Matarazzo J, Weiss S, Herd J, Miller N (eds) Behavioural health: a handbook of health enhancement and disease prevention. Wiley, New York

Green L W, Raeburn J 1990 Community wide change: theory and practice. In: Bracht N (ed) Health promotion at the community level. Sage, California

Hadley A 1992 Unplanned teenage pregnancies. Community Outlook 2(3):35–36

Hall D 1991 Health for all children (The Hall report). Oxford Medical Publications, Oxford

Health Education Authority 1996 Folic acid and the prevention of neural tube defects. Guidance for health service purchasers and providers. HEA, London

Health Visitors' Association 1991a The health of the nation: the HVA responds. Health Visitor 64(11):365–367

Health Visitors' Association 1991b Project health: health promotion and the role of the school nurse in the school community. HVA, London

Hudson F, Ineichen B 1991 Taking it lying down. Sexuality and teenage motherhood. Macmillan Education, Hampshire

Hunt S M, McKenna S P, McEwen J 1986 Measuring health status. Croom Helm, London

Lalonde M 1974 A new perspective on the health of Canadians. Information, Ottawa

McBride A 1995 Health promotion in hospital. Scutari Press, London

McCleod-Clark J, Haverty S, Kendall S 1990 Helping people to stop smoking: a study of the nurse's role. Journal of Advanced Nursing 16:357–363

McKnight S 1994 Ethical issues in health promotion. Unpublished MA dissertation (Philosophy and Health Care). University of Wales, Swansea

Naidoo J, Wills J 1994 Health promotion. Foundations for practice. Baillière Tindall, London

National Curriculum Council 1990 Curriculum guidance No5 Health education. National Curriculum Council, York

NHS Executive 1996 GP health promotion, Circular FHSL(96)35. NHSE, Leeds

Noack H 1987 Concepts of health and health promotion. In: Abelin T, Brzezinski Z J, Carstairs V D L (eds) Measurement in health promotion and protection. WHO Regional Office for Europe, WHO Regional Publications, European Series No 22, Copenhagen

Pavitt J, Clark S 1992 Service review of women's health and contraceptive services. Forest Health Care Trust, London

Ross M 1995 Community organisation: theory and principles. Harper and Brothers, New York

Royal College of Nursing 1991 The health of the nation. A response from the Royal College of Nursing. RCN, London

Royal College of Nursing 1994 Public health: nursing rises to the challenge. RCN, London

Royal College of Nursing 1995 Community health care nurses. Challenging the present, improving the future. RCN, London

Seedhouse D 1986 Health. The foundations for achievement. John Wiley, Chichester

Tolley K 1995 Health promotion: how to measure cost-effectiveness. Health Education Authority, London

Townsend P, Davidson N, Whitehead W 1992 Inequalities in health. Penguin, London

Walton I 1989 The health of nations. Open University Press, Milton Keynes, ch 5, p. 27

Working Group of the Coronary Prevention Group 1991 British Medical Journal 303:748–750

World Health Organization 1946 Constitution. WHO, New York

World Health Organization 1978 Report of the international conference on primary health care, Alma Alta. WHO, Geneva

World Health Organization 1984 Health promotion. A discussion document on the concepts and principles. WHO, Copenhagen

World Health Organization 1985 Targets for health for all. WHO, Copenhagen

FURTHER READING

Brown T 1996 South Thames Regional Health Authority. Opportunities for health and education to work together. Linking the health of the nation targets to the national curriculum. NHSE, London

The Crown 1993 Better living, better life. Knowledge House, Henley-on-Thames

Department of Health 1994 Negotiating school health services. DOH, London

Ewles L, Simnett I 1992 Promoting health: a practical guide, 2nd edn. Scutari Press, London

Luft S, Smith M 1994 Nursing in general practice. A foundation text. Chapman and Hall, London

11 Quality

Carmel Blackie

The issue of assuring quality in health care delivery has assumed significance for all professionals since the creation of the internal market in the NHS and the emergence of the client or patient as consumer. Community health care nurses, who as a group work very closely with clients and do so predominantly in the client's own home, must be able to engage in the process of quality assurance with their multidisciplinary colleagues. They must, therefore, have knowledge of the range of quality assurance tools available for this purpose and some of the issues which surround the subject: standard setting; the development of clinical guidelines; audit and evaluation: the management of quality; the link between cost and quality; and change through quality assessment. The community health care nurse should be able to apply this knowledge to practice through problem solving and reflection.

Attempts to ensure quality in healthcare systems have been made since the times of the ancient societies in Egypt, Assyria, China, Japan and Mexico. These cultures had ways of ensuring that what the doctors (or medicine men – nurses were not mentioned in those times) did to patients was legitimate and that patients did not die too frequently. This often involved an apprentice system for training 'doctors' with candidates learning the trade through watching a respected elder practitioner. Hippocrates identified methods of analysing the outcome of diseases, the beginnings of audit. In ancient Greece, the Hippocratic Oath was a public statement relating to acceptable standards in medical practice and which, if breached, would lead to punishment. Lack of quality in care usually brought severe penalties such as death or mutilation of the surgeon. The first recognised standards of care were introduced in the sixteenth century by Juan Ciudad Duarte, later known as St John of God, and related to the humane treatment of the mentally ill. In 1518, the Royal College of Physicians in England designed a charter to uphold their honour and that of the public, an early reference to the concept of accountability and consumerism in health care. In 1859, Florence Nightingale published her notes on nursing at Scutari in the Crimea – the first standards of care for nursing.

The concept of quality care, therefore, was present in the ethos of the earliest healthcare systems, and in 1948 the fledgling NHS also embraced the concept. What has become apparent more recently is the desire to develop systematic methods of setting, implementing, maintaining, ensuring and auditing the quality of care provided, and to adapt practice as a result. Quality issues gained impetus as a consequence of the market reforms of the health service in the 1980s. As such, it is a concept borrowed from industry where it is linked to increased efficiency, output and better use of resources. For a health service operating an internal market and with limited resources, this is a highly desirable goal.

QUALITY IN HEALTH CARE

WHY IS QUALITY NECESSARY?

Health care is a set of complex, systematic activities that people perform for and with other people. It is dependent on many factors, including interpersonal skills, culture, expectations, clinical skill, technology and available resources, for successful delivery. Healthcare professionals need to understand each other and share views with society and individuals about what constitutes quality in health care, why it is important, how it is decided and how to ensure that it is maintained. It is only through engaging in this debate that the health service can provide society with acceptable and appropriate services.

The demand for health care is increasing in the UK and other western economies. There are many reasons for this, but the most significant are:

• Social deprivation
• Advances in science which have increased treatment options
• An increasingly elderly population which requires more care into an older age than experienced by previous generations
• Changing morbidity patterns associated with elderly people
• A greater awareness of what is possible and a more vocal public which asserts its claims to health care encouraged by education and the media, which has created the 'healthcare consumer'
• Changing lifestyle. As people live longer into very old age, conditions such as arthritis and dementia can afflict them, increasing morbidity. In previous generations, many people died before very old age.

The health service must now meet greater demand from an increasingly articulate population of potential clients and patients, and do so with dwindling resources and in the face of increasing marketisation of healthcare services.

Health care is expensive. Regardless of how it is organised or what is offered it remains true that expectation and demand exceed available resources. The challenge to governments, healthcare planners, commissioners, providers and the public who use and fund the NHS, is how to make best use of available resources to meet demand as effectively as possible. This requires open debate at all levels about the values and ethics involved in shaping the nature of the health service. At a practical level, quality initiatives including quality assurance (QA) or continual quality improvement (CQI) as it has become known, are an attempt to achieve cost-effective options in health care which are beneficial and yield health gain, through using resources wisely in the reformed NHS. The quality and nature of the service to be provided is now often made explicit in contracts between commissioners/purchasers and providers of health care. In the past, quality was largely implicit.

In 1985, the World Health Organization (WHO) working group on QA identified four reasons to emphasise quality in health care: economic; social; political; and professional. These four categories are interlinked and influence each other, but are discussed separately here.

Economic. Resources and the supply of health care cannot match actual and potential demand. Balancing resources against demand requires agreement from society about how money is best spent. During this process quality initiatives are one way to ensure that resources currently available are spent to best effect.

Social. People expect to be healthy and live long, fulfilled lives. Therefore, they expect healthcare services to maintain their health and provide a panacea for every disease and complaint. These expectations range from simple things such as antibiotics for a sore throat or a district nurse to support palliative care, to more complex treatment such as transplant surgery. The population also expects treatment options and services for conditions which are not life threatening, but which do reduce the quality of life for the individual, such as infertility treatment or cosmetic surgery.

As services such as social services are depleted and take on a crisis function, primary health care workers are left to deal with problems which affect health but are, arguably, not necessarily the responsibility of the health service; for example, misery caused by poor housing or unemployment can lead to people consulting primary care professionals.

The demand for health through universal health care reflects values and attitudes which have developed throughout the twentieth century and which are linked to the philosophical principles on which the NHS was founded (see Ch. 2). Increasingly, however, successive Conservative governments have encouraged people to be responsible for themselves in all aspects of life. In addition, the market reforms of the health service (see Ch. 2) and the consequent rise of the patient as consumer, supported by initiatives such as the Patients' Charter (DoH 1993), have placed extra emphasis on a demand-led health service. Patients and users of healthcare services now expect to be told explicitly what they will receive.

As in the USA, the patient, user or healthcare consumer is increasingly likely to demand compensation, either through negotiated settlement or through litigation, should healthcare services fall below an expected standard. This has increased the need to make services and the expected level of quality explicit to the consumer and to ensure that standards are consistently achieved. Health cannot be purchased but health care can and consumer views play a large part in shaping services. The data generated through quality initiatives enable the health service to exercise its duty in a publicly accountable manner, and increasingly in response to litigation.

Political. Central government spending is derived from taxation in one form or another. Resources are limited for all public spending and governments are obliged to balance resources. Health care is just one state provision competing for money from the same source. Competing interests include education, social security and defence among others, and all have a legitimate claim to funding in a democracy.

In the UK, government departments compete for funding in the run up to the annual budget statement by the Chancellor of the Exchequer. It is the responsibility of ministers to put the case for increased resources for their department to the Chief Secretary to the Treasury. It is the goal of the Chief Secretary to limit spending and broker compromise between departments so that an acceptable balance is struck.

Spending on health care in the UK is approximately 5% of the gross national product (GNP). In the USA it is 10%, and in Scandinavia as much as 20% of the GNP is devoted to health. When spending on health rises above 10% of GNP there is public outcry over costs and calls for cost containment (Rodriguez 1988, Donabedian 1989) resulting from concern that dwindling resources should be spent to best effect to maximise quality. Whatever the driving force behind the call for savings, resources must be managed (Ellis & Whittington 1993). Imposing an internal market economy on the NHS and linking this to quality through contracting, commissioning and consumer choice, is an attempt by the government to manage the situation. The NHS, through its management executive, now requires improvements in healthcare delivery, outcome and the promotion of health.

Professional. Healthcare professionals of all disciplines need to know that the service provided to patients and clients is of a high standard, offering the best care possible. They have a responsibility to the public through codes of conduct and ethics to strive towards this goal and to be publicly accountable. QA methods therefore have great relevance for healthcare professionals. They are one way a profession can explicitly communicate its standards of service to the public. Managing cyclical quality initiatives, setting standards and guidelines, auditing care and changing practice are ways of retaining internal control over the profession's own regulations, and they set a standard by which acceptable professional service or conduct is measured.

WHAT IS QUALITY?

Large amounts of resources are invested in the pursuit of quality in the delivery of health care; how to achieve and improve it and how to implement and manage the concept. However, there is no unequivocal definition of quality. Laughlin (1993) points out that there is little or no attempt in the literature to shape and define a core idea of quality which stands up to scrutiny. He states that 'while there is widespread agreement that "quality matters" there is little agreement over what this thing is that matters so much'.

The notion of what constitutes quality in any environment is often subjective and differs dramatically depending upon the perspective of the individual concerned. In health care this relates to whether the individual is a patient, provider of care, manager or purchaser of care and is affected by local issues and priorities.

One important issue for practitioners is that they know what they mean by quality: it is something which could be said to relate to 'the goodness' of their care (Lawrence & Schofield 1993). This perspective is linked to ethical principles of beneficence and non-maleficence (see Ch. 13). However, this concept must be made explicit to professional colleagues and to the public.

DEFINING QUALITY

Black (1990) defines the nature of quality in primary health care by suggesting four dimensions of quality which should characterise the service; effectiveness, equity, humanity and efficiency.

These categories blend the perspective of the professional with that of patient or client and also encompass social issues. He suggests that professionals are largely, but not exclusively, concerned with clinical effectiveness as a measure of quality. Clients and patients view this from a different perspective and are concerned with the way care is carried out as well as the outcome. Society has a different viewpoint again and Black asserts that this is linked to cost and equity.

Hill et al (1990) state that 'Quality is taken to refer to one or more attributes or characteristics of a service which are important enough to be identified and specified'. One factor around which there is some degree of consensus is that quality is a recognisable concept in the perception of clients or customers.

Kelly & Swift (1991) assert that health professionals should recognise quality issues as being integral to any system or department and should contain elements which recognise the importance of services appearing attractive to customers or patients. Viewed in this way, quality requires management to ensure that it is achieved. Total quality management (TQM) is a concept for managing quality issues which holds that the quality of a service is more important than the individual practitioner and to be achieved, it must be managed. This is particularly relevant to the complex issue of health care; how do health professionals ensure that nursing operates standards which integrate with medicine and with social services, if this is dependent upon an individual acting autonomously? Success is more likely to be achieved through a co-ordinator or manager.

Management or co-ordination of quality does, however, pose problems. Professionals will be required to work to standards being set by outside agents for previously autonomous professional groups. This could limit the power and control of individual professions over their own internal regulations, weakening their influence over the direction of health care and the growth of that profession. To balance the effect of management the professions need to engage in quality activities, such as standard setting, guidelines and audit, which lead to professional self-regulation and the adaptation of practice as a consequence.

Inherent in the concept of quality is quality assurance (QA). Williamson (1978) states that 'QA is the measurement of the actual level of the service provided plus the efforts to modify where necessary the provision of these services in the light of the result of the measurement'. Schmadl (1979) adds another dimension: 'The purpose of QA is to assure the consumer of nursing of a specified degree of excellence through continuous measurement and evaluation'.

QA is a straightforward concept. Standards are set for a product or service; production or delivery of the service is organised so that the standards can be achieved consistently, and the system is monitored, evaluated or audited making sure that the standards are achieved. If not, adjustments are made thereby assuring quality (Ellis & Whittington 1993).

The activities involved in QA are known as a quality cycle; the process constantly repeats itself in a dynamic action. The quality cycle exists as part of TQM. QA is a developing concept and is evolving into continuous quality improvement (CQI), the difference being that the emphasis placed in CQI is on changing practice.

Nearly a decade earlier, the World Health Organization (WHO) established a working group on QA which reported its findings in 1985. The group highlighted difficulties in formulating a generally acceptable definition of quality; each organisation tends to have its own understanding of the meaning of quality. The WHO concluded that this has hampered the development of quality systems because the design of a system relies in part upon an agreed operational definition of quality.

In spite of the lack of definition, the WHO working group (1995) gave a statement of intent regarding the nature of quality, which states that quality health care means:

To ensure that each patient receives such a mix of diagnostic and therapeutic services as is most likely to produce the optimal achievable health care outcome for that patient, consistent with the state of the art of medical science, and with biological factors such as the patient's age, illness, concomitant secondary diagnoses, compliance with the treatment regimen and other related factors; with the minimum expenditure of resources necessary to accomplish this result; at the lowest level of risk of additional injury or disability as a consequence of treatment; and with maximal patient satisfaction with the process of care, his/her interaction with the health care system, and the results obtained.

This should be achieved through a process of continuous and cyclical monitoring, assessment and improvement of services throughout primary, secondary and tertiary care including health promotion activities at all three levels of the service. It is also worth noting in the statement of intent how quality is linked to social, political, professional, societal and individual issues.

The quality cycle

The quality cycle contains the following elements:

- Quality assessment, which involves evaluating the current level of performance of the service
- Quality improvement, which combines an element of assessment, but is essentially a process of changing practice
- QA, to ensure that the high quality achieved through the first two phases is maintained.

The quality cycle involves a series of stages and depends for its success upon good communication and education as well as management support and professional commitment (Box 11.1).

Box 11.1   Stages in the quality cycle

1. Establish a quality steering group and identify and agree values and a philosophy. Reach a consensus about what you are trying to achieve, the nature and purpose of the health service you are offering, the organisational context and the philosophy under care. At this stage, knowledge about your own value system and beliefs is important as well as professional and contractual obligations such as your contract of employment, the UKCC Code of Professional Conduct (1992) and initiatives such as the Patients' Charter (1993).
2. Review the literature. Seek out examples from other units and nationally about what constitutes quality and best practice. Remember, you do not have to start from scratch.
3. Analyse the literature you have found and examples of good practice locally. What can be used; what is inappropriate; what can be adapted; what is unique for your local area?
4. Select the quality programme most appropriate for your area.
5. Establish criteria and standards of care, possibly using Donabedian's approach to standard setting (Donabedian 1966) which involves structure, process and outcome. Remember, standards must be realistic, achievable and measurable.
6. Agree and ratify the standards set. This involves communication with colleagues and the other professions involved in care, and with managers.
7. Evaluate or audit current practice against the defined standard.
8. Analyse the audit and identify factors which contribute to the result.
9. Select appropriate actions to maintain or improve care.
10. Implement actions to improve or maintain the standard. This involves knowledge of the process of change.
11. Evaluate the whole process. Is the QA programme you are using doing what you intended it to do? If not change it.
12. Repeat from point one.

Achieving consensus and applying ideas

In health care, there are numerous different but interrelated people and interests to consider. These can be identified as groups related to the market system of the reformed NHS (Yorkshire RHA et al 1994); purchasers, providers, recipients of care and services (patients or clients) and the general public who are potential recipients of care and services. This complexity in the nature and structure of health care means that applying quality assurance to health care is a difficult task.

Quality is a multidisciplinary concept. This complicates its definition within a health context. Health care encompasses individual interactions with clients as well as a community or public health emphasis within a global strategic overview. Each facet needs to be considered in terms of quality. In many instances, the idea and perception of quality depends upon the expectations of both the individual provider and the consumer of care. This can derive from many issues such as past experience, cultural background, education and gender. The perception of quality has a subjective as well as an objective element. Because it is socially constructed, it depends on who measures it and the values they employ (Rodriguez 1988).

WHAT IS QUALITY IN HEALTH CARE?

Maxwell (1984) and Shaw (1986), using a similar approach, suggest that quality in health care, whether strategic and at a population level or whether at the level of individual practice, can be considered in terms of:

- Appropriateness/relevance, that is, the service offered is actually what the recipients of that service want and need
- Equity, where every user or potential user has a fair distribution of resources available
- Accessibility, so that users/consumers can reach services and service providers and are not constrained or disadvantaged by unreasonable limits of time or distance
- Effectiveness, that is, services achieve the intended benefit for the population or the individual patient/client
- Acceptability, or providing services in such a way as to satisfy the reasonable expectations of patients, providers and the community. This includes elements of social, cultural and ethical perspectives
- Efficiency, which means that resources are not wasted on one service or patient to the detriment of another. It links a service to its production costs in terms of time, money and human and physical resources.

These categories, however, conflict with each other. For example, if services are to be efficient, and in the terms given this relates to not wasting resources on one person to the detriment of another, how does this balance with the idea of equity when decisions are made about who is offered treatment? Who is more 'valuable', a father of three needing bypass surgery or an 85-year-old lady needing a hip replacement?

Equity demands that every user and potential user of the healthcare system has access to an equal share of resources, but how can this be the case when there are insufficient resources to go around? Criteria must be set regarding the delivery of services. These are currently based on need associated with maintaining life and the quality of life. In most cases, this is decided by health care providers.

How decisions are made about people and how the needs of a population are balanced against the needs of an individual, are decisions made on a daily basis by practitioners. Increasingly, the population using the healthcare system is becoming involved in decisions about rationing, and in a democracy, this is appropriate.

Wilkinson (1990) suggests seven categories of healthcare quality which are similar to Maxwell's (1984) and Shaw's (1986). He omits equity but adds efficacy (is the care or procedure useful?) and continuity (was care carried out without interruption, with follow-up and appropriate exchange of information?), thereby concentrating on the nature of the process rather than the distribution.

Other factors which can be considered in relation to a quality service relate to the competence of the person who delivers that service. The UKCC (1994) have identified standards for post-registration, education and practice which stipulate a number of criteria the nurse must fulfil to maintain registration and demonstrate competence. Attributes which may describe a competent practitioner could include (Wright & Whittington 1992):

- Committed, caring, communicative
- Accountable, autonomous, approachable

- Reliable, respected, resourceful
- Expert, efficient, ethical.

Similarly the service itself could be described as having several features which enhance quality (Wright & Whittington 1992):

- Comprehensive, cost-effective, contractual
- Accessible, accredited, acceptable
- Relevant, reliable, resourced
- Efficient, equitable, effective.

The WHO working group on QA (1995) states that there are 3 general positive benefits to implementing a quality programme:

1. It provides a vehicle for public accountability by providing objective evidence that public funds are being used wisely and to best effect, in other words efficiently and effectively. Definitions of 'efficiently' and 'effectively' may vary depending upon whether you are a purchaser, provider, health service planner or consumer.
2. It gives a managerial tool for problem solving in healthcare systems and as such should be integral to every level of management.
3. It should facilitate the process of innovation in healthcare delivery. This should include technological, organisational and interdisciplinary advances.

The benefits which quality initiatives confer to community health care (CHC) professionals are many and include:

- Linking education to service needs
- Helping to develop primary health care teams through the interactive process involved
- Helping to establish a primary, secondary and tertiary care link
- Contributing to the development of incentives for staff involved in care
- Providing a framework for service development.

Guidelines for clinical practice

Guidelines are defined by the Institute of Medicine in the USA as 'Systematically developed statements to assist practitioner and patient decisions about appropriate health care for specific clinical circumstances'. Lohr (1994) suggests that implicit within this definition are the ideas that guidelines are based on evidence; that decision making about health care involves patients and professionals equally; that there is a focus on clinical intervention, implying the full range of care options which are available in primary health care; and that there is an assumption that guidelines will be practical and easy to follow to allow professionals to use them in everyday practice. In other words, guidelines disseminate evidence-based practice.

Over recent years the development of clinical guidelines has become popular in relation to professional education and quality. Clinical guidelines give a framework within which practice may be learned and refined and through which standards, particularly replicable standards, are ensured. They are developed in the belief that health outcomes and health gain are improved and efficiency and effectiveness increased.

Much of the work in relation to clinical guidelines has been undertaken in relation to medicine, although other professionals implement guidelines and are affected by them. This is particularly true in relation to general practice where practice nurses support the management of chronic disease such as hypertension. An evaluation of the suitability, acceptability, impact and effect of guidelines in all healthcare practice is lacking, particularly in relation to the use of guidelines by nurses and within a multidisciplinary context; research is necessary and timely as the overlap of roles between doctors and nurses increases.

Clinical guidelines have the potential to make significant contributions to health care, particularly in relation to assessing and improving the quality of care which is offered and as a means to rationalising the health service and so containing costs (Lohr 1994).

The way in which guidelines are developed and disseminated influences their acceptance by professionals and whether or not they are used. Guidelines are only able to achieve their potential in health care if practitioners put them into practice.

There are two general approaches to developing guidelines. Consensus guidelines depend upon experts in the field debating and arriving at agreement about what constitutes good practice. The result is formulated in a guideline and shared with healthcare professionals. Consensus guidelines rely on the acknowledged prestige of the experts and their opinion is paramount. Evidence-based guidelines rely upon systematic review of the literature and seek out research to back up recommendations. Evidence-based guidelines are now being preferred to consensus guidelines. Whichever way they are developed, clinical practice guidelines should possess certain attributes (Table 11.1).

Standard setting

A standard is an acceptable or approved example or statement of something against which measurement and judgement takes place. It is a level of quality deemed to be relevant to the activity. Setting standards involves writing and agreeing statements which describe achievable and desirable levels of quality of care. These represent the professionals' expectations of the service and are a statement of intent to the public.

Standard setting is a central component of any quality system. Practitioners can identify and develop their own standards or can adopt and adapt standards which have been developed by other practitioners in similar care settings. In most cases standards are derived from a mixture of local initiatives and borrowed ideas. This is of no consequence as long as the standards are achievable and measurable, locally appropriate and acceptable to practitioners and users of the healthcare service. Visser & de Bekker (1993) developed the mnemonic 'RUMBA' (Relevant, Understandable, Measurable, Behavioural, Attainable) to symbolise the criteria which make up a good standard.

In health care, professional bodies and interest groups for all disciplines are traditionally involved in standard setting in a broad sense; for example, the UKCC produced the Code of Professional Conduct for Nurses, Midwives and Health Visitors (1992) which sets out what is

Table 11.1 Desirable attributes of clinical practice guidelines (Field M J, Lohr K N 1992 Guidelines for clinical practice: from development to use. Institute of Medicine, National Academy Press, Washington. Copyright 1992 National Academy of Sciences, USA).

Attribute	Explanation
Validity	Practice guidelines are valid if, when followed, they lead to the health and cost outcomes projected for them. A prospective assessment of validity will consider the substance and quality of the evidence cited, the means used to evaluate the evidence, and the relationship between evidence and recommendations
Strength of evidence	Practice guidelines should be accompanied by descriptions of the strength of the evidence, and the expert judgements behind them
Estimated outcomes	Guidelines should be accompanied by estimates of the health and cost outcomes expected from the interventions in question, compared with alternative practices. Assessments of relevant health outcomes will consider patient perceptions and preferences
Reliability/reproducibility	Guidelines are considered reliable and reproducible if, given the same evidence and methods for guideline development, another set of experts produces the same statements, and if, given the same clinical circumstances, the guidelines are consistently interpreted and applied by practitioners
Clinical applicability	Guidelines should be as inclusive of appropriately defined patient populations as evidence and expert judgements permit. They should also state the population to which the guideline applies
Clinical flexibility	Guidelines should identify the specifically known or generally expected exceptions to the guideline and discuss how patient preference should be identified and considered
Clarity	Language used should be unambiguous, define terms precisely and use logical, easy to follow modes of presentation
Multidisciplinary process	Guidelines must be developed by a process that includes participation by representatives of key affected groups. Participation may include serving on panels that develop guidelines, providing evidence and viewpoints to the panel and reviewing draft guidelines
Scheduled review	Guidelines must include statements about when they should be reviewed to determine whether revision is warranted, given new clinical evidence or professional consensus
Documentation	The procedures followed in developing guidelines, the participants involved, the evidence used, the assumptions and rationales accepted, and the analytic methods employed must be meticulously documented and described

acceptable behaviour and conduct for a practitioner. Contravention of the code can lead to disciplinary action ranging from suspension to removal from the register. The UKCC have also recently published the PREPP report (1994) which sets standards for post-registration education and practice and which is enacted in the Nurses, Midwives and Health Visitors Act (1995). The RCN as a professional body is involved in developing guidelines and standards for nursing through focused professional forums, such as the Diabetes Nursing Forum. The ENB gives guidelines in relation to the nature and content of education for practice, and validates courses.

In this way professional bodies and interest groups provide both a source of ideas and ready made standards and advice, and support for practitioners developing their own.

Setting local standards which are related to healthcare delivery, is a more recent initiative than national standards and it is logical for local standards to be set by the healthcare professionals who deliver care and who are accountable for it (DHSS Holland 1991). Professionals at this level are sensitive to the needs of the users/consumers of the health service and also possess specialist knowledge. Involvement in quality through standard setting and evaluation of those standards gives ownership to the group. This makes the standards more achievable as well as more locally relevant.

Most activity in this area is related to specific professional groups, such as district nurses or health visitors, although multiprofessional standards are beginning to emerge, for example covering care offered in a general practice setting between a doctor and a practice nurse. Standards for the emerging specialty of CHC nursing are being developed and address areas of overlap between different themes in the umbrella specialty.

Quality is also being specified in contracts between purchasers and providers of health care. What will actually be provided and to what standard is linked to payment. Purchasers are becoming increasingly interested in methods to evaluate care, and in the outcome or health gain resulting from it. In this sense, the market reforms of the NHS exert a powerful influence in determining quality. In response to this, professional bodies such as the RCN and BMA have established working parties or research groups to set overall or central standards, which most consider as providing a framework from which local healthcare providers can devise their own local standards. Local standards should develop out of central standards which draw upon current knowledge, are research-based and ensure that evidence-based practice is incorporated into all episodes of care. In measuring standards, target standards reflect the intended quality of care, and achieved standards reflect what is actually delivered.

How to set standards

The steps involved in setting a standard are:

- Select a topic of relevance
- Select indicators of quality for the care
- Develop criteria and a level of performance which is acceptable
- Identify standards for each criteria; these may be broken down into ideal, average, minimum, unacceptable.

In 1995 the RCN established its Standards of Care Project which set out a programme of research, education and development (Kitson 1986, 1990) which has had a major impact upon the profession. This work led to the publication in 1990 by the RCN of the Dynamic Standard Setting System (DySSSy).

The DySSSy is based on a cyclical approach to quality which originated in the American Nurses' Association model of quality (ANA 1982, Lang & Clinton 1984). The cycle consists of three elements, each further subdivided into four actions

Box 11.2	**Elements in a quality cycle (RCN 1990)**	
Describing	Select a topic for quality improvement	
	Identify a care group	
	Identify criteria in relation to Donabedian's structure, process and outcome definitions (1980)	
	Agree the standard	
Measuring	Refine criteria	
	Select or design an audit tool	
	Collect data	
	Evaluate the data	
Taking action	Consider action to be taken	
	Plan the action	
	Implement the plan	
	Audit	

which are required to achieve the main element to which they relate (Box 11.2).

The DySSSy has its origins in acute health care and was intended for implementation at ward level. It proved to be a useful tool, however, for any nursing activity. It places a strong emphasis on locally relevant and specific standards. It assumes that the results of standard setting will be shared through a quality network with others in similar local settings. Standards developed as a result of DySSSy are automatically subject to review and audit. DySSSy has been adapted for use in community settings (Poulton 1990).

Another example of an approach to quality in relation to community health care is AMBUQUAL, developed by Benson & Miller (1989). AMBUQUAL is a set of quality initiative activities which apply to ambulatory care, community care and outpatient care in the USA which equates roughly to community health care in the UK.

AMBUQUAL takes a multiprofessional approach to quality but can be used by single as well as multiprofessional groups. It could, therefore, be a method for assuring quality in services offered by the PHC teams centred around general practice in which care is a complex mix of nursing, medicine and social care.

AMBUQUAL stipulates 10 measurable dimensions of care:

- Provider performance, relating to either the individuals or the organisation or both
- Support staff performance
- Continuity of care
- Records system
- Risk management in relation to practitioner error or environmental hazards
- User / client satisfaction
- User compliance with health care treatment or advice
- Accessibility
- Appropriateness
- Cost of the provided service.

In practice, each aspect is subdivided into measurable mini-standards. For example, user compliance could be broken down into aspects such as whether the user was part of developing the plan of care and whether he was encouraged to trust the provider of care. These mini-standards are devised locally and each unit using the system has control over the content of the standards.

Debate and agreement on standards are important issues in the support and involvement of clinical staff as providers of care. They can contribute invaluable data to improve clinical standards and access to services and could be linked to staff members and individual performance review (IPR).

Audit

Appraising achievements involves comparing what happens in practice with the defined standard using measurement criteria, which is known as audit. The purpose of audit is to develop practice by identifying elements that are succeeding, to encourage consolidation and improvement, and to identify areas for development. Audit is a critical element of the quality cycle and is the catalyst for dynamic growth and changing practice. It is essential that planning for improvement and taking appropriate action must follow the audit process.

The process of audit offers numerous benefits to primary care if executed as part of the quality cycle.

- It encourages change and service development.

- It makes the most of resources.
- It promotes efficiency.
- It promotes effectiveness.
- It targets care and services to where need is greatest, linked with needs assessment.
- It provides evidence of good care and care which requires action.
- It addresses clients' needs and expectations.
- It raise standards.
- It is a vehicle for communication.
- It provides data for professional defence.
- It makes a case for resource allocation.

Judgements made regarding quality often rely on opinion (Roberts 1987). Regardless of the method of audit or evaluation selected, once the data is gathered a judgement must be made about whether the quality of care is good, requires some development or adaptation or whether it is so poor that the whole process is to be scrapped and recreated.

There are two approaches to exercising judgement about quality, namely implicit and explicit review systems, and the relative merits of each method have been debated (Roberts 1987).

Implicit review systems. An implicit review requires the auditor to use a high degree of inference when a decision is made regarding quality or lack of it. Use is made of consensus amongst groups of experts or peers. Consensus guidelines are designed and appraised in this way. The expert groups can be utilised to actually review care. The decisions they make rely on implicit understanding and agreement. The rationale behind the decision is not articulated to the group under review and in the absence of their decisions being made explicit to outsiders, the leap from observation of care or review of audited data to a decision on quality must be made on inference alone.

Explicit review systems. Explicit review systems purposely try to minimise the amount of inference which is included in a decision about quality. To do this requires very careful specification of what constitutes acceptable quality by professionals involved in care before the care is given or audited. This means standards of care must be designed, agreed and implemented and their means of review agreed in advance. This is what the WHO (1985) meant in its conclusion that the lack of definition of quality hampered the development of quality systems. This system is more acceptable to professionals involved in care as it is more aligned to managed and integral QA programmes. The standards of care may be set by expert groups, but should be agreed by local practitioners.

Who should carry out audit?

There are a number of contenders for the role of auditor in the healthcare setting.

The standard writing group. This group understands the issues in detail, but they may introduce a bias to the audit in favour of the system they have created and ignore different but equally valid perspectives.

Managers. Managers may be able to bring a wider perspective but may be biased or viewed as such. They are perhaps responsible overall for quality, and this might threaten staff. This is particularly true if achievement of quality goals is linked to incentives or IPR.

Peer review. Peers are involved in a similar care setting and are of a similar level of expertise and experience. They have relevant clinical qualifications and experience to understand subtlety within the process perhaps lost by those who have been divorced from the particular subject for a while. They have no vested interest and are usually accepted by colleagues under review. They could be biased in favour of colleagues and may also lack the necessary power or influence to effect change where required.

Outside consultants. Outside consultants are usually acceptable to staff depending upon their background. There is no institutional bias; however, they may lack the relevant expertise and could be expensive.

Audit committee. A group offering multi-representation could involve providers, users and other stakeholders in the audit process. Disadvantages could be the lack of time, training etc. provided by the organisation.

Methods of audit

The complex nature of health and health care – a mix of physical, intellectual, emotional and social aspects of human life – makes quality difficult to measure.

Some aspects and effects of health care are relatively easy to gauge, for example biological changes as a result of medication, but how can a change in values, attitudes and beliefs be measured effectively in relation to health promotion activities? How can prevention be measured? How can a health visitor know, for instance, that an incidence of child abuse has been forestalled because time was spent building up the confidence of a young, disadvantaged mother? This dilemma affects other aspects of CHC nursing practice in relation to health promotion and disease prevention.

Another dilemma in relation to healthcare evaluation is how to separate the effects of technical interventions from other variables such as the interpersonal elements of interaction between the provider of health care and the client? How is the influence of the environment on treatment efficacy or outcomes assessed? Diet, housing, poverty, and health-related knowledge, attitude and expectations all influence the outcome of care (Klien 1980, Donabedian 1986, Whittington 1989). How can health professionals decide whether client improvement is a direct result of the health care offered to them or whether it is due to another variable within their life which enhances or confounds the intervention? These are important questions, particularly because in CHC nursing much of what is offered to clients falls within the hard to measure and intangible categories.

Another issue in relation to measurement of healthcare quality relates to the type of measurement carried out and which aspects of health care are reviewed. Roberts (1987) points out that it is inefficient and impractical to measure everything all of the time and to do so creates a deadlock. There must be prioritisation of what is evaluated. In the USA for instance, evaluation is focused on cost and risk due to a litigation oriented user group (Williamson 1978).

How to audit

Evaluation priorities can be arrived at in a variety of ways, including the tracer method, the sentinel approach and an 'as-it-happens' evaluation.

The tracer method. Kessner (1973) suggests an approach in which a representative view of healthcare activity is sought through tracing the quality of care for certain conditions throughout an episode, the tracer method. It is based on the assumption that the way healthcare professionals routinely manage care for the common conditions and issues presented to them by clients, reflects the way health care is offered throughout the system. The method does not take account of variations in approach between healthcare professionals.

Suitable situations for tracing, according to Kessner, are those which exhibit the following characteristics.

- They are easy to define.
- Healthcare intervention is likely to deliver a positive outcome.
- High and low quality of care are easily identified.
- The confounding or enhancing variables of poverty, diet, housing, attitude, etc., are well understood and can be eliminated.
- The issue to be traced has a high incidence.

Examples of tracer situations include birth visits carried out by health visitors, assessment of patients discharged into the community by district nurses and new patient screening carried out routinely by practice nurses.

Kessner developed the tracer method specifically for use in a primary health care setting, and traced care for visual disorders, otitis media, iron deficiency anaemia, hypertension, UTI and cervical cancer. In 1990, an audit of general practice by the Health Care Research Unit at the University of Newcastle Upon Tyne used a tracer methodology, but added criteria.

Traced situations should:

- Cover the range of mortality and morbidity experienced by the practice population
- Be amenable to treatment or intervention given the range of skills at the disposal of the primary care team

- Be amenable to treatment if there were enough resources at the disposal of the PHC team.

The sentinel approach. Roberts (1987) defined the sentinel approach, which is a retrospective review of healthcare records in which certain 'red flag' incidents identified beforehand are targeted.

Sentinel evaluation is relatively easy to accomplish; the records are a captive resource. However, the data gathered about the episode of care is only as good as the record keeping ability of the person making the records. What is recorded or omitted colours the findings and the evaluation may be biased or skewed.

This approach targets poor quality practice and as such could inhibit the innovative development of good practice. Staff involved in audits such as these tend to view them as punitive, which brings a negative element to the whole process.

The 'as-it-happens' method. Another often used method is to audit care as it happens. This has the advantage that it happens at the same time as the care episode. It does, however, review only one practitioner with an individual client and may not be representative of all care given in similar circumstances. The scale of reviews necessary to make the observation valid is quite large.

A disadvantage of this method is that it can intrude into the healthcare transaction between practitioner and client and this in itself could affect the quality of the service. There is also the issue of confidentiality for clients receiving care and for the practitioners involved in care delivery.

Donabedian's model

Donabedian (1966) categorises the measurement of health service quality into three areas, structure, process and outcome.

Structure. This relates to the infrastructure elements which must be in place to allow care to be organised and offered. These include personnel to carry out care, equipment, supplies and facilities, buildings to house staff and services, record systems to document care and treatment, to follow up clients appropriately and to operate legally, finance to pay staff, maintain and purchase buildings, equipment and so on.

Process. This is planning, implementing, evaluating and adapting care to a community, family or individual. Process is concerned with all of the activities which are involved in the delivery of healthcare services.

Outcome. This is the end result of the care or the service offered. It includes whether the client's condition improved, whether he adapted to a chronic condition, the numbers of cervical cytology specimens taken and so on. Some outcomes are easily measured, for example in cytology results, but others are difficult to quantify, such as client adaptation to chronic illness. Both are the outcomes of health care.

The relationship between structure, process and outcome must be identified if the health service is to be evaluated in those terms (Donabedian 1980). The quality of the structure and process for a given service may be a poor indicator of health outcome. The relationship between health care and outcome for the client is uncertain due to the influence of the interpersonal, cultural and environmental confounding factors.

Berwick & Knapp (1987) suggest that understanding of the relationship between health care and health outcome is so poor, that this is not a useful means of measuring the quality of the health service and is in fact a means of paralysing progress.

Maxwell's (1984) model attempts to measure quality through dividing health care into several areas, some of which relate to concepts of quality expressed earlier in this chapter:

- Timeliness; this includes access, waiting time and action time
- Information clarification; that is, answering what, why, how, when and who
- Technical competence
- Medical and nursing knowledge, skills, expertise, ethics, technology, completeness and treatment success
- Personal interaction between practitioners and

clients; involving courtesy, respect, appropriateness, partnership
- Environment, buildings and infrastructure, cleanliness and amenities.

SUCCESSFUL QUALITY INITIATIVES

For quality initiatives to be successful, commitment from both senior management and operational personnel, clear responsibilities for quality activities, willingness to change if necessary, accurate documentation, effective communication at all levels of the organisation, ongoing training in relation to the concept of quality, ongoing skills training and reflective practice are all required.

The effectiveness of quality programmes is measured by the overall effect and influence they have upon improving the delivery and outcome of health care. A criticism of current quality systems is that they place a heavy emphasis on the audit element of the process and discovering poor performers. There is some emphasis on standards and guidelines and little or no emphasis on developing and advancing practice. The vast majority of practitioners whose care is acceptable could generally develop and improve services (Sisman 1990, O'Leary 1991). In this respect, current quality techniques could be seen as mechanistic (Ellis & Whittington 1993). Barter (1988) suggests that there is currently no evidence to suggest that any of the current activities undertaken at great expense to the health service, gives any tangible long-term benefits to improving care. Audit must result in changes to practice so that previous low standards of care do not recur.

There is a movement towards developing CQI because most quality initiatives do not appear to yield practice improvements. This matches the current philosophy of audit for primary health care which has developed out of medical audit advisory groups (MAAGs). The CQI model encourages organisational development and has its roots, as does much of the quality culture, in industry (WHO 1985, Roberts 1987, Buckland 1989, Keyser 1989, Williams 1989, Wong 1989, Dagher & Lloyd 1991).

Box 11.3 **The Pier model**

P   Planned principal functions
I   Identification of performance indicators and
    important components
E   Evaluation/audit
R   Response with feedback leading to identified
    action

CQI is a structured system for creating organisation wide participation in planning and implementing a continuous improvement process to meet and exceed customer needs, and this is illustrated in the Pier model (Box 11.3).

O'Leary (1991) suggests that the distinction between QA and CQI lies in the recognition in CQI of the human element in health care, and that it takes account of the diversity and complexity of what is essentially a multidisciplinary enterprise. This acknowledgement, O'Leary suggests, leads to greater emphasis on the individual and upon developing interdisciplinary networks. Prevention of problem situations and service development are paramount.

THE COST OF QUALITY

A complex relationship exists between quality and the cost of health care. Health care does not produce an easily quantifiable product the way industrial processes do. Therefore, a strict relationship between cost and outcome is difficult to define. Health economists have debated this issue and the arguments discussed earlier regarding defining quality are similar to those regarding cost and quality. Different kinds of costs can be identified.

Failure costs. These costs are a consequence of lack of quality within the system. Not meeting agreed standards, not having standards at all, or having inappropriate standards are causes of diminishing quality and rising costs. Incompatible treatment through failure to communicate, plan and co-ordinate, late treatment of curable conditions, inappropriate treatment or drugs and indemnity costs if the client sues, are only some of the possible but potentially disastrous results.

Utilisation costs. When resources, human and other, are not used to best effect, utilisation costs are incurred. These include inappropriate use of skills, for example, personnel being asked to carry out tasks for which they are either under-, over- or not qualified; under-utilisation of available skill, over-utilisation of drugs and treatments and over-utilisation of personnel, for example, inappropriate repeat appointments, poorly maintained equipment.

Appraisal costs. Operating a quality service leads to appraisal costs incurred by administering and monitoring a system to appraise and assess the quality of care.

Prevention costs. These costs are incurred by performing activities aimed at keeping failure to a minimum, including development and maintenance of a quality system, developing and improving standards, education and training.

A certain level of cost is inevitable, but the aim is to keep costs to a minimum. Paramount within this objective is the creation of an effective and efficient workforce. Primary health care is provided by groups of teams which will help to create and maintain a well-organised system. The requirements for teams to function effectively are the creation of a leader, frequent informal as well as formal meetings, interaction on a personal level, similar attitudes and values, agreement on the purpose for the group, agreement, implicit or explicit, about the division of labour, and effective discussion skills (Argyll 1969). A poorly functioning team system incurs extra costs due to loss of morale and goodwill. Every penny lost is lost to direct client care. As much as 40% of operating costs may be lost, linked directly to poor quality (Jones & Macilwaine 1991).

Change

Successful quality initiatives are characterised by the extent to which practice develops as a result of the whole process. Delivery of good quality care depends upon four factors: knowledge, skill, attitude and organisation (Lawrence & Schofield 1993).

In a survey carried out by Ashbough &

McKean (1976), 95% of poor results in primary health care audits were the result of inadequate performance rather than lack of knowledge. Lawrence & Schofield (1993) suggest that as a consequence the first action to take is to ask whether making organisational change will enhance practice.

Change is a complex process and in order to manage change effectively as part of CQI it is necessary to understand the process. Lewin (1951) identified three stages of change: unfreezing, cognitive redefinition and refreezing, described in detail in Chapter 7. It is important that everyone involved in the change process is included at each stage.

Strategies for achieving planned change include:

- An empirical, rational approach which assumes that all human beings are rational and will act in accordance with rational self-interest
- A normative re-educative approach which considers that change will only be effected if individuals within the structure adapt their normative orientation and commitment to old patterns and become loyal to new structures. This relies upon attitudinal change fed by information over a period of time.

Most people view change as a crisis situation. There are several stages which individuals experience as they adapt to new circumstances:

- Shock; an inability to plan, reason and make decisions
- Retreat; when there is an unwillingness or inability to face the situation. This is characterised by a tendency to trivialise it
- Acknowledgement of the reality of the situation is accompanied by the beginning of a search for a solution
- Adaptation; change is now evident

There are also several reasons why change may be resisted:

- Inconvenience; the working environment may become more difficult or existing working practices may be exposed as inadequate
- New ideas and new learning may have to be acquired. Perhaps the individual feels threatened or assumes her knowledge is undervalued
- Change brings uncertainty and this gives rise to irrational fears
- Social and working relationships may change and the individual may feel her status within the team or with colleagues is devalued
- Change may be imposed and this causes resentment.

Summary

Quality issues are integral to providing primary health care. There are many elements relating to quality but practitioners should be encouraged to use quality assurance techniques to try to improve the care of patients and advance practice. The key to this is understanding why quality issues are important in today's healthcare environment. The delivery of health care is a complex process that involves a number of factors such as interpersonal skills, culture, expectations clinical skill, technology and available resources. Reforms of the NHS have tried to shift the balance of power to clients so that they are able to demand and receive the services they require to meet their needs. Practitioners of all disciplines must engage with clients to ensure the services offered meet the needs of clients and that nurses and their professional colleagues continue to assess and meet need appropriately.

REFERENCES

American Nurses' Association 1982 Nursing quality assurance management learning system. ANA, Kansas
Argyll M 1969 Social interaction. Methuen, UK
Barter J T 1988 Accreditation surveys: nit picking or quality seeking. Hospital and Community Psychiatry 39(7):707
Benson D, Miller J 1989 AMBUQUAL: an ambulatory quality assurance and quality management system. In: Ellis R,

Whittington D (eds) Quality assurance in health care: a handbook. Edward Arnold, UK
Berwick, Knapp 1987 Theory and practice for measuring health care quality. Health Care Financing Review Annual Supplement 49–55
Black N, 1990 Quality assurance of medical care. Journal of Public Health Medicine 12(2):97–104

Buckland A E 1989 In search of quality. Journal of the American Medical Record Association 60(3):27–31

Dagher D O, Lloyd R J 1991 Managing negative outcome by reducing variances in the emergency department. Quality Review Bulletin 17(1):15–21

Department of Health 1993 The patients' charter. HSG (93)27 HMSO, London

Department of Health and Social Security (Holland) 1991 Policy document on health care quality. In: Visser G, de Bekker J 1993 Quality requirements in nursing departments: development and use of general framework. Quality Assurance in Health Care 5(3):255–259

Donabedian A 1966 Evaluating the quality of medical care. Millbank Memorial Fund Quarterly 44(2):166–206

Donabedian A 1980 Explorations in quality assessment and monitoring, volume 1. Ann Arbour, Health administration pack

Donabedian A 1986 Quality assurance: corporate responsibility for multihospital systems. Quality Review Bulletin 12(1):3–7

Donabedian A 1989 The quest for health care: whose choice? Whose responsibility? Mount Sinai Journal of Medicine 56(5):406–422

Ellis R, Whittington D 1993 Quality assurance in health care: a handbook. Edward Arnold, UK

Field M J, Lohr K N 1992 Guidelines for clinical practice: from development to use. Institute of Medicine, National Academy Press, Washington DC

Fine R B 1986 Conceptual perspectives on the organisation design task and the quality assurance function. Nursing Health Care 7(2):100–104

Health Care Research Unit 1990 North of England study of standards and performance in general practice. Setting clinical standards with small groups, final report no 4. Health Care Research Unit, Newcastle Upon Tyne

Hill, Russel M, Gill S, Marchment M, Morgan J, Everett T 1990 Introducing TQM – a training manual. South East Staffordshire Health Authority

Jones J, Macilwaine H 1991 Diagnosing the organisation: the health authorities' experience of total quality management. Journal of Health Care Quality Assurance 4(4):22

Kelly P J, Swift R S 1991 Total quality management – getting started. International Journal of Health Care Quality Assurance 4(5):27

Kessner D M 1973 Assessing health quality – the case for tracers. New England Journal Of Medicine. 228:189–194

Keyser W 1989 Health care: is TQM relevant? Total Quality Management 110–115

Kitson A 1986 The methods of assuring quality. Nursing Times 27(8):32–34

Kitson A 1990 Quality matters and standard setting. Nursing Standard 4(44):32–33

Klien R 1980 The politics of the NHS. Longman, UK

Lang N M, Clinton J F 1984 Quality assurance: the idea and its development in the USA. In: Willis L, Linwood M (eds) Measuring the quality of care. Churchill Livingstone, UK

Laughlin M 1993 The illusion of quality health care analysis. Journal of Health Philosophy and Policy 1(1):69–73

Lawrence M, Schofield T 1993 Medical audit in primary care. In: Lawrence M, Schofield T (eds) Primary health care. Oxford GP Series 25, Oxford

Lohr K N 1994 Guidelines for clinical practice: applications for primary health care. International Journal for Quality in Health Care 6(1):17–25

Maxwell R J 1984 Quality assessment in health. British Medical Journal 288:1470–1471

Nurses, Midwives and Health Visitors Act 1995 HMSO, London

O'Leary D S 1991 CQI – a step beyond QA. Quality Review Bulletin 17(1):4–5

Poulton B 1990 Evaluating health visiting practice. Nursing Standard 5(3):36–39

Roberts J S 1987 Reviewing the quality of care: priorities for improvement. Health Care Financing Review Supplement 69–74

Rodriguez A R 1988 The effects of contemporary economic conditions on availability and quality of mental health services. In: Stricker G, Rodriguez A R (eds) Handbook of quality assurance in mental health. Plenum, New York

Royal College of Nursing 1990 Dynamic standard setting system. RCN, UK

Schmadl J C 1979 Quality assurance: examination of the concept. Nursing Outlook 27(7):462–465

Shaw C D 1986 Introducing quality assurance. The King's Fund, UK

Sisman B 1990 Quality assurance: myth? Quality Review Bulletin 16(8):278

United Kingdom Central Council for Nursing, Midwifery and Health Visiting 1992 The code of professional conduct. UKCC, London

United Kingdom Central Council for Nursing, Midwifery and Health Visiting 1994 The future of professional practice – the council's standards for education and practice following negotiation. UKCC, London

Visser G, de Bekker J 1993 Quality requirements in nursing departments: development and use of general framework. Quality Assurance in Health Care 5(3):255–259

Whittington D 1989 Performance indicators and quality assurance in the NHS. In: Ellis R, Whittington D (eds) Quality assurance in health care: a handbook. Edward Arnold, UK

Williams S A 1989 Total quality management. In: Spath P (ed) Innovations in health care quality measurement. American Hospital Publishing, Chicago

Williamson J W 1978 Assessing and improving health care outcomes: the health accounting approach to quality assurance. Ballinger, Cambridge, Massachusetts

Wong H 1989 Quality measurement and customer service. In: Spath P (ed) Innovations in health care quality measurement. American Hospital Publishing, Chicago

World Health Organization 1985 The principles of quality assurance. In: European Reports And Studies, 1994. WHO, Copenhagen

WHO Working Group on Quality Assurance 1995 WHO, Copenhagen

Wright C, Whittington D 1992 Quality assurance – an introduction for health care professionals. Churchill Livingstone, UK

Yorkshire RHA, Northwest Region, South Thames Region West, NHS in Scotland, NHS in Wales, NHS Training Division 1994 Using information in practice management – setting the context – quality and audit. Greenhalgh, HMSO, London

12 Research informing practice

Pam Smith

The NHS research and development strategy emphasises epidemiology and randomised controlled trials as means of producing evidence on which to base health care delivery. Therefore there is a need for community health care nurses to re-examine the role of natural sciences as a model for research and practice. This also involves considering the debate over descriptions of research as qualitative or quantitative. There is a range of philosophical and methodological approaches to research which nurses must assess critically for their applicability to their own practice. To be able to carry this out, nurses must understand the major influences within social sciences which, together with the natural sciences, have shaped health care, nursing and community healthcare research. They must also be aware of associated issues such as ethics, research proposals, funding, validity and reliability.

CONTEXT OF NURSING AND HEALTHCARE RESEARCH

The current context of nursing and healthcare research can be assessed by reviewing key documents issued by the professional bodies and the NHS Executive.

Key nursing documents

The International Council of Nursing (1990) stated that there is 'no health without research' and that research should be promoted in all countries; the ICN is in the process of developing an international agenda which emphasises the role of governments and professional nursing bodies in focusing on and implementing research.

The United Kingdom Central Council for Nursing, Midwifery and Health Visiting's (1992) Code of Professional Conduct emphasised the need for practice to be based on up-to-date knowledge.

The Department of Health's (1993) taskforce report emphasised the need for nurses, midwives and health visitors to participate in multidisciplinary research, as well as for academic nursing departments to develop research programmes in specialist fields and organise research training. The shift from small-scale projects to systematic, generalisable research was recommended. The need for dedicated funding and scholarships to pay for nursing research and research training, from the national research councils such as the Medical Research Council (MRC) and Economic and Social Sciences Research Council (ESSRC) as well as the Department of Health, was expressed. The ultimate aim of research was to inform and improve practice.

The then National Health Service Management Executive (1993) in its document 'New Worlds, New Opportunities: Nursing in Primary Health Care', places general practice populations at the heart of community nursing. Nurses are identified as key players in health profiling, commissioning, purchasing, policy formation, auditing, monitoring and service provision. Research, primary health care and public health are clearly interdependent in supporting these activities.

Key NHS research and development documents

It is important to place nursing and primary health care research within the broader context of the Department of Health research and development strategy, launched in 1991.

The NHS research and development strategy marked the first national framework for setting research priorities. One of the prime aims of the strategy was to promote a research culture within the NHS which moved the base of clinical practice from ritual to evidence and improved the quality of patient care. The strategy took into account the newly organised purchaser/provider health service (Department of Health 1989) and the 'Health of the Nation' policy document (Department of Health 1992) which specified five priority areas for improving the nation's health, namely:

- Coronary heart disease and stroke
- Cancers
- Mental illness
- HIV/AIDS
- Accidents.

Research and development programmes were set up for each of these areas in order to document and reduce the incidence of disease and investigate treatment outcomes. In turn, it was suggested that the findings of such investigations could be used to develop audit tools. The responsibility for these programmes was devolved to the regional health authorities which, in 1996, were incorporated into the Department of Health.

Harris (1993) believes that the changes within the NHS offer opportunities to redress the balance between the hospital dominated research programmes of the past and population-based primary health care (PHC) research of the future. Certainly in the field of community nursing there has been a dearth of research in favour of topics associated with the care of hospitalised adults.

Further developments have taken place in the NHS, particularly in relation to research that contributes to 'evidence-based practice'. Health service purchasers setting up contracts with providers are more likely to purchase a service or treatment if research has 'proved' its effectiveness. Systematic reviews of clinical trials, including nursing interventions, are being undertaken to provide evidence for improving health care. Centres at Oxford and York have been established to review trial findings and disseminate their results nation-wide.

More recently, the Culyer report (Department of Health 1994), concerned with addressing potential threats to research funding and support associated with the NHS market reforms, contained proposals to prevent this happening. The report recommended closer collaboration between the NHS and the academic research communities so that service oriented research would not be squeezed out by the traditionally more prestigious medically-led scientific research. One set of recommendations were specifically aimed at improving the chances of 'Cinderella settings and disciplines' (including nursing, midwifery and health visiting) to secure research funding (Culyer 1995). In this way, health-based research was seen as having a double benefit by both preventing people becoming clients in the first place and improving the treatment and care of those who did. Finally, it provided 'knowledge that may benefit all' (Culyer 1995).

DEFINING TERMS

What is research?

The definitions discussed here were selected and summarised by Czuber-Dochan et al (1997) while preparing a seminar on research mindedness.

In 1989, Macleod Clark & Hockey defined research as 'an attempt to increase the body of knowledge, that is, what is currently known about nursing, by the discovery of new facts and relationships through a process of systematic scientific enquiry'. For Macleod Clark and Hockey, 'the essential characteristic of research is its scientific nature'. The Department of Health's (1993) definition saw research as the acquisition of knowledge which includes 'gaining information, clarification and illumination as well as translating it [research] directly into policy or practice'. This last point suggests the important role practitioners play in assessing critically the relevance of research for practice.

Drawing on these and other texts, Czuber-Dochan et al (1997) characterise research as:

- A process
- Scientific
- Objective
- Systematic
- Problem solving
- Advancement of knowledge

- Exploration of facts and relationships
- An enquiring attitude.

The authors conclude:

As the list of features indicates, we adopted a broad concept of research because we saw it as being representative of the 'real world' of nursing. We believed that conceptualising research in this way would provide opportunities to embrace both the art and the science of nursing knowledge. It would also support the notion that nursing, like research, is a diverse activity that takes place in a variety of settings.

The research process

Czuber-Dochan et al (1997) refer to research as a process. The research process offers a conventional but convenient and useful framework in which to fit the paradigms, approaches and methods of research that are explored throughout this chapter.

The research process refers to the different stages involved in undertaking a research project. Like any process, however, although research is represented as being divided into distinct stages which follow on from each other, often they are not mutually exclusive.

The research process involves identifying a topic, specifying underlying theories, formulating questions, selecting a suitable approach, specifying methods and devising a plan to take the study forward.

An important part of the research plan includes the careful consideration of time and financial budgeting, secretarial support and obtaining ethical clearance. Time spent resolving outstanding organisational, political and ethical issues at the planning stage can have significant benefits over the rest of the study.

The stages of the research process can be grouped as shown in Box 12.1.

The way in which researchers take the research process forward will depend to some extent on whether a qualitative or quantitative research approach is adopted. Many researchers involved in studying health and its delivery prefer to see the so-called distinction as more of a continuum in which, as Bell (1993) suggests, 'no approach

Box 12.1   Stages of the research process

- Identifying the research problem
- Selecting an appropriate research approach
- Designing the study
- Developing data collecting methods and techniques
- Collecting the data
- Organisation, analysis and interpretation of the data
- Writing and presentation of research findings

prescribes nor automatically rejects any particular method'. It is common in social science to see the use of a multi-method research approach or 'triangulation' by which more than one method is used and/or group of people studied within the same project (Denzin 1989).

Research mindedness

Ever since the Briggs report (DHSS 1972) recommended that nursing and midwifery should become a research-based profession, research has been on the educational and practice agendas. This does not mean that every practitioner and teacher is actually engaged in research projects, but it is quite likely that at some stage in their pre- and post-registration education, they either have undertaken, or will be required to undertake, research-based assignments. Community nursing programmes expect participants to undertake neighbourhood profiles and family case studies which incorporate aspects of the research process. A recent Post Registration Education Project (PREP) factsheet on continuing education (UKCC 1995) identifies research as an integral component of education and practice which contributes to and enriches advanced clinical practice as a whole. In turn, an increase in nursing research and research-based practice was identified as an outcome of advanced clinical practice.

The first step to undertaking research and incorporating it into practice is to become research minded. The Royal College of Nursing's (RCN 1982) Research Society defined research mindedness as 'a critical and questioning

approach to one's work, the desire and ability to find out about the latest research in the area and apply it as appropriate'.

For the community nurse practitioner who shares many similar work experiences with social workers, the elements of research mindedness identified by Everitt et al (1992) seem appropriate (Box 12.2).

Box 12.2   The characteristics of the research minded practitioner (Everitt et al 1992)

- Constantly defining and making explicit their objectives and hypotheses
- Treating their explanations of the social world as hypotheses, that is, as tentative and open to be tested against evidence
- Aware of their expertise and knowledge and that of others
- Bringing to the fore theories that help make sense of social need, resources and assisting in decision making with regard to strategies
- Thoughtful, reflecting on data and theory and contributing to their development and refinement
- Scrutinising and analysing available data and information
- Mindful of the pervasiveness of ideology and values in the way we see and understand the world

Their definition of research mindedness reflects an integrated approach to research-based practice. The emphasis for the authors is clearly not on doing research but on using its theoretical perspectives and methods to think analytically about and inform practice. Research mindedness also allows practitioners to identify their own knowledge and expertise which would otherwise be unrecognised and undetected. Being research minded, therefore, encourages us to think critically, challenge current situations and construct arguments to defend resources and assist decision making.

Another way of thinking about research is as an 'enterprise' that dares practitioners to think creatively and take risks. This view is not dissimilar to Medawar's (1984) view of science:

The word 'science' itself is used as a general name for, on the one hand, the procedures of science – adventures of thought and stratagems of inquiry that go into the advancement of learning – and on the other hand, the substantive body of knowledge that is the outcome of this complex endeavour.

The relationship between knowledge and research

Since one of the purposes of research is to discover and produce new knowledge about the world, it is important to have reached a working understanding of what knowledge is. The ways in which researchers do this depend to some extent on their own theories of knowledge, referred to as 'epistemology'. Knowledge tends to be synonymous with the facts and theories drawn on to teach and practice. Smith (1994) defines epistemology as a 'knowledge producing system' that each individual learns to develop from early childhood.

Defining epistemology in these different ways distinguishes between formal knowledge which guides and is produced as part of scientific research, and the common sense or informal knowledge which develops from early childhood. Practitioners also develop 'on the job' knowledge about community nursing through caring for patients and clients.

Carper's (1978) framework of knowledge is useful for looking at the patterns or processes by which nursing knowledge is produced. Carper describes four patterns of knowing:

- The formal approaches associated with traditional scientific methods, which she refers to as 'empirics' or 'empirical' as in the sense of systematic, scientific observation
- The knowledge associated with the art of nursing, described as 'aesthetics', of which empathy is a key component
- The personal knowledge unique to each individual and the use of 'self' in relationships with others
- The type of knowledge associated with moral decision making and ethics.

Traditionally, scientific or empirical knowledge, which tends to predominate in medicine, possesses more credibility than aesthetic or personal knowledge. One reason for the high status of scientific knowledge is its association with facts and theories; but, on closer scrutiny, these facts and theories can change. This is particularly apparent in the literature on risk factors in health.

One recent example is the view of stress as a risk factor in the development of peptic ulcers being replaced by a bacterial model of disease causation. Researchers have now shown that there is a strong association between the organism *Heliocobacter pylori* and the occurrence of the condition (Moore 1995).

In the context of changing facts and theories, Rees (1992) writes 'We must accept that the information and research we talk about today is based on yesterday's understanding'. We need, therefore, 'to understand the limitations of our present knowledge' and acquire 'skills to evaluate new information and research findings and to apply this to tomorrow's situations' (Rees 1992).

It is clearly important for practitioners to think about different types of knowledge and how they are valued. Exploring the links between knowledge, reflection and research as part of becoming a reflective practitioner, is one way of developing and validating personal knowledge.

Knowledge, reflection and research

Benner (1984) and Schön (1987) explore the close association between knowledge, reflection and research. Benner's research illustrates the use of reflection in the nurse's skills acquisition as she moves from being a novice to an expert. According to Schön (1987), this process takes place through 'reflection in action' as practitioners develop 'professional artistry' to bridge the theory–practice gap. Reflection may also be retrospective as practitioners think back on situations after they have occurred. They may then use their feelings to evaluate the situation and gain new insights, understandings and knowledge. One way to do this is to keep a reflective diary as a record of the situations experienced and the insights gained over time.

Reflective practice assists the practitioner to become more research minded. Similarly, researchers who use interviews and participant observation work in a reflective and analytic way, moving between the research field and their data to guide their future research, make interpretations and develop findings.

It is possible to see how the researcher who is also a practitioner, can draw insights from his own knowledge of the field both to reflect on practice, and also to develop research findings.

In a series of papers compiled by the Health Visitors' Association (1994) the contribution of community nurses to healthcare commissioning, monitoring and evaluation was emphasised, with regard to their knowledge of local populations. This knowledge was described as 'qualitative' and 'anecdotal'. In this context the reflective diary is a powerful tool available to the practitioner for the purpose of accumulating qualitative and anecdotal evidence for commissioning and evaluating health care.

The relationship of knowledge to paradigms and theories

Carper (1978) suggests that practitioners produce different types of knowledge according to four patterns or processes of knowing that are aligned with particular views of the world, assumptions or values. These are referred to as paradigms.

The term paradigm, first used by the physicist turned philosopher of science Kuhn (1970), is defined in two basic ways: first, as the range of beliefs, assumptions, values and techniques shared by a scientific community; and second, as the procedures used to solve specific problems and take theories to their logical conclusions. Positivism, the interpretive tradition, critical theory and feminism are all examples of paradigms.

Theory, a term often used in the context of research and associated with the formalisation of knowledge, can be described as a set of concepts which highlight and explain the world about us. Often a theory is the answer to a 'Why?' question: why, for example do some people develop lung cancer and others not; or why do some women have low birth weight babies and others not? By looking at the distribution of lung cancer or low birth weight babies in a number of differ-

ent populations, it may be possible to construct a general theory about the factors affecting these conditions. Theories may also provide predictions. Smoking, for example, has emerged as an important predictor of both lung cancer and low birth weight.

Feminist social work practitioners and researchers Everitt et al (1992) hold a more sceptical view of the role of theory in research. They see theory as a provisional set of explanations that at any time may be reformulated and revised.

Approaches, methodologies and methods

The research approach to a study usually refers to the approach adopted by a researcher working within a specific paradigm (Haase & Myers 1988). Methodology is defined by Silverman (1993) as a general approach to studying research topics and as such can be used interchangeably with 'approach'. The concept of methodology or approach as opposed to research method, concerns the philosophy and theory that drives the research rather than the practicalities of data collection and analysis in the field.

Methods, therefore, are the techniques of doing research: asking questions, observing people and groups, analysing case records, sifting through historical documents and local newspapers (Everitt et al 1992). A variety of research methods can be used within a study, irrespective of the underlying paradigm and approach.

Choosing research paradigms and approaches

Novice researchers begin to develop a preference for particular philosophies, paradigms and approaches as they become exposed to the range of options available to them.

Qualitative or quantitative research? Research may be described as 'qualitative' or 'quantitative'. Bryman (1988) suggests that these terms have come to 'signify much more than ways of gathering data: they came to denote divergent assumptions about the nature and purposes of research in the social sciences'.

For behaviourial psychologists, epidemiologists studying the distribution of diseases in populations and clinicians conducting clinical trials, the methodology of choice is likely to involve experimentation, careful observation, measurement and control. Because this type of methodology is associated with numbers and counting, it is described as quantitative.

Anthropologists, however, are more likely to use interactive methodologies which involve participant observation and in-depth interviewing, to describe and explain qualities of phenomena. This is described as 'qualitative'.

For nurse researchers, there is still a tendency to describe their research as qualitative or quantitative when referring to methods rather than underlying paradigms and approaches. According to qualitative researchers Guba & Lincoln (1994), research methods can be described as qualitative or quantitative irrespective of paradigm. For them, questions of method are secondary to questions of paradigm. They state, 'Paradigm issues are crucial; no inquirer, we maintain, ought to go about the business of inquiry without being clear about just what paradigm informs and guides his or her approach'.

Haase & Myers (1988) make the case for nurses to value and integrate a range of paradigms and approaches by reconciling rather than choosing between qualitative and quantitative research. Their framework is useful for thinking about the feasibility of developing combined approaches to research in a market-led health service that emphasises both quality and cost-effectiveness.

An example of this approach can be found in Pound et al's (1995) paper which describes the use of qualitative in-depth interviews as an alternative to large-scale surveys to explore the components of hospital care valued by people having had a stroke. The authors explain that previous studies have assumed that patients prefer to stay at home following stroke, but using a different approach, this study revealed otherwise. Patients were shown to use both technical and psychosocial criteria to evaluate both the process and outcome of their care.

To some extent the choice of particular paradigms, approaches or methods will depend on the researcher's preference but also on the purpose of the research, the topic under study, the subject discipline and the funding body.

HISTORICAL ACCOUNTS OF SCIENCE, RESEARCH AND KNOWLEDGE

The dictionary definition of science, and its association with knowledge, observation, experimentation, testing and general principles, represents a common account of how scientific research is conducted. It has its origins in seventeenth century Europe when new ways of thinking, referred to as 'enlightenment thought' were emerging. One of the famous names associated with the new thinking was René Descartes (1596–1650) a French philosopher and mathematician whose claim 'I think, therefore I am' emphasises the importance afforded to rational thought and the idea that the mind and body are two separate entities operating in distinct ways. For Descartes, the body was made up of lifeless matter that reduced it to a series of mechanical operations subject to the same laws as the physical world.

Descartes' reductionist and mechanistic view of the body being separate from the rational mind and his emphasis on thinking rather than feeling, is characterised as 'Cartesian dualism' or the mind–body split. Descartes has exerted a significant influence on science in general and medical and nursing research in particular. Lock & Gordon (1988) suggest that the mind–body split 'limits our understanding not only of illness, but also of what we accept as knowledge'. They suggest that seeing the world in this Cartesian way marginalises intuition, emotions and experiences. They also suggest that the medical research perspective fits closest to the notion of 'pure science'.

'Enlightenment thinking' allowed nature and the physical world to be presented as orderly, lawful and predictable and hence amenable to systematic observation and experiment. Isaac Newton used this approach to derive mechanistic laws and theories about the nature of the universe, including gravity, on which modern physics is based. According to Chalmers (1982) and Nielsen (1990), physics has become the 'gold standard' by which scientific research is judged, based on the assumption that its methods are reliable and can produce 'hard' facts.

This view of science, by which the factual basis of scientific knowledge is established through systematic observation and measurement rather than relying on intuition or subjective experiences, is referred to as empiricism. The traditional empirical method has two stages:

1. Gathering of data directly through our external senses (i.e. sense data), with no preconception as to how it is ordered or what explains it
2. Induction of patterns and relationships within the data.

Induction means that the researcher moves from individual observations about data to statements about general patterns within it (Coolican 1990).

Deduction is the next stage in the scientific process, going beyond induction to develop and test formal theories. Although induction and deduction are often explained as two separate processes, in reality they are often used alongside each other.

Empiricism is based on the notion that 'facts speak for themselves' and Smith (1994) cautions that it can lead to 'mindless fact gathering' if researchers have no theoretical expectations for their data. It may also lead to an assumption that facts are value free. This is a particularly important point when considering the wide use of surveys in health service and social research.

Empiricism is integral to positivism, which is attributed to the work of the French philosopher Comte (1789–1857). Positivist philosophies of science assume the discovery of a body of independent, objective knowledge able to explain, predict and control the phenomena under study.

The most extreme form of positivism is characterised in the early part of the twentieth century by the hypothetico-deductionism of the logical positivists referred to as the Vienna Circle of scholars. Hypothetico-deductionism closely resembles the formula familiar in epidemiological studies:

hypotheses are devised and tested in order to verify theories and make predictions. An hypothesis is a tentative proposition by which the researcher formalises the research question into a statement about the expected relationship between phenomena. Often the hypothesis is stated in terms of causality such as 'smoking causes lung cancer'. The phenomena (smoking and lung cancer) are broken down or reduced to smaller components known as 'variables' which are assumed to have some explanatory value which will contribute to theory testing and prediction. Smoking, for example, may be broken down into variables such as type and number of cigarettes smoked and over how many years; lung cancer may be examined in relation to variables such as the patient's age and class status.

The hypothetico-deductive research approach is characterised as logical, rational, objective, value free, based on ultimately verifiable truth, laws, and measurement. This approach has been criticised by many social researchers as inappropriate for the study of people because it is 'reductionist'. In other words, complex phenomena are reduced to small unrelated units rather than putting them in the context of whole systems or persons.

Epidemiology, the cornerstone science of public health, is underpinned by positivism and the hypothetico-deductive approach to research. It is concerned with 'the occurrence, distribution and determinants of states of health and disease in human groups and populations' (Abramson 1990). Epidemiological studies include descriptive surveys, explanatory surveys and experiments, and serve three main purposes: for community diagnosis, aetiology, and the evaluation of health care. The purpose of these studies is to answer the 'cardinal questions that face practitioners of community medicine' (Kark 1981, cited in Abramson 1990). These questions are listed in Box 12.3.

Epidemiological studies contribute to family and community oriented primary care which integrates individual and community care (Fig. 12.1) (Abramson 1990).

As Figure 12.1 indicates, primary care researchers recognise the need to move away from reductionist studies which test hypothe-

- What is the state of health of the community?
- What are the factors responsible for this state of health?
- What is being done about it by the healthcare system and by the community itself?
- What more can be done, what is proposed, and what is the expected outcome?
- What measures are needed to continue health surveillance of the community and to evaluate the effect of what is being done?

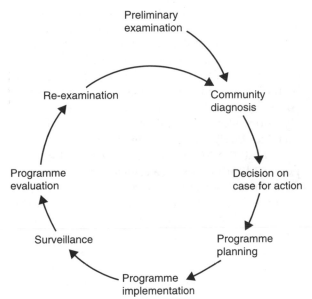

Figure 12.1 Stages of community-oriented primary care (Abramson 1990). (Reproduced with kind permission.)

ses to holistic, participative studies of communities.

Popper (Magee 1973), an influential philosopher of science, was also critical of positivism. He argued that no matter how many times we observe that A follows B we can never be sure that the next time we make an observation B may not follow A. Even though we know the sun rises every day we can never be sure that this will be the case tomorrow. Popper devised the notion of falsification by which the spirit of the research enterprise was to strive constantly to falsify theories by retesting them.

At the same time as the logical positivists rose to prominence, advances in physics, such as quantum theory and Einstein's theory of relativity, were incorporating principles of uncertainty and unpredictability within the physical world. These theories are very different from Newton's mechanistic views and it is interesting that they are not incorporated into the popular view of science. The logical positivists were seemingly untouched by the changes taking place in physics (Chalmers 1982). Furthermore, their views of science and research and their association with deductive reasoning and reductionism continued to have enormous influence. In Watson's (1981) view, until recently it was the logical positivists who exerted the main influence on nursing research.

THE SOCIAL, POLITICAL AND PERSONAL RESEARCH CONTEXT

The dominant accounts of science, medicine, nursing, research and knowledge represented in textbooks and journals are likely to be represented as objective and value free.

Lock (1988) takes issue with this representation, pointing out that:

- Medicine and science are permeated by social forces
- Medicine and science are social enterprises
- Researchers are interrelated with their scientific community
- The scientific community is located within broader religious, social and political currents.

Lock (1988) describes researchers as interrelated with their scientific communities through their shared knowledge 'and the broader religious, social and political currents within which the community exists'.

The impact of these religious, social and political currents on the scientific community are graphically illustrated in Shilts' (1987) account of the discovery of the AIDS virus in the USA. He describes the concealment of and lack of interest in researching what was seen as 'a gay plague' as a combination of the effects of government budget cuts and the homophobia of certain sections of the social, political and religious community.

Smith (1994) suggests that financial considerations played a part in delaying the uptake of the bacterial theory proposed for peptic ulcer formation, despite the major flaws in the dominant stress model, because the pharmaceutical companies stood to lose large amounts of money when the drugs they had produced to control the secretion of hydrochloric acid were seen no longer to play the key role in the treatment of peptic ulcers.

The influence of Kuhn (1970) is evident in the writings of both Lock and Smith. In a major critique of science, Kuhn debunks a number of assumptions including the myth of objectivity. Rather, science is identified as a social activity rooted in the scientific community and a part of the wider society. Kuhn also challenges the idea that science follows a neat linear process by which theories are refuted when they no longer stand the rigour of scientific testing. In reality, their survival (as the peptic ulcer theory suggests) depends on whether they continue to be supported by members of the scientific (and business) establishment. Kuhn argues that scientific progress depends on a revolution by which one paradigm is replaced when no longer compatible with another. The changes which took place in theoretical physics from Newton's mechanistic laws to Einstein's theory of relativity described above are examples of a paradigm shift.

An article in the *New York Times* presented a new theory of menstruation, proposed by Profet, a young woman scientist (Angier 1993). The proposal illustrates the interplay of personal as well as social and political factors in the context of science. In contrast to male biologists, Profet's personal situation as a young woman led her to ask a different set of questions and pose new hypotheses about the role of menstruation. In time, her new theory may have the potential to trigger a paradigm shift within the biological sciences.

By drawing attention to the social, political and personal component of the philosophies, theories and assumptions that drive the research enterprise, the importance of recognising that research is not neutral but takes place within a social context informed by underlying values, assumptions and a belief system has been demonstrated. It follows, therefore, that the knowledge produced is shaped by our belief systems. However, the predominant view in science, medicine and health care is that objective knowledge can be produced.

SOCIAL SCIENCE, RESEARCH AND KNOWLEDGE

So far research has been viewed in the context of science in general and natural sciences in particular. It is important to consider research in relation to the social sciences. To what extent, for example, have the social sciences been influenced by the philosophies of science already discussed? Are social scientists, who study people and society, more likely to concern themselves with the social and cultural context of research? 'Pure' science and the scientific research paradigm are powerful influences in western society in general, and medicine in particular.

There have been reactions within the social sciences, however, to 'traditional' scientific approaches which have resulted in the adoption of research paradigms and methods that incorporate a different set of assumptions which value subjectivity, meaning and consciousness. These reactions have been particularly apparent among sociologists, anthropologists and psychologists. Over the last two decades, nurse researchers have also been influenced by disciplines such as sociology, anthropology, psychology and philosophy. A number of these scholars and their associated theories have influenced healthcare practice and research and therefore are relevant to community nurses.

In sociology the work of Weber (1947) has been very influential. In particular, Weber identified the importance of studying meaning in social interaction which is the essential difference between the social and natural sciences. Weber worked within the interpretive or hermeneutic tradition defined by Nielsen (1990) as 'a theory and method of interpreting meaningful human action'.

During the mid-twentieth century the 'Chicago School' of sociologists, based at the University of Chicago, were an important group who reacted against the continued dominance of traditional scientific approaches within the social sciences. The Chicago School scholars were influenced by the theory of 'symbolic interactionism' first developed by George Herbert Mead, a philosopher and social psychologist. His objective was to incorporate psychoanalysis and go beyond behaviourism with its focus on measurement and control, to describe the process of social interaction during which individuals make interpretations about their world and decide their future course of action (Blumer 1966). Symbolic interactionism informed the development of qualitative methods referred to as 'naturalistic research'.

In 1967, sociologists Glaser and Strauss, in the spirit of 'naturalistic research', proposed grounded theory as a means of closing the gap between social theory and empirical research. They suggest that one of the problems with social research had been forcing data to fit theories rather than using data inductively to generate and/or confirm existing theories (Hammersley 1989). One of the first major community nursing studies incorporated symbolic interactionism and grounded theory into an examination of the care of stroke patients by district nurses (Kratz 1978).

Anthropology, with its commitment to the study of human culture as a way to understand the nature of human existence, was the social science least dominated by 'traditional' science. Even so, anthropology was not immune to contextual factors. It grew as a discipline during the period 1880–1950 when anthropologists such as Evans Pritchard provided detailed information about the colonies and their peoples.

Ethnography developed as a sub-discipline of anthropology and is a popular research approach for the study of health care. An ethnography can be summarised as the detailed study of small groups such as gangs, drug users, nurses, patients and their subcultures, in a range of settings such as housing estates, villages, classrooms and residential homes. Ethnographers focus on interactions taking place between group members, and the meanings of these interactions, in an in-depth study (micro). They may then examine how people amid their settings reflect the wider society (macro) (Burawoy et al 1991).

Other influences came from philosophers such as Husserl, who developed phenomenology, a research methodology which focuses on the study of consciousness. Husserl introduced the concept of 'life-world' or 'lived experience'. Husserl's pupil Heidegger, who inspired the writings of Benner, was more concerned with how people interpreted being in the world through their understanding of the 'lived experience', a theory known as existential phenomenology.

Heidegger used the concept of 'hermeneutics' to focus on the question of how people come to understand their lived experience. Hermeneutics concentrates on the experience of understanding and accepts that the observer can never be objective. Heidegger was a senior academic during the Nazi period in Germany and some social theorists have questioned the integrity of his work because of this association.

The original sources of phenomenological philosophy represented by Husserl's and Heidegger's writings are complex and abstract and have undergone many interpretations and applications by a variety of writers, which may lead to confusion when applying them in the field (Koch 1995).

Critical theory

The critical theorists of the Frankfurt School were influenced by Marx's central critique of capitalism and the class system. They were also open to a range of theories and methods from across the social sciences, philosophy and humanities, challenging the wholesale use of the scientific model for social enquiry which 'they pejoratively labelled 'positivism'' (Morrow 1993).

Critical theory originated in 1920s Germany from a research institute in Frankfurt. Because of their critical stance, the group was forced into exile by Hitler in the 1930s. Many went to the USA where they continued to exert their influence on the development of the social sciences in that country.

The concept of 'standpoint epistemology' (Nielsen 1990) which is central to critical theory, differentiates it from other research perspectives because it addresses such issues as power relations and what counts as knowledge within society in general, and the research enterprise in particular:

Standpoint epistemology begins with the idea that less powerful members of society have the potential for a more complete view of social reality than others, precisely because of their disadvantaged position. That is, in order to survive (socially and sometimes physically) subordinate persons are attuned to or attentive to the perspective of the dominant class (for example white, male, wealthy) as well as their own.

For community nurses, standpoint epistemology is particularly important because they are more likely to be in contact with marginalised, disenfranchised members of society (Everitt et al 1992). Social workers in contact with a similar client group, believe that 'articulating and analysing the experiences of the less powerful in society reveals a more complete knowledge'. They also believe standpoint epistemology allows a more complete picture of the subjective views and perceptions of those at every level of society. 'Nina's story' (adapted from Harper and Hartman 1997) illustrates this point (Case study 12.1).

This example demonstrates that standpoint epistemology is about asking questions, looking at the world from different standpoints, which in turn allows us to discover diverse, alternative forms of knowledge.

Feminism

Feminism challenges dominant male perspectives including critical theory, to focus on women's perspectives. Nielsen (1990) suggests that in the spirit of Kuhn's scientific revolution, feminism is an alternative way of thinking, knowing and doing, and represents a major paradigm shift. It is worth noting that the majority of scholars referred to in this chapter are men, confirming feminists' claim that the dominant philosophical and scientific discourse is male.

Nielsen (1990) refers to a number of feminist

Case study 12.1 Nina the midwife's story

'For most of our professional history the predominant philosophy in nursing and midwifery (represented by positivism) did not allow us to discover diverse, alternative forms of knowledge'.

For Nina standpoint epistemology offered that alternative. She continues: 'While pondering on the practical application of standpoint epistemology for me as a midwife, I had an illuminating experience in the classroom...We were discussing neonatal care and parent support as described in various textbooks and articles [during which] we got onto the topic of how parenting and particularly mothering is defined.

One of the students told us that she had looked after a baby in the Special Care Baby Unit (SCBU) whose mother (who was black) was labelled 'a bad mother'...because she hardly ever visited her baby.

The student, who was also black, noticed that on the rare occasions the woman visited she appeared quiet and withdrawn. On talking to the mother the student discovered she had had nine previous miscarriages. Nina continues:

'She was of course now afraid to invest in this new, intensely longed for, patiently, passionately awaited relationship with her tiny baby. As the student recounted the woman's story, the classroom was silent, the textbook examples set aside.'

Nina reports that sadly the student had felt unable to tell the mother's story to the ward staff because she assumed they would not take her seriously because of her student status and racial difference.

A number of standpoints relevant to both research and clinical practice are demonstrated by this story. First, there are the textbook definitions of parenting and mothering which may differ from practice-based examples. Then there are the values and assumptions which inform our standpoints. The unit staff did not find out why the mother behaved in a certain way possibly attributing it to her race and culture; the student assumed the staff would not listen to her because she was 'different' from them and too junior to be taken seriously.

Nina concluded that 'this emotional connection to an experience, to a topic...generates questions and a desire to look at things anew'.

scholars who, during the 1970s and 1980s, reinterpreted the world from women's rather than men's points of view. Feminist scholars come from disciplines in natural as well as social sciences. Nielsen notes that topics such as housework, childbirth, rape, sexual orientation and prostitution which were formerly invisible and often sensitive, have been included on the research agenda. Feminist inquiry looks for anomalies and theories that best fit data rather than starting with the theories and anomalies and seeking data to confirm them.

Women's work, health care and nursing

The contribution of feminist perspectives to nursing research is particularly pertinent, given that it is a practice-based, predominantly female occupation in which nurses are involved in traditionally female roles and work activities prescribed by the predominantly male medical profession.

How can feminism be applied to the research process and what is its relevance for studying women's work, health care and nursing? Nielsen (1990) refers to Oakley, a British sociologist who studied motherhood and housework in the 1970s, as 'a good starting point for understanding feminist research'. In an influential paper on interviewing, Oakley (1981) criticises traditional research for the way in which it mystifies 'the researcher and the researched as objective instruments of data production' and condemns 'personal involvement as dangerous bias'. For Oakley, the use of subjectivity in research was essential to both the collection and production of data (Oakley 1974, 1980).

Oakley's contribution of a feminist perspective to the research enterprise in the early 1980s was described by Webb (1993) as a 'landmark'. Since then, however, her approach has been criticised. The notion of 'personal involvement', which Oakley describes as 'reciprocity', and friendship with research participants, has been characterised as naïve. Webb (1993), citing Ribbens (1989), identifies issues which were thrown up by Oakley's discussion of 'personal involvement': the importance of maintaining boundaries and the difficulty of redressing the power imbalance between 'researcher' and 'researched' during the interview process and, indeed, in practice situations.

Carrying on this theme, Stanley & Wise (1983) draw attention to the potential power of the researcher over the group being studied (the 'researched'), when information is extracted without reciprocity or responsibility. These observations are equally relevant to practitioners

and researchers of nursing and health care where nurses and patients can be especially vulnerable to external structures of authority. For community nurses, much of whose work takes place in the home, behind closed doors, away from the public gaze, men may continue to dominate women especially within the 'sanctity' of marriage. Research undertaken by two nurse researchers in the USA on the highly sensitive topic of marital rape, highlights the importance of nurses as confidantes to women who had endured this ordeal (Campbell & Alford 1989). Not only was a hitherto invisible topic brought to both public and professional attention, the research findings were used to help make rape within marriage unlawful in the State of Michigan (Trevelyan 1991).

In the UK, Webb (1984) introduced explicitly feminist perspectives to nursing research. She describes feminist research as 'critique' which 'aims specifically to work towards defining alternatives and understanding everyday experience in order to bring about change. Analysis and critique of research methods leads on to analysis and critique in the research context through consciousness raising for both researcher and researched'. In her 1993 update, Webb suggests that a 'shorthand definition (of feminist research) perhaps could be phrased as 'research *on* women, *by* women, *for* women'. What is distinctive about feminist methodology is its engagement with issues of concern which are particular to women and its acceptance of a variety of methods'.

In summary, feminist perspectives can be seen to value and also develop interpretivist and critical research traditions, by making gender visible at the level of both researcher and researched and putting women at the centre of the study. Being aware of feminist perspectives encourages practitioners to view the world in different ways.

Natural and social sciences and the study of nursing

The Royal College of Nursing's 'Proper Study of the Nurse' is an example of systematic research undertaken to investigate various aspects of nursing care (McFarlane 1970, Inman 1975). What is important about this project is that nurses were provided with their first large-scale opportunity to investigate practice. The majority of the studies were supervised by psychologists and took place during the early 1970s.

In the 1980s, a critique of the project appeared, suggesting that it had been too much rooted in conventional science to be able to address the life and death issues that confronted nurses and patients (Spencer 1983). The critique, which was delivered to a national nursing research conference and then appeared in a popular nursing journal, subsequently reached a wide audience. The critique neatly divided research into two categories, describing it as either quantitative or qualitative. Spencer (1983) was particularly critical of what he described as the dominance of 'positivistic' medical science (that is, biomedicine), yielding statistical 'objective' results rather than the subjective qualitative findings more appropriate to nursing.

Salvage (1990) suggests that nursing has shifted from a biomedical model to the 'new' nursing. The 'new' nursing involves problem solving and transforming relationships with patients into active, holistic partnerships. Community nurses, however, might ask what is so new about this approach, since assessment, problem solving and partnership have always been integral to the practice of district nursing and health visiting.

It may be that because of this interest in holistic partnerships, nurses, like social workers, feel uneasy with the so-called and assumed objectivity of quantitative scientific research, which categorises and numbers clients as opposed to capturing the warmth and spontaneity of their relationships (Everitt et al 1992). Everitt et al suggest that social work as a practice discipline has disengaged from research because of its association with positivist science. Such an approach is seen as inappropriate in a world that is 'uncertain, complex, spontaneous and concerned with individual difference' (Everitt et al 1992). Qualitative approaches, therefore, are seen as more appropriate for capturing nuances.

In Spencer's critique of the RCN research studies, it is interesting to speculate as to why these projects were designed in this way. At that time relatively few nurses had degrees, and even fewer were undertaking doctoral studies. Thus, nurses were relative newcomers to research and as such were likely to embrace methodologies that were familiar to them, acceptable to doctors who were their main professional colleagues and academic role models, and deemed fundable by the former Ministry of Health.

Despite Spencer's criticisms, many of the studies have become classic works, making major contributions to nursing knowledge and patient care, such as Hayward's study of pain management (1975), Stockwell's The unpopular Patient (1972) and Hawthorne's research into the care of children in hospital (1974).

However, the late 1970s and early 1980s marked a turning point in nursing research when many nurses became increasingly interested in qualitative methodologies. McFarlane (1977) discussed the need for methodologies appropriate to nursing as a practice discipline and recommended the use of grounded theory to conduct research and develop theory. McFarlane was, therefore, publicly encouraging the use of the qualitative methodologies endorsed by Kratz (1978) in her study of the district nursing care of stroke patients.

It is interesting to note that of the 12 RCN studies included in the Proper Study of the Nurse, only one of them, the study of hospital discharge, had direct relevance for community nurses (Roberts 1975). Although important, the topics of the other studies such as pain management (Hayward 1975), surgical dressing techniques (Hunt 1974), nurse reporting and communication systems and their relevance for patient care (Lelean 1973), were conducted in a hospital setting.

As mentioned earlier, in the market-led health service of the 1990s there is a renewed emphasis on systematic experimental research to provide evidence for better practice and cost-effective purchasing, and this is where future funding lies. It is likely, therefore, that nurses will find themselves involved increasingly in randomised controlled trials. However, as Oakley discovered, even this most medical of methodologies can be combined with a feminist framework.

APPLYING COMMUNITY NURSING RESEARCH TO PRACTICE

Research approaches and findings selected for their particular relevance to community nursing research and practice are now examined. Key issues of validity, reliability, ethics, proposals and funding are also considered here.

SURVEYS

Most people are familiar with the survey, either as an investigator or respondent. Surveys purport to collect social facts using value free methods and 'in such a way that our fingerprints do not leave any trace on them' (Everitt et al 1992). This approach is said to be informed by 'empiricism' where the facts are said to speak for themselves (Smith 1994). Conducting surveys has been very popular amongst epidemiologists, nurses, psychologists and sociologists.

Social surveys in Britain date back to the nineteenth century when social reformers were keen to accumulate evidence on the living and working conditions of the 'labouring classes'. Social workers trace their research origins to these roots (Finch 1986). Policy research, for example, can be traced to the nineteenth century statistical societies, and to poverty studies by Booth (founder of the Salvation Army), the philanthropist Rowntree, and the social reformers Sidney and Beatrice Webb.

The Office for National Statistics, formerly the Office of Population Censuses and Surveys (OPCS) regularly conducts a whole range of routine and special surveys. The prime example is the 10-yearly national census which aims to include the total population resident in the UK. More commonly, surveys target a sample rather than the total population, using techniques to ensure that the sample is 'representative'. A recent example of a special survey is the investigation of sudden infant deaths (OPCS 1993).

Even though the aim of the census is to include the total population, problems can still occur. The 1991 census 'lost' a number of groups which did not appear on the electoral register because in doing so they would have been forced to pay the unpopular poll tax. The Office for National Statistics stated that 20% of men in their twenties in inner London and another 36 British cities (this fell to 9% when calculated for the UK as a whole) and 6% of women over 85 were estimated to have been 'lost' (Simpson 1994, Thompson 1995). This situation led to the cutting of resources in the inner cities, particularly in inner London, because budgets were calculated according to the apparent rather than the actual social need of the population (Hanlon 1994).

Surveys can be broadly divided into two types; descriptive and explanatory. The descriptive survey's primary aim is to collect 'facts' in response to questions such as 'What'?, 'Where?', 'When?' and 'How?'. Techniques used to collect this information include questionnaires, interviews and observation. Typically, surveys are used to collect biographical, demographic and attitudinal information. The explanatory survey goes beyond descriptions to ask 'Why?'. Explanatory surveys are often conducted to follow up descriptive surveys (Bell 1993).

The explanatory survey can be used to test hypotheses in order to explain differences and similarities between two groups. In order to make the explanatory survey as close to a controlled environment as possible, the researcher chooses subjects and settings with limited heterogeneity, thereby restricting variables from the outset. For example, one study investigated health visitors' and social workers' attitudes to cases of violence and neglect towards children (Dingwall & Fox 1986). This small-scale study asked 20 participants from each profession to rate what they thought was happening in 20 vignettes which described a set of circumstances or incidents related to child neglect and violence. The findings suggested there were many areas of overlap between the social workers and health visitors and that organisational rather than training differences might account for their reported difficulties in working together.

The case control study is the closest medical equivalent of the explanatory survey. Case control studies are set up to investigate particular conditions, for example lung cancer, among a patient population. All cases, or a random sample of all the existing cases, must be included. An appropriate control sample must be identified, drawn from the same population as those with the condition. In this way, comparisons can be made between the two groups in order to draw inferences as to why the sample of cases developed the condition and the control group did not.

The explanatory survey and case control trial adopt the hypothetico-deductive research approach associated with the traditional scientific method. Hypotheses are set up to identify causal links between variables. In the example of smoking and lung cancer, the difference between an independent and a dependent variable would need to be specified. In short, the independent variable precedes the dependent one and is assumed to 'cause' or explain it. In the case of smoking and lung cancer, smoking is the independent variable that is shown to 'cause' lung cancer. This, of course, is an oversimplification of how causality is established in survey research

Lewontin (1993), a geneticist, describes the separation of causality into individual variables as a major prejudice within modern biology, which is:

nowhere more evident than in our theories of health and disease. Any textbook of medicine will tell us that the cause of tuberculosis is the tubercle bacillus. Modern scientific medicine tells us that the reason we no longer die of infectious diseases is that scientific medicine, with its antibiotics, chemical agents, and high-technology methods of caring for the sick, has defeated the insidious bacterium.

Countering the dominant medical view of causality, McKeown (1979), a public health doctor, used the decline in mortality from tuberculosis to demonstrate the importance of social factors over and above treatment. The disease had already declined dramatically before the discovery of streptomycin in 1948. On face value, without looking at the trends in the mortality statistics, the decline of the disease might have been attributable to the discovery of that drug. McKeown, by looking at the trends, attributed the decline to an improvement in living conditions and nutrition rather than to medical intervention.

When setting up a survey, design is important at all stages from formulating the question to selecting the respondents in order to minimise variability from outside sources, such as the researchers themselves, and the validity and reliability of the research techniques they use. One source of variability may be from the respondents themselves. If surveys are retrospective, the respondents may have problems in recalling past information accurately.

It is necessary to draw attention to a number of issues related to the validity and reliability of survey findings. One issue relating to validity is the extent to which the sample being surveyed is representative of the total population who might have been eligible to be included in the study; another relates to the validity of the techniques used to collect data. Since many surveys set out to measure variables, researchers need to ask if the techniques being used really do measure what they claim to.

A much more fundamental question is why certain populations are chosen for study over and above others. The famous epidemiological studies in Framingham, USA, which studied the incidence of cardiovascular disease in white, middle-aged men, might be regarded as biased towards that sector of the population (Kannel et al 1961). Great care was taken to ensure representativeness within the population under study, drawing on a random sample of middle-aged males in Framingham, Massachusetts, but why, for example, were non-white subjects and women not chosen? The results of the study have provided detailed knowledge of risk factors associated with heart disease, but it may be argued that these findings are limited to one section of the population who were seen to be at particular risk of heart disease and, because they were white men, more worthy of study than other groups. Thus researchers may hold biases that influence their studies even before they begin selecting their samples.

Sampling procedures can be broadly divided into two types: 'probability' and 'non-probability' sampling. Probability sampling is the technique used to ensure representativeness. The basic requirement for probability sampling is that the researcher has a list of the entire population from which the sample will be drawn. Sapsford & Abbot (1992) recommend the random sample as the best choice for survey work, stating that through the use of tables of random numbers the researcher can be sure of picking a systematic, bias-free sample.

Some of the non-probability techniques can lead to bias for two reasons. First, the samples they generate are not drawn from the general population and second, sample selection may depend on the preferences, however unconscious, of the researchers. In particular, neither the convenience nor the purposive sample common in qualitative studies is considered suitable for survey research.

Statistics play an important role in survey analysis and the strength of relationships between variables is tested using statistical significance tests. Bernal (1969) states that it was during the Second World War that British social researchers were exposed to the statistical techniques that had been developed by biologists and agriculturalists, and applied them on a large scale to social surveys. He also observed that each discipline benefited from being in contact with the other because they learnt about different research methods and techniques. For the social scientists he wrote:

The most powerful and general of the new methods was the statistical. Whatever names they go under – social survey, opinion polls, social and industrial psychology, market and operational research – they all consist essentially of a more or less statistical analysis of data about thinking, working or living situations extracted by systematic enquiry.

EXPERIMENTS AND RANDOMISED CONTROLLED TRIALS

In medicine the experimental approach referred to as the randomised controlled trial (RCT) has been widely applied to the study of interventions on human subjects. As with the explanatory survey and case control study, experiments are under-pinned by the hypothetico-deductive approach to research.

The use of randomisation for recruiting subjects for research studies gives all members of a given population an equal chance of being selected and reduces the risk of bias.

In order to decide on the specific design for the trial, researchers need to be clear from the outset what their aims are. A study should have one or two clearly stated objectives (Crichton 1990). Study design incorporates every stage of the study, including decisions about sampling, size, the techniques by which the subjects will be allocated to a treatment (or non-treatment) group, how the intervention will be introduced, statistical applications required and the methods for evaluating the outcome of the study.

Patient selection

The way in which patients are recruited to take part in a study is important, to ensure that they are representative of the population from which they are drawn. They must also bear some similarity to the type of patients who are likely to benefit from the study findings. An important aspect of recruiting subjects for clinical trials is to have a clear set of inclusion criteria to ensure their suitability.

Some researchers add a placebo group to the experimental and control groups. The placebo group receives a modified version of the treatment or intervention. A placebo group may be introduced into the study design for two reasons. First, it helps to discount any bias on the part of researcher or patient in their judgement, whether favourable or otherwise, of the experimental intervention. Second, it provides a control for the frequency of spontaneous changes that may occur in the patient independently of the intervention under study.

Oakley (1989) combines the experimental approach of the RCT with a feminist perspective. Citing the case of random allocation of subjects to experimental and control groups, Oakley shows how midwives' intuitive judgements were sometimes in conflict with objective sampling techniques. She attributes this to health professionals' ideology, which previous researchers had shown led 'to discriminatory stereotyping of women, based on such characteristics as working class or ethnic minority' (Oakley 1989). This example is a further illustration of how a feminist approach differs from the more usual 'objective' approach of RCTs. Midwives were responsible for recruiting and randomly sampling the women who attended antenatal clinic. It was only because Oakley kept in close contact with the midwives that she was able to discuss how they felt about random sampling. In the end she probably obtained a more accurate sample than she might have done if she had not engaged with them. This combined approach gives added insights on issues such as ethics and informed consent before agreeing to enter the study.

Oakley suggests that by rejecting quantitative methods out of hand, feminists, like qualitative nurse researchers, are not open to the possibilities these methods offer within their own paradigms. Using Daly's (1973) term, she calls for the abolition of 'methodolatry' and the need to take a critical stance on methodologies, recognising that there are only a limited number of methods available to investigate a wide range of research questions.

In the process of data analysis, a number of variables affecting the dependent variable, other than the independent variable, may be identified in the causal chain. These variables are referred to as antecedent or intervening variables. Confounding variables are two variables which vary with each other in a systematic way, making it difficult to discover the independent effects each has on a third variable. Height and weight are good examples of confounding variables, since height and weight tend to vary systematically. As previously noted, the strength of relationships between variables is tested using statistical significance tests.

As McKeown's (1979) example of causality and tuberculosis illustrates, sometimes there may appear to be a relationship between variables but this may be 'spurious' and have no explanatory value.

Evaluation

Evaluation is closely associated with experimen-
tal approaches. Sapsford & Abbott (1992) confirm this view by stating, 'the overall logic of experimental design underlies all serious attempts to evaluate policy or practice ... and is not particularly tied to one method of data collection'. Oakley (1989) also notes that 'the RCT has been increasingly promoted over the last twenty years as the major evaluative tool within medicine'.

The Department of Health's research and development strategy demonstrates a close association between evaluation and experimental logic in research. For example, the strategy identifies the RCT as one of the most important ways of finding out whether treatments are effective or not. The Cochrane Centre in Oxford has been set up to review trial findings critically and disseminate them among clinicians and purchasers. The NHS Centre for Reviews and Dissemination (1995) has also been established at the University of York. The aim of the centre is 'to promote the application of research-based knowledge in health care'. This knowledge relates to information on not only the effectiveness of treatments but also the delivery and organisation of health care.

Meta-analysis

In addition to systematic reviews of clinical trials, there is also a commitment to meta-analysis within the current health service research and development strategy. Meta-analysis refers to the systematic review of both the methodologies and the findings of clinical trials on a given topic. Crichton's (1990) point that the larger the study the more confident we can be of the findings, has been complemented by the recognition that the findings of many clinical trials are often inconsistent or inconclusive because of their small size. Meta-analysis deals with this issue by combining the populations and findings of many trials of a given intervention, such as a drug, treatment or educational procedure, to draw firmer conclusions about its effects on such outcomes as mortality, recovery and survival rates. For each trial being reviewed in the meta-analysis, the characteristics of the sample and setting and the methods used are examined. Statistical methods are used to analyse the significance of the combined results (Abramson 1990).

In the context of the reformed health service's internal market, meta-analysis is seen as an important initiative to encourage the use and purchase of 'tried and tested' health care. Cullum, a nurse researcher, undertook a critical review of community nursing management of leg ulcers, as part of the Department of Health initiative. Although she found that a number of RCTs demonstrated the effectiveness of a number of leg ulcer treatments, further studies were required to provide more conclusive evidence (Cullum 1994a,b).

Getting Research into Purchasing and Practice (GRiPP) is an initiative first devised by public health doctors and the director of research and development in Oxford regional health authority (Dunning et al 1994). The initiative was designed to inform clinicians and purchasers about the effectiveness or ineffectiveness of certain treatments, based on evidence provided by clinical trials. Four areas were identified: management of services for stroke patients; dilation and curettage (D & C); grommet surgery for children; and the use of cortico-steroids in pre-term delivery. Each of these areas showed a range of appropriateness and effectiveness with implications for future purchasing and practice.

The Oxford Health Authority also publishes a monthly journal, entitled 'Bandolier', which contains the latest information on evidence-based health care. Its logo reads, 'What do we think? What do we know? What can we prove?', in the spirit of traditional scientific enquiry.

The factors affecting the implementation of evidence-based practice were reviewed by Oxman (1994) in a systematic review of 102 trials, entitled 'No Magic Bullets'. He concludes that 'there are no magic bullets for improving the quality of health care, but there is a wide range of interventions available which, if used appropriately, can lead to substantial improvements in the application of research'.

ACTION RESEARCH

Action research is presented by Sapsford &

Abbott (1992) as the simplest example of an experiment 'in its crudest form', in that the researcher makes a change and sees what happens. This is an interesting perspective given that the experiment is clearly located within the positivist perspective, whereas action research can also be underpinned by critical theory and be committed to emancipation and empowerment. In action research the participants are equal partners with the researcher and share and control the interventions, findings and feedback.

Action research is a good example of research which integrates a variety of methods beyond experimental interventions. It is particularly popular amongst nurses, teachers, social workers and community development workers (Everitt et al 1992). Many accounts of action research show the researcher in the role of active participant working closely with the subjects, identifying problems, implementing solutions and evaluating their effectiveness as part of a cyclical process (see Fig. 12.1, p. 225). Bell (1993) concludes 'The essentially practical, problem-solving nature of action research makes this approach attractive to practitioner–researchers who have identified a problem during the course of their work, see the merits of investigating it and, if possible, of improving practice'.

ETHNOGRAPHY

Burawoy et al (1991) describe the ethnographic enterprise in a compilation of studies undertaken by students during a qualitative methodology class. The studies describe how each researcher, acting as a participant observer, focused on one in-depth case study (the micro) in order to make connections between the everyday activities of the participants and the wider social context (the macro).

Fox's (1991) account of an AIDS prevention project is an example of a researcher's use of data to demonstrate how external forces such as political and social structures and finance and policy decisions were handled by the participants. The twin aims of the project were to prevent AIDS among intravenous drug users, and also to research its progress. The project was funded by the local state and federal governments in the USA and Fox's paper is useful for thinking about funding issues in the context of the NHS research and development strategy: what types of studies will funders find most attractive? It is interesting to note, for example, that simple survey research, showing the effectiveness of the AIDS prevention project in raising awareness about using bleach to clean needles, seems to have been the reason why policy makers gave further funding. On the other hand, the project was directed by professional ethnographers and an ethnographic approach to both research and practice was adopted.

Rather than expecting clients to attend clinics, outreach workers walked the streets in neighbourhoods inhabited by at-risk populations, handing out bleach to sterilise syringes, condoms and advice on prevention. One aspect of their strategy was to learn about and become part of the subculture they were trying to access.

For the community nurse, Fox's study demonstrates the impact of national policies and funding on local initiatives; the application of the ethnographic approach to practice whereby outreach workers brought condoms and bleach to the drug users on the streets rather than using a treatment model of care which expected users to come to clinics. Fox's study also demonstrates the ethical dilemma of using practitioners to collect data. Outreach workers (practitioners) were asked to gather data about the 'culture of drug users', raising the issue of whether researchers should have access to data about practice and how it would be used?

Fox disliked what she observed concerning the organisational structures and power relations between the project directors, workers and clients, but felt powerless as a researcher to do anything about it. She also experienced the tensions of what she described as floating 'between the two worlds' of academia and the subject field. This study demonstrates the real dilemmas that occur at the interface between practice and research.

GROUNDED THEORY

In keeping with the grounded theory approach to research, Kratz's (1978) study objectives emerged over time. These objectives were: to investigate the problems of people in the community following a stroke; to observe district nurses' motivation to give different levels of care; and to describe the structure of the district nursing services which contributed to the care. Kratz's principal method was participant observation, but many grounded theorists also use interviews. Detailed fieldnotes and transcripts must be kept.

Grounded theory is a strategy for collecting, handling and analysing data from fieldwork in order to devise working hypotheses. The hypotheses then guide ongoing fieldwork from which theory can be developed. Conceptual categories and properties are developed as part of this process. 30 patients were selected for study, although 14 died during the data collection. Kratz used random sampling to select the patients. Usually in grounded theory, theoretical rather than random samples are selected. Sampling is described as theoretical because the participants are selected for particular characteristics which will contribute to the emerging theory. In-depth literature reviews are suspended until the theory development stage. Grounded theory is often used in situations where little has been written about a given topic, as in Kratz's study in the early 1970s.

Figures 12.2 and 12.3 demonstrate how Kratz generated theory from the data in relation to care. Figure 12.2 presents a model for the analysis of care delivered to patients by the district nurses. Figure 12.3 illustrates the refinement of the model in relation to the different categories of care the patients were receiving.

These figures give some idea of how material from reflective diaries can be used to transform anecdotes into systematic accounts.

On the basis of her findings, Kratz (1978) found that district nurses did not have sufficient knowledge to care adequately for stroke patients. She recommended a change in the education and training of district nurses to address this problem, a recommendation subsequently implemented. She also indicated the relative isolation of district nurses and proposed their integration

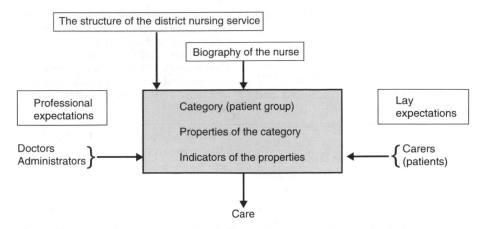

Figure 12.2 A model of care (Kratz 1978). (Reproduced with kind permission.)

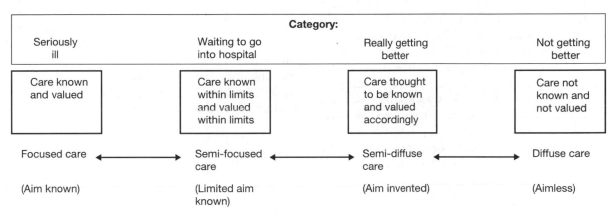

Figure 12.3 The continuum of care (Kratz 1978). (Reproduced with kind permission.)

into the PHC team at the same time as maintaining peer support. In a recent evaluation of elderly care, Smith and colleagues (Smith et al 1996) found that peer support is still an issue for general practice-attached district nurses who work closely with staff nurses and auxiliaries, but rarely with qualified district nurses who are based elsewhere. It is interesting to take the findings of Kratz's 20-year old research and evaluate them in the current context.

ETHICS AND RESEARCH

Irrespective of paradigm, approach or method,

research proposals should be submitted to ethics committees for approval prior to the commencement of the study. Research subjects should be fully informed of the implications of the study before giving their written consent and be able to withdraw without prejudice at any time. Participant observation should not be covert and researchers using this method should be clear about their role.

The Tuskegee syphilis study (Caplan et al 1992), set up in 1932 as a case control study, 'satisfied none of the requirements for ethical research, least of all in relation to informed consent'. The subjects were 400 black men in Tuskegee, Alabama, USA. The unethical conduct of the study still has repercussions for the

African-American community today which, not surprisingly, profoundly distrusts the motives of both public health services and research.

The study was set up to 'determine the natural history of untreated syphilis' (Caplan et al 1992). 400 black men with syphilis were recruited and matched against 200 black men who were not infected with the disease. Subjects underwent spinal taps to investigate the neurological effects of syphilis under the guise of 'special free treatment'. Informed consent was not obtained from the recruits. They were given the standard heavy metal treatment for syphilis, available when the study began, but they were denied penicillin when it became available as an effective treatment for the disease in the 1940s because it would interfere with its 'natural' history. The study, which was funded by the federal government, continued until 1972 when a public health official expressed his deep concern about the morality of it to a newspaper reporter. Following media exposure, the study was finally discontinued and a series of law suits followed on behalf of the subjects.

A number of ethical issues are raised by the Tuskegee study, including two key questions. First, should the results of an unethical study continue to inform the clinical knowledge base of syphilis? Second, how can groups already discriminated against be protected from such unethical invasions while also being adequately represented in and benefiting from clinical trials?

The exposure of the study in the USA led to the setting up of a National Commission for the Protection of Human Subjects of Biomedical and Behaviourial Research in 1974. The Commission laid down rigorous ethical requirements which continue to serve as guidelines for the conduct of present day research on human subjects.

Proposals

Monkley-Poole (1997) suggests:

There can be many reasons for writing a proposal apart from 'pure' research. For example, similar principles can be applied to writing proposals to obtain resources to introduce change into clinical practice or undertake an audit of services. Proposals can also be submitted to request funding to support study leave or attendance at a conference. In the health service, the move to the market with its emphasis on evidence-based health care suggests the need for practitioners to attract monies to fund research and to clearly identify and document research activities being undertaken in the clinical areas.

A proposal supports the argument for carrying out a research study by explaining how it will add to the body of knowledge and the plans and procedures necessary to complete it successfully. The applicant also includes a short curriculum vitae to demonstrate that he has the necessary experience to undertake the study. When writing any proposal, it is important to consider the membership of the panel or committee who will be making decisions based on its content, since each member will have different backgrounds and biases. It is important to be clear and explicit when putting together the proposal, especially if the people making decisions about it are likely to be unfamiliar with its approach.

Funding

Researchers with an interest in particular topics will apply for funding in response to tenders advertised in a variety of publications such as nursing journals, including the Nursing Times or Nursing Standard. Newspapers like the Guardian or the Times Higher Education Supplement are also good sources of information about funding. In addition, there are a number of publications which contain information about funding sources and their purposes, such as the Charities Aid Foundation's annual publication, the Directory of Grant Making Trusts.

Guidelines supplied by funding organisations contain relevant information for the applicant, such as the recommended philosophical and methodological approach.

Individual funding bodies invite submissions at different times of the year and may offer varying degrees of financial support. It is important, therefore, for the project proposer to be realistic when estimating the budget and to request resources which will satisfy anticipated need, as 'top-up' funds after the event may not be forthcoming. In addition to the Department of Health, funding bodies include the English National Board for Nursing, Midwifery and Health Visiting, and the United Kingdom Central Council for Nursing, Midwifery and Health Visiting. Funding is also available through higher education establishments. Most universities have a research committee which will allocate funds to local staff. It is also worth investigating health service opportunities for funding since most trusts will have a research budget.

Professional organisations such as the Health Visitors' Association (Pearson 1995) and the Royal College of Midwives (RCM 1989) publish guidelines on proposal writing and funding sources. The Foundation of Nursing Studies (1996) is committed specifically to funding projects which disseminate and implement research rather than those which set up new studies.

Summary

Research is the combination of systematic inquiry and a personal journey. The personal interests and style of each researcher and practitioner influence the questions asked and the approaches adopted.

The key NHS and nursing documents and statements identified in this chapter show that research within nursing and health care is important. Research in its various forms is no longer an optional extra in the new look health service of the 1990s. CHCNs need to shape a role for themselves in order to meet both their own professional and personal needs and those of their patients and clients.

Terms such as approach, methodology, method, qualitative and quantitative are used to describe research, and are related to the relationship between paradigm, theory and epistemology and the way in which they inform the nature and purposes of research. By viewing research as an enterprise or 'complex endeavour' we can dare to think creatively.

The final section of the chapter discussed some of the approaches and findings used for the study of community nursing and health care and their application to practice. It also raised issues associated with research, such as ethics, proposal writing and funding, in order to assist CHCNs to make their own choices about how to use research in their everyday practice.

REFERENCES

Abramson J H 1990 Survey methods in community medicine. Churchill Livingstone, Edinburgh

Angier N 1993 Radical new view of role of menstruation, New York Times, September 21

Bell J 1993 Doing your research project. Open University Press, Buckingham

Benner P 1984 From novice to expert. Addison-Wesley, Menlo Park

Bernal J D 1969 Science in history, vol 4. Penguin Books, Harmondsworth

Blumer H 1966 Sociological implications of the thoughts of George Herbert Mead. American Journal of Sociology 71:535–544

Bryman A 1988 Quality and quantity in social science. Routledge, London

Burawoy M et al 1991 Ethnography unbound: power and resistance in the modern metropolis. University of California Press, Berkeley

Campbell J C, Alford P 1989 The dark consequences of marital rape. American Journal of Nursing 89(7):946–949

Caplan A, Edgar H, King P A, Jones J H 1992 Twenty years after – the legacy of the Tuskegee syphilis study. Hastings Center Report 22(6):29–40

Carper B A 1978 Fundamental patterns of knowing in nursing. Advances in Nursing Science 1(1):13–23

Chalmers A F 1982 What is this thing called science? 2nd edn. Open University Press, Milton Keynes

Coolican H 1990 Research methods and statistics in psychology. Hodder and Stoughton, London

Crichton N 1990 The importance of statistics in research design. Complementary Medical Research 4(2):42–49

Cullum N 1994a Leg ulcer treatment, part 1. Nursing Standard 9(1):29–31

Cullum N 1994b Leg ulcer treatment, part 2. Nursing Standard 9(2):32–36

Culyer T 1995 Cure at a cost. Synthesis, Times Higher Education Supplement January 20:i

Czuber-Dochan W, McBride L, Wilson J 1997 The media and research. In: Smith P (ed) Research mindedness for practice. Churchill Livingstone, Edinburgh

Daly M 1973 Beyond God the Father. Beacon Press, Boston

Denzin N 1989 Strategies of multiple triangulation. In: The Research Act: a theoretical introduction to sociological methods. McGraw Hill, New York

Department of Health 1989 Working for patients: the health service: caring for the 1990s. HMSO, London

Department of Health (Research and Development Division) 1991 Research for health. HMSO, London

Department of Health 1992 The health of the nation. HMSO, London

Department of Health (Research and Development Division) 1993 Report of the taskforce on the strategy for research in nursing, midwifery and health visiting. Department of Health, London

Department of Health 1994 Support for research and development in the NHS. HMSO, London

Department of Health and Social Security 1972 Report on the committee on nursing. HMSO, London

Dingwall R, Fox S 1986 Health visitors' and social workers' perceptions of child care problems. In: While A (ed) 1986 Research in preventative community nursing care. John Wiley, Chichester

Dunning M, McQuay H, Milne R 1994 Getting a GRiPP. Health Services Journal 104(5400):24–26

Everitt A, Hardiker P, Littlewood J, Mullender A 1992 Applied research for better practice. Macmillan, Basingstoke

Finch J 1986 Research and policy: the uses of qualitative methods in social and educational research. Falmer, Lewes

Fox K 1991 The politics of prevention: ethnographers combat AIDS among drug users. In: Burawoy M et al Ethnography unbound: power and resistance in the modern metropolis. University of California Press, Berkeley

Glaser B, Strauss A 1967 The discovery of grounded theory. Aldine, New York

Guba E G, Lincoln Y S 1994 Competing paradigms in qualitative research. In: Denzin N, Lincoln Y (eds) Handbook of qualitative research. Sage, London

Haase J, Myers S T 1988 Reconciling paradigm assumptions of qualitative and quantitative research. Western Journal of Nursing Research 10(2):128–137

Hammersley M 1989 The dilemma of qualitative method. Routledge, London

Hanlon J 1994 Ghost of the poll tax. Red Pepper June:33

Harper M, Hartman N 1997 Research paradigms and associated philosophies: values, assumptions and research approaches in nursing and midwifery. In: Smith P (ed) 1997 Research mindedness for practice. Churchill Livingstone, Edinburgh

Harris A 1993 Developing a research and development strategy for primary care. British Medical Journal 306: 189–192

Hayward J 1975 Information – a prescription against pain. RCN, London

Hawthorne P 1974 Nurse I want my mummy! RCN, London

Health Visitors' Association 1994 Mix and match. HVA, London

Hunt J 1974 The teaching and practice of surgical dressings in three hospitals. RCN, London

Inman U 1975 Towards a theory of nursing care. RCN, London

International Council of Nurses 1990 How the ICN is promoting nursing research. International Nursing Review 37(4):295–298

Kannel W, Dawber T, Kagan A, Revotskies N, Stokes J 1961 Factors of risk in the development of coronary heart disease: six year follow-up experience, the Framingham study. Annals of Internal Medicine 55:33–43

Koch T 1995 Interpretive approaches in nursing research: the influence of Husserl and Heidegger. Journal of Advanced Nursing 21:827–836

Kratz C R 1978 Care of the long-term sick in the community: particularly patients with stroke. Churchill Livingstone, Edinburgh

Kuhn T 1970 The structure of scientific revolutions, 2nd edn. University of Chicago Press, Chicago

Lelean S 1973 Ready for report nurse. RCN, London

Lewontin R C 1993 The doctrine of DNA biology as ideology. Penguin, Harmondsworth

Lock M 1988 Part I: Introduction. In: Lock M, Gordon D (eds) Biomedicine examined. Reidel, Boston

Lock M, Gordon D 1988 Relationships between society, culture and biomedicine: introduction to the essays. In: Lock M, Gordon D (eds) Biomedicine examined. Reidel, Boston

Macleod-Clark J, Hockey L 1989 Further research for nursing. Scutari Press, London

McFarlane J 1970 The proper study of the nurse. RCN, London

McFarlane J K 1977 Developing a theory of nursing: the relation of theory to practice, education and research. Journal of Advanced Nursing 2:261–270

McKeown T 1979 The role of medicine. Blackwell, Oxford

Magee B 1973 Popper. Fontana/Collins, Bungay

Medawar P 1984 The limits of science. Oxford University Press, Oxford

Monkley-Poole S 1997 Research proposals and funding. In: Smith P (ed) Research mindedness for practice. Churchill Livingstone, Edinburgh

Moore R A 1995 Heliocobacter pylori and peptic ulcer – a systematic review of effectiveness and an overview of the economic benefits of implementing what is known to be effective. Cortecs, Isleworth

Morrow R A 1993 Critical theory and methodology. Sage, London

NHS Centre for Reviews and Dissemination 1995 Practice and service development. University of York, CRO, York

NHS Management Executive 1993 New worlds new opportunities: nursing in primary health care. HMSO, London

Nielsen J (ed) 1990 Feminist research methods – exemplary readings in the social sciences. Westview Press, Boulder

Oakley A 1974 The sociology of housework. Martin Robinson, London

Oakley A 1980 Women confined: towards a sociology of childbirth. Schocken Books, New York

Oakley A 1981 Interviewing women: a contradiction in terms. In: Roberts H (ed) Doing feminist research. Routledge & Kegan Paul, London

Oakley A 1989 Who's afraid of the randomised controlled trial? Some dilemmas of the scientific method and 'good' research practice. Women and Health 15(4):25–59

Office of Population Censuses and Surveys 1993 Sudden infant deaths 1988–92. OPCS Monitor No. 2, DH3 93/2

Oxman A 1994 No magic bullets. North East Thames Regional Health Authority, London

Pearson P 1995 The health visitor guide to research. HVA, London

Pound P, Bury M, Gompertz P, Ebrahim S 1995 Stroke patients' views on their admission to hospital. British Medical Journal 311:18–22

Rees C 1992 Practising research-based teaching. Nursing Times 8(88):55–57

Ribbens J 1989 Interviewing – an unnatural situation? Women's Studies International Forum 12(6):579–592

Roberts I 1975 Discharged from hospital (study 12). In: Inman U (ed) Towards a theory of nursing care. RCN, London

Royal College of Midwives 1989 Writing a research proposal and applying for funding. RCM, London

Royal College of Nursing 1982 Research mindedness and

nurse education: an RCN research society report. RCN, London

Salvage J 1990 The theory and practice of the 'new' nursing. Nursing Times 85(4):42–45

Sapsford R, Abbott P 1992 Research methods for nurses and the caring professions. Open University Press, Buckingham

Schön D A 1987 Educating the reflective practitioner. Jossey Bass, San Francisco

Shilts R 1987 And the band played on – people, politics and the AIDS epidemic. Viking, New York

Silverman D 1993 Interpreting qualitative data – methods for analysing talk. Text and interpretation. Sage, London

Simpson S 1994 Editorial: coverage of the Great Britain census of population and housing. Journal of the Royal Statistical Society. 157(3):313–316

Smith P, Towers B, Mackintosh M, Jennings P 1996 The integration of health and social care for the elderly in one local authority. Unpublished consultancy report

Smith S L 1994 Using information – an open learning module. Kingston University, Surrey and UK National Health Service

Spencer J 1983 Research with a human touch. Nursing Times 79(12):24–27

Stanley L, Wise 1983 Breaking out. Routledge and Kegan Paul, London

Stockwell F 1972 The unpopular patient. RCN, London

Thompson E 1995 The 1991 census of population in England and Wales. Journal of the Royal Statistical Society 158(2):203–240

Trevelyan J 1991 Marital rape. Nursing Times 87(13):40–41

United Kingdom Central Council of Nursing, Midwifery and Health Visiting 1992 Code of professional conduct, 3rd edn. UKCC, London

United Kingdom Central Council of Nursing, Midwifery and Health Visiting 1995 PREP and you: maintaining your registration; standards for education following registration. UKCC, London

Watson J 1981 Nursing's scientific quest. Nursing Outlook 29(7):413–416

Webb C 1984 Feminist methodology in nursing research. Journal of Advanced Nursing 9:249–256

Webb C 1993 Feminist research: definitions, methodology, methods and evaluation. Journal of Advanced Nursing 18:416–423

Weber M 1947 (Translated by Henderson and Parsons.) The theory of social and economic organisation. William Hodge, London

FURTHER READING

Campbell J C, Bunting S 1991 Voices and paradigms: perspectives on critical and feminist theory in nursing. Advances in Nursing Science 13:1–15

Smith P 1996 Research methodology (MSc in nursing MIM61U): study guide. RCN, London (See, especially, Units 1 and 2.)

Smith P (ed) 1996 Research mindedness for practice. Churchill Livingstone, Edinburgh

Thorne S E 1991 Methodological orthodoxy in qualitative nursing research: analysis of the issues. Qualitative Health Research 1(2):178–199

Ethics

Yvonne T. Morris

Community health care nurses (CHCNs) are confronted by ethical issues on a daily basis in their practice and also in relation to policy making. In order for them to be equipped to deal with these issues as they affect caring for clients and the overall provision of services, CHCNs should be able to:

- Distinguish between the terms 'ethics' and 'morals'
- Understand why the subject of ethics is important to health care and clients
- Demonstrate knowledge about the ethical dimension of their work as it affects autonomy and responsibility for health, the right to health care, the principle of justice as it relates to the distribution of healthcare resources, the principle of respect for persons and the principles of beneficence and non-maleficence
- Reflect upon the ethical conflicts raised by their professional role
- Understand how to apply a model of ethical decision making
- Appreciate the use of ethical theories of utilitarianism and deontology in decision making
- Provide a model of ethical decision making that can assist them in clarifying aspects of ethical conflict

DEFINING ETHICS AND MORALS

Any discussion concerning healthcare ethics raises fundamental questions about what constitutes ethics, values and morals. The terms 'morals' and 'ethics' are frequently confused or misused. Morals, and hence morality, relate to the difference between right and wrong; they often correlate to customary rules and the accepted standards prevalent in society. Morals 'are the composite result of life experiences, family, friends, culture, education and personal crises' (Fenner 1980). Morality is learnt but becomes an intrinsic part of who a person is. It is not an unchangeable force; each person has the capacity to make moral choices and to invoke moral action to change for the better. According to Tschudin (1996), morality:

starts with the self and ends with others. We tend to think of morality as that which we do at home – or at least under the duvet. But morality is far wider than that; it may start with personal courage, but it will possibly end with compassionate action, intelligently done and always considering what matters. (Tschudin 1996)

ETHICS

In academic terms, ethics involves the study of morality and morals, which can also be referred to as moral philosophy. It is a means of striving to understand the nature of human values, how humans ought to live, and what constitutes right conduct, that is, what is a good reason for acting in one way rather than another? This encompasses decision making, personal values and behaviour, and means 'thinking and reasoning about morality' (Rowson 1990). Jackson (1992) suggests that ethical study 'asks questions about the content of morality, such as how we should live our lives; what we owe one another in the way of help and non-interference; and what is to be admired, or despised, in human behaviour and attitudes'.

The importance of ethics in health care

Health care is essentially a moral activity with enormous potential for both harm and good. The good relates to the benefits people gain from enjoying an optimum state of health and how this affects their well-being and the quality of their lives, and the harm relates to the detrimental effects of being denied access to the resources and care necessary to create a state of being healthy. Health care carries with it a sense of duty and responsibility towards others and relies on a series of interpersonal relationships spanning a variety of situations and involving a diverse range of interactions. Powerful moral implications arise from health care because it relates directly to the great ethical ideals of goodness, justice, freedom, equality and respect for others. In making decisions relating to health care, such ideals can and often do conflict, resulting in a tension between differing human values and priorities. For example, tension exists in trying to balance good or harm for the individual and good or harm for the wider society.

An understanding of ethical issues can help to resolve problems of relating human values to policy decisions by making explicit the reasoning behind the decisions that have been made. The study of ethics helps people to examine the moral values that govern decision making at both the macro and micro levels of health policy and service delivery, in order to determine what ought to be in an individual's and/or society's best interests and whether decisions made are 'fair' and 'right'.

Ethical challenges for community nurses

Community health care (CHC) professionals are developing greater sensitivity to the ethical dilemmas facing them as they care for people. Complex ethical dilemmas have always existed in this area of health care, but the factors influencing the delivery of care in the community setting are a new dimension. Duncan (1992) argues that although the challenges and conflicts experienced by community health care nurses (CHCNs) are in the main similar to those experienced by nurses in other areas of nursing, 'the ways in which these nurses experience them is influenced by unique features of this nursing role'. The uniqueness of the CHCN's role lies in the primary contact between the nurse and the clients needing health care, and the fact that contact occurs mainly where clients live and work. As a result CHCNs are more likely to encounter the social, political and economic influences that give rise to ethical dilemmas. For example, in the area of community and primary health care, nurses are faced with dilemmas that are the direct result of radical government policy and reform. Such changes mean that CHCNs face ethical challenges on two broad levels.

First, at a policy making level, recent changes have emphasised cost effectiveness, primary health care, health promotion and the shifting of care from institutional settings to the community. This means that community and primary health care nurses face an unprecedented challenge in 'marshalling resources, sharing responsibilities and combining skills to achieve good quality modern services to meet the actual needs of real people in ways that those people find acceptable and in places which encourage rather than prevent normal living' (DHSS 1985). Delivering care in line with government policy has heightened ethical considerations as policy issues affect all areas of people's lives and are present in issues such as the right to and the context of the delivery of health care.

Second, health professionals face ethical challenges and dilemmas arising from their practice when caring for vulnerable individuals and families. Healthcare providers must show concern for individuals' rights, accessible health services and extensive collaborative relationships. According to Duncan (1992), 'Nurses' concerns for human autonomy, accessible health and social services, and collaborative relationships result in conflicts as they care for people in their homes, places of work, clinics and on the streets'.

The many areas that are central to the emergence of moral challenges for community and primary health care nurses can be summarised in three categories (Aroskar 1980, Schrock 1980, Duncan 1992).

1. Clients' rights: the right to health care, the right to autonomy and freedom, the right to justice, the right to respect, the right to competent care
2. Resource allocation
3. Family-centred care.

CLIENTS' RIGHTS
The right to health care

Nowadays, society places great emphasis on rights, in particular the right to health care (Department of Health 1991). This stems from a strong tradition; indeed, the NHS was founded on the principle that health care should not be the privilege of the few but freely available at the point of need to everyone. The World Health Organization (WHO) in 1978 stated that 'Health, which is a state of complete physical, mental and social well-being, is a fundamental human right', and the ultimate thrust of its health policy, the main purpose of which is to set goals in the national and international contexts, is to achieve health for all by the year 2000. The WHO definition of health, which has been widely accepted, implies that there is an obligation on governments to provide the means by which individuals can acquire, maintain or restore their health.

The United Nations Declaration of Human Rights (1978) explicitly recognises people's entitlement to receive health care, in the holistic sense, as a human right, and makes clear that provision of health care is a prerequisite of a moral and just society committed to social justice:

Everyone has the right to a standard of living adequate for the health and well being of himself and his family, including food, clothing, housing and medical care and the necessary social services, and the right to security in the event of unemployment, sickness, disability, widowhood, old age or other lack of livelihood in circumstances beyond his control.

In 1994 the WHO European member states reaffirmed the protection of human rights in health care.

The right to health care is a moral right and not a legal right, and yet it is a right claimed as part of their citizenship by sufficient numbers of people in society to be considered a 'claim right'. It is a justified entitlement which carries correlative duties and obligations and as such it places on society an obligation to provide health care. An ethical obligation results when a relationship based on a commitment relating to an ethical duty is established. A duty is a requirement that some action be performed and a right is fulfilled when the correlative duty is carried out. It is important to make clear that rights do not exist in a vacuum; a right implies a corresponding duty – one cannot exist without the other (Bandman & Bandman 1978).

The belief in a right to health care is complex and controversial, charged with ethical as well as political concerns centred around the individual's right to health care and society's sense of justice and fairness in allocating resources to meet individual healthcare needs. The issue of resource allocation is an important one in relation to people's claim to health care. For some, the dominant argument is that where human life is concerned, decisions about health care should not be dominated by economic considerations and that it is simply a matter of reordering society's priorities, for example by diverting funds from other areas such as defence into the provision of health care. Others accept the argument that it is impossible and indeed undesirable to provide all citizens with equal health care. According to Buchanan (1984), all that can be realistically expected is 'a decent minimum' that makes life 'tolerable'.

Society emphasises the rights of individuals to health and education for the benefit of all in society. Johnstone (1989) asserts that philosophers who criticise the idea of health care rights do so mistakenly because they equate health care with medical care. She goes on to argue that the right to health care is easier to accept if health care is viewed as an holistic enterprise which encompasses all aspects of healthcare provision. If health workers believe that health care is a moral enterprise, then it becomes increasingly impossible to deny that claims to it are valid, and this is certainly so when it is considered in relation to the ethical principles of care, justice and autonomy.

The nature of the right to health care

Having discussed some of the substantive argu-

ments supporting the legitimate moral claim of citizens to healthcare provision, we must now distinguish the nature of that claim. Johnstone (1989) suggests three broad facets that comprise such a claim:

- The right to equal access to health care
- The right to have access to appropriate care
- The right to quality care.

Even if the argument that society has a duty to provide its citizens with health care is accepted, it still remains a fact that such a duty creates ethical tensions between obligations to society and obligations to individual clients and their rights (Fry 1985). Hence, it is necessary to explore further the concepts of individual freedom and responsibility for health in order to understand the conflict between the individual's rights and society's duties and responsibilities.

The right to autonomy and freedom

Defining freedom

Concepts of individual and social freedom are part of general social theories relating to ethics, politics and morality. Philosophers since the time of Socrates have attempted to define individual rights in the context of social duties in civil society (Matthews 1991). The ideal of freedom is a relative concept and begs the question 'What is genuine freedom?'. This is pivotal to theories about the nature of self, autonomy, justice and equality. Hollis (1991) proposes that there are positive and negative aspects of freedom. By 'negative freedom', he means that an agent is free if there are no obstacles or constraints to his doing what he wants. His notion of 'positive freedom' stems from the idea that there is a state of existence in which humans can live to their maximum potential and freedom can be defined as the ability to live in this state. The libertarian ideal of freedom is the ability of each person to pursue freedom in his own way. John Stuart Mill, the 19th-century philosopher, wrote that the individual is the person most interested in his own well-being and is thus in the optimum position to direct his own future. The assumption here is that all individuals have the prerequisite personal, intellectual and social attributes to do this. Mill would argue further that the only justification for the removal of someone's liberty is the threat of harm to himself or to others. This issue of how far and in what areas of an individual's life it may be justified to interfere is examined later in the chapter.

Defining autonomy

One of the basic assumptions of society is that, within legal parameters, people have the freedom to make choices about their own lives and those things which affect them. This freedom, based on the ethical principle of autonomy, was reaffirmed in 1994 by the WHO. Human autonomy relates to the ability of a person to be self-determining, and Gillon (1986) defines this as 'the capacity to think, decide and act on the basis of such thought and decision freely and without let or hindrance'. To be autonomous, then, depends on a person's competence and capacity to think and act on the basis of his reasoning, and means that a person is able to choose and make decisions for himself as long as those decisions do not adversely affect others. The right to autonomy and free choice is based on the ethical principles of respect for persons, beneficence (doing good) and justice and means that society should uphold and honour the choices competent people make because they are the best judges of their own interests.

It is important not to refute wholly the argument for individual autonomy and freedom where it is appropriate; but to portray these principles as absolutes in themselves and to view society as being based on autonomy with no individual obligations to others, is to create a selfish and uncaring climate and a society which does not consider its well-being to be linked closely to that of its members. A society which supports an individualistic approach has been described aptly by Loewy (1990) as 'a minimalist community', a society which is devoid of moral fibre and based on egoism. Accepting that society has some moral obligation to its members, whose well-being is interdependent, implies that we should as a society protect those who are ill or weak, as this protects society as a whole (Margolis 1982, Jensen & Mooney 1990). To achieve this requires what Jensen & Mooney (1990) call 'social autonomy', which they define as a rejection of individualism and a concern with society as a whole. They argue that people are 'embedded in relationships of interdependence and power' and that weaknesses such as illness may undermine our individual autonomy at any time, but can be 'compensated for or overcome by support from our fellow beings, who have it in their power to support us and liberate us from our weaknesses'. In other words, humans are by nature inherently bound by a sense of kinsmanship and have a sense that the well-being of others is related to their own. The provision of health care then becomes part of a social contract where the concern is to promote a social 'good' based on mutual needs and interdependence. This supports the view of community as bound by acknowledgement of its obligations to others. In the light of this position, society must at least provide equally for the basic needs of all its citizens.

Loewy (1990) defines basic needs as those relating to bio-psycho-social existence and contends that there are first order and second order necessities. By first order necessities, he means those things which sustain normal biological life, such as food and water. Second order needs are those required to sustain an acceptable level of existence, amongst which Loewy places education and health care.

Autonomy in health education and promotion

Debate about the WHO (1994) declaration on the promotion of human rights is a prerequisite for those working in community settings, in particular those involved in educating individuals about their health, as it raises particular ethical concerns about the individual's right to self-determination.

If society invests in the individual the right to control his own destiny and the onus is on nurses and allied professionals to educate the client as to his rights and to respect him as a self-care agent who is rational and autonomous, then this has implications for community nurses as health educators and health promoters. As health educators CHCNs are confronted by the ethical challenge of promoting the health of society as well as protecting individual freedom and autonomy (McCormick 1981).

Health is promoted as being of value to all, and individuals are encouraged to be responsible for their own health; that is, they have a moral obligation to live a lifestyle that accords with the maintenance of health. The rationale for this is that health is in itself desirable, and positive health has benefits for the individual; it enables him to reach his potential and to make a full contribution to society. In this context health is viewed as a moral duty, synonymous with moral goodness, and ill-health is seen as a moral failing, indicative of a lack of control and autonomy, and therefore something which rational beings should avoid.

Public health education measures, such as immunisation and screening, are undertaken by community nurses in order to promote the health of society as a whole; but why should members of society be interested in the health and lifestyles of others? The answer lies in the fact that we are all interdependent. We all contribute to society, and ill-health is costly to society as a whole and makes unfair demands on those who follow more healthy lifestyles. This places a moral obligation on individuals not to make unnecessary demands on limited resources through deliberate health-damaging behaviour. Clients must be educated in making choices about their lifestyles.

The principle of autonomy in relation to health education requires that clients have the necessary information, the capacity and the freedom to make choices. The autonomy model of health care is one in which nurses inform patients about care and treatment and patients determine whether the proposed intervention is appropriate to their needs; but nurses must also assist clients to acquire the internal and external skills and resources to act on the information, and recognise why clients might not feel able or ready to do so. This approach is appropriate for community nursing with its emphasis on empowering clients and maximising their autonomy.

For health educators, the idea of autonomy raises fundamental questions relating to the extent to which it is morally permissible to intervene in people's personal lives. If it can be legitimately argued that a person is responsible for his own health and lifestyle, then ethical problems arise from interfering with individual autonomy when the individual is capable of making choices regarding his own body.

If education fails, coercion may be necessary, but if so, how far may nurses go (Glover 1990)? What happens when the client, for whatever reason, makes decisions that act against his own best interests? Do nurses have the right to coerce and in so doing, override a person's autonomy and act in a paternalistic manner? Paternalism means making decisions about the lives of others irrespective of their wishes in the belief that it is for their own good.

Pellegrino's (1984) response to coercion is that where coercive measures are unavoidable they should be strictly limited to matters which have direct public impact, for example seat belt legislation, and not be aimed at specific individuals. According to Thompson et al (1992), the ethical justification for compulsory public health measures 'is an appeal to the common good on the basis of beneficence and justice and to protect the rights [to health and safety] of the majority'.

Seedhouse (1995) appears to offer health educators a solution to this problem when he talks about 'the autonomy flip'. He suggests that it may well be useful for health professionals to create the conditions under which a patient can exercise his autonomy, for example by giving information about treatment interventions and their implications. This creates for the individual a position 'where it means something to say of him that he can and ought to exercise a right', in this case his right to be an autonomous agent. After creating the necessary conditions for autonomy, the health educator must respect the client's decision even if he disagrees with it, as not to do so 'renders the whole idea of creating autonomy meaningless' (Seedhouse 1995).

Health and society's moral responsibility

According to Kleining (1983) many health problems could be significantly reduced if individuals altered their lifestyles; for example by giving up smoking, which has been linked to heart disease and to cancer of the lung. Adopting this stance assumes that increased knowledge enables individuals to act rationally in relation to their own well-being. Freedom then becomes an act of rational consciousness. Of course, education is necessary but education for conscious freedom is not enough. Society is organised in such a way that a person's desire to be in charge of his own health and destiny is compromised by social and economic constraints.

The extent of freedom depends upon the range of possibilities over which an individual has choice (Hunt 1990). National health education campaigns frequently emphasise the notion of individual freedom in the choice or rejection of healthy lifestyles. In essence their approaches centre on the conventional individual behaviour-oriented approach to health education, which largely ignores the role played by the the social environment and ultimately reduces a campaign's chances of being effective. For example, Rayner et al (1990) showed that the population knew about the importance of exercise and had positive attitudes to exercise, but individuals were constrained by lack of facilities and money. The extent to which individuals can be considered free to choose healthy lifestyles is determined by the distribution of assets such as class and wealth. If individuals are to be held responsible for their own health, then they must be free to make real choices about their lifestyles.

The premise that individuals are responsible for their health implies that they are also responsible for their ill-health; in other words, if they behave and act appropriately they can prevent disease. This is a convenient approach to health as it effectively absolves government of any responsibility. This over-emphasis on individual behaviour often results in 'victim blaming'. As Beauchamp (1987) points out, 'It is a short step from a position of individual autonomy to a position of social responsibilty to the larger society, and from a position of individual autonomy to social stigmatisation'.

The underlying assumption is that individuals have real freedom to comply with behaviour in a way that is conducive to health, so that ill-health is solely the responsibility of the individual. Such an approach fails to understand that health is inextricably linked to and heavily influenced by social and political structures and the prevailing moral and cultural values. This is not to disregard the responsibility individuals have for their own health, but if health promotion and education are to succeed they must be successfully integrated with other influences on health.

Health is experienced in a social context; it is grounded in the experiences of people in their everyday lives and, therefore, reflects the crises often found there. If individual responsibility for health is to be emphasised, then more attention must be paid to the criteria that determine and evaluate living environments. These criteria should be used to build healthy communities and reduce feelings of social isolation, anonymity and alienation for the benefit of society.

The only acceptable target for health care is the highest level of well-being for all members of the community. Based on this premise, responsibility for health is the concern of individuals, governments and communities (Hollis 1991). Government clearly has a prominent role to play in instigating measures to improve the social and environmental conditions which constrain individual choice. This is a legitimate expectation under the ethical principle of beneficence, a principle which is enshrined in the WHO programme Health for All by The Year 2000 (WHO 1994) with its expressed aim of securing justice and equity in health care.

Government has a moral responsibility to maintain the general health and well-being of the wider population. It was this philosophy that enabled substantial parts of the Beveridge Commission's findings (Beveridge 1942) to be implemented in 1946. Subsequently, responsibility has shifted from the state to the individual.

The belief that education and information

alone are enough to induce healthy behaviour depends upon the assumption that all members of society have equal health choices; and the idea that health educational activities aimed at an individual level can promote change places responsibility firmly on the individual and ignores the environmental and socio-economic aspects of an individual's life. Without the necessary economic conditions, there can be no value in the concept of individual freedom.

The right to respect

Respect for persons is an ethical principle widely recognised in nursing. It acknowledges the personal worth and dignity of the patient, his autonomy, and the need for justice in the nurse–patient relationship. The principle of respect for persons challenges CHCNs to consider how they act towards clients. In community nursing, as well as in other areas of health care, practitioners are required to attempt to maintain an ongoing relationship with an individual so that that person does not become an object to whom things are done. Practitioners are precluded from practising in a manner which violates the sanctity of others.

Respect is deeply rooted in the caring ethic and is associated with nursing's humanistic and holistic philosophies. It is distinguished by being unconditional in nature, that is, it involves caring without being judgemental. Respect requires that people should be treated as having intrinsic worth and value irrespective of their ability to be autonomous, their lifestyles or their achievements (Harris 1966, Rumbold 1993).

This has implications for CHCNs. For example, nurses who work in the community care for increasing numbers of patients who have AIDS. This can pose moral problems for nurses in relation to the patient's right to respect as nurses confront their own personal values, fears and prejudices about this disease. As members of society, nurses may reflect society's values and fears and thus, for some, AIDS may be associated with a particular lifestyle and patients may be blamed and victimised for their illness. Such judgements impose the nurse's own moral values on the patient, and she can be accused of

treating the patient as being of less value and thus worthy of less respect than others. The UKCC Code of Professional Conduct (1992) makes it clear that nurses must care for all clients regardless of their lifestyles and must always act in such a manner as to promote and safeguard the interests and well-being of patients and clients. This means that AIDS patients have the same right to care and respect as other client groups.

For some, a necessary condition of being a person worthy of respect includes a person's right to autonomous self-determination. To respect a person is to respect his right to autonomy (Gillon 1986). However, other ethical problems are raised for health promoters and educators by the idea of each individual being autonomous and therefore worthy of respect.

As previously discussed, an individual may not be able to act autonomously if he or she lacks the necessary knowledge or resources to do so. Mental impairment or immaturity can also undermine the capacity for autonomy. Examples in practice include children, clients diagnosed as having a mental illness or Alzheimer's disease, or the unconscious patient.

When a client is considered incapable of exercising rational choice and acting in his own best interests, CHCNs are confronted with the dilemma of who should decide what is in the client's best interests. Any decision should, where possible, be based on the values and beliefs of the patient and be a genuine attempt to choose a course of action which, had he been competent, the client would have chosen for himself.

Professional responsibilities and duty of care

In any situation regarding care options the CHCN must take into account her professional reponsibilities. According to Thompson et al (1992), the nurse has four different but interrelated areas to consider:

- Personal responsibility – this is responsibility for one's own actions.
- Fiduciary responsibility – this involves accepting responsibility for someone who

places their trust in you, on the assumption that you know more than they do. Fiduciary responsibility includes a duty of disclosure (of relevant information).

- Professional accountability – this involves accountability to the UKCC as nursing's professional body and it includes the nurse's legal accountability.
- Public accountability – this involves a nurse's responsibility to society.

If nurses consider that clients do not have the necessary capacity and knowledge to meet the criteria for competent, autonomous decision making and they do not know what their wishes would be, then the options have to be decided upon with reference to the nurses' responsibilities as healthcare professionals and their duty of care. This duty means upholding the client's right to competent care under the ethical principles of beneficence and non-maleficence. In such circumstances using the principle of beneficence to override the principle of autonomy can be morally justified on the grounds that such acts 'are for the benefit or welfare of those who are being interfered with' (Gorovitz 1976). In other words, CHCNs may, at times, have to deal with conflict between moral principles.

Beneficence and non-maleficence

Beneficence means to do good and non-maleficence means to do no harm and these ethical principles underpin the moral obligation that doctors have towards their patients, and are enshrined in the Hippocratic Oath (replaced by the Declaration of Geneva) in which doctors swear that treatments 'will be for the benefit of the patient according to my ability and judgement and not for their hurt or for any wrong' (cited in Melia 1992). They are also part of a nurse's duty of care, based on the premise that the nurse will provide care that is competent and morally sound. The potential for nurses to inflict harm and suffering on patients is immense and it requires nurses to be alert to individuals who are vulnerable and who need support. The UKCC

Code of Professional Conduct (1992) cites beneficence as the prime motive for any healthcare intervention undertaken by nurses in whichever setting they practise.

According to Melia (1992), beneficence requires the CHCN to:

- prevent evil or harm
- remove evil or harm
- promote good.

Non-maleficence requires the CHCN to eliminate or reduce the risks to patients she cares for. However, it is important to emphasise that primarily, healthcare interventions should be aimed at 'promoting the welfare of patients not merely avoiding harm' (Beauchamp & Childress 1983).

Clearly, the implications of the principles of beneficence and non-maleficence have ethical significance for CHCNs, who must decide which nursing actions will produce the least harm and the most benefit for clients and also which actions follow the professional and legal constraints imposed by professional responsibilities.

Case study 13.1 is designed to encourage the reader to apply the knowledge gained so far from reading this chapter.

The right to justice

If patients' rights, such as the right to health care, are to be upheld, then society and healthcare practitioners are obliged to regulate and justify these rights for all citizens regardless of sex, race or religion. Upholding people's rights with equity and fairness is a moral imperative of the principles of respect for persons and justice, and requires that all individuals have an equal opportunity to access and to benefit from health care. This includes preventive health care as well as healthcare treatments.

Principle of justice

The concept of justice is poorly defined in the literature and therefore open to a multiplicity of interpretations. In general, it seems that justice is an ethical principle regulating the distribution of

---

Case study 13.1   Applying ethical principles

There is strong evidence to suggest that smoking has serious detrimental effects on an individual's health, and has major implications for society as a whole. CHCNs, amongst others, have a duty to educate patients about the effects of smoking, but how far is it justifiable to intervene in an individual's freedom and what are the ethical considerations in doing so?

The scenario

Mr Barnes is 66 years of age. He has recently been discharged from hospital into the care of his general practitioner following extensive surgery for cancer of the lung. Prior to his admission to hospital Mr Barnes smoked 40 cigarettes a day. On discharge he was strongly advised to stop smoking. The CHCN, with a professional duty to promote optimum health, notes that Mr Barnes is ignoring this advice and is still smoking heavily. After lengthy discussion and consultation with Mr Barnes, it is clear to the nurse that he has chosen to exercise his right to smoke despite the obvious implications.

The situation causes the CHCN particular concern. To deal with this, she will have to identify the ethical problems raised by Mr Barnes' attitude, particularly relating to respect for persons, beneficence, and non-maleficence. The CHCN must also explore the ethical basis of the health promotion activities she can use to try to change Mr Barnes' attitude to health and his lifestyle.

But does Mr Barnes have the right to be 'unhealthy' if he so chooses? Does his right to autonomy have consequences for other individuals and society in general?

These considerations will influence how the CHCN responds to the situation. It is worth considering at this stage, how the situation would be affected if Mr Barnes was deemed to be mentally incompetent and therefore unable to make a rational decision about his lifestyle.

---

social benefits and burdens (Beauchamp & Childress 1983). It is closely linked to the idea of law and people receiving their fair share of an item. The central characteristics of justice are fairness, equity and equality, desert and entitlement. Beauchamp & Childress (1983) offer the view that 'one acts justly toward a person when that person has been given what is due or owed, and thus what he or she deserves and can legitimately claim'.

The difficulty with this approach is that the task of determining who deserves what and how much is highly subjective and could be based on misplaced value systems, such as eco-nomic deserts (Johnstone 1989). How can what a person can legitimately claim be measured? Are there, for example, morally relevant properties, such as being a productive member of society (deserts) or being in need, which an individual must possess in order to lay claim to benefits?

Nature of justice

There are two broad approaches:

- Retributive
- Distributive.

Retributive justice is based on the premise that the way to balance the claims and burdens amongst individuals in society is according to an individual's deserts, i.e. giving each his due. This derives from the idea of meritocracy, the view that one should give individuals differing amounts of a benefit such as health care, based on their contribution to society or to the community in which they live.

Distributive justice has three main, but conflicting, facets: each according to his rights; each according to his needs; and to each an equal share.

In contrast to retributive justice, distributive justice appears to imply a morally sound approach to the allocation of social benefits. If taken at face value, the supposition that all people should share equally in society's benefits and burdens is an appealing one, yet this position, which readily accepts the notion of equality, and is often interpreted to mean everyone receiving the same, is open to criticism. If the principle of equality is to be realised, then there must be equal access and opportunity to gain that access in terms of health, wealth and power, but this, as discussed earlier, is not the case. It is surely preferable and more just to use the idea of equity, which is the distribution of a commodity according to need following equal consideration. The implication of this is that more might be given if it is decided that more is needed. Although this approach has much to offer, it still leaves the question of how to balance people's needs and desires with the decision regarding which needs take precedence, given that they cannot all be met.

Theories of justice

The divergent approaches to the concept of justice might be resolved by examining various theories of justice. These may offer a systematic approach to determining how goods and services can be distributed justly across society as a whole.

Rawls' theory of justice. Rawls (1971) attempts within his treatise to secure the basis for a just society. His theory of justice makes a clear connection between politics and morality. He extrapolates that the level of morality that exists for people is linked to the structures that govern the society in which they live. Rawls' theory attempts to deal with those inequalities related to power, wealth and social class, and he argues that such inequalities are unacceptable to a just society unless they work specifically to the benefit of the worst-off members of that society.

According to Rawls, everyone should have basic liberties, and no differences in wealth should be tolerated unless it is for the overall good of others. For Rawls, justice is equated with the notion of fairness and is part of a social theory of rational choice.

His approach is an appealing one because it asks us to make fair choices from a neutral position, and because it attempts to nullify social advantages and is based on a belief in equality in the assignment of basic rights and duties. However, Rawls makes it clear that the overriding ethical principle that governs his just society is that of liberty, and it is for this that he has been criticised (Seedhouse 1992). Seedhouse argues that ranking the principle of liberty above that of equality is inappropriate and flaws Rawl's theory. Seedhouse argues that 'the best way of ensuring justice within a society is to guarantee equal distribution of resources even at the cost of a lower level of personal liberty in the populace'. What is being proposed here is that if nurses and health workers are obligated by ideas of freedom, equality, justice and the 'good' of society as a whole, then these principles may justify the limiting of the freedom of others in order to meet the needs of the more disadvantaged in society.

Utilitarian theories. The appeal of utilitarianism lies in its relative simplicity. Utilitarian thinking focuses on serving and maximising benefit for the greatest number. Utilitarianism commonly portrays justice as a process 'involving trade-offs and balances' and offers the belief that 'we must balance public and private benefit, predicted cost savings, the probability of failure, the magnitude of risks and so on' (Beauchamp & Childress 1983). In utilitarianism, the most moral acts are those which produce the greatest good or happiness. Furthermore, where no obvious good can be produced, then any decision made should be that which produces the least amount of harm.

The proponents of utilitarianism argue that the approach is morally justified because it follows the principle of utility. However, in terms of the principle of justice in resource allocation, the approach is deeply flawed because, as Melia (1992) rightly points out, 'if actions are to be judged according to the amount of happiness produced it must be possible to calculate how much happiness will result from a particular action, and it is not'. More importantly, it raises some fundamental ethical questions such as 'what is good?' and 'what is happiness?'.

According to Rawls, utilitarianism is incompatible with the notion of a just and fair society and with the idea of reciprocity implicit in the notion of social co-operation or contract. As a method of determining how health services should be organised, this approach is pragmatic but it does not fit with the concept of justice as fairness, because it penalises minority groups and probably the most needy in society. It does not acknowledge individuals and their needs; for example, it would be very hard for healthcare professionals employing a utilitarian approach to advocate sustaining the life of a mentally handicapped child (Campbell 1984).

Libertarian theories. Libertarians are concerned essentially with the idea of free choice and regard this as the foundation of justice. Perhaps the prime example of this can be found in the US where health care is left to the market place and to individual choice. Proponents of this approach argue that 'social intervention in the market in the name of justice perverts true justice by placing unwarranted constraints on individual liberty' (Beauchamp & Childress 1983). Libertarians espouse the view that all rights to social goods based on unconsented and enforced beneficence violate the principle of respect for autonomy.

RESOURCE ALLOCATION

The ethical principle of justice is one means of addressing the questions of how resources should be allocated, whose need is the greatest and which approach would yield the best result in terms of health care for all.

In the 1990s there has been a dramatic escalation in people's expectations of health care, fuelled by:

- The NHS reforms (Department of Health 1989), which have led, in theory, to a redistribution of resources from one area to another more needy area and to healthcare provision being shifted from acute hospitals to community-based services
- The rise in consumerism with its emphasis on patients' rights (Patient's Charter, DoH 1991)
- Advances in health care both at a preventive level, such as screening patients for potential health problems, and at the curative/ treatment level.

These changes have led government and health care policy makers to focus on the problem of resource allocation in order to manage spiralling expectations and costs in the face of severe fiscal limitation. For CHCNs, the issue of how to use healthcare resources justly is a thorny one, because they have conflicting obligations: to meet the individual needs of clients and families and to meet the health needs of the community as a whole.

The different interpretations of the principle of justice raise ethical as well as practical issues for the CHCN, in two areas in particular. First, if, as has been argued, the principle of justice requires that all individual claims to health care be treated

equally, then this raises the moral question of balancing the rights of all individuals to have their needs met against the needs of the 'general good' (or the community as a whole). For example, is it more justifiable to fund expensive in vitro fertilisation for couples who are unable to conceive a child or to increase funds for caring for the increasing number of elderly being nursed in the community?

Achieving a balance amongst competing needs has always been controversial and, as Jones (1990) points out, 'the just division of resources is a major moral problem in a service where need is so apparent'. If justice can be said to mean the opportunity to benefit from and have access to health services according to need, then Jones (1990), citing Aristotle, reinforces what was discussed earlier, that 'equals should be treated equally, and unequals unequally in proportion to their inequalities'. In other words, justice is about ensuring that healthcare resources are allocated to those who are most socially and/or clinically disadvantaged. This is very different from the notion that all individuals, regardless of their need, should be treated equally, and is an approach which seems to lend itself to ethical decision making as it relates to CHCNs and individual clients' needs. Clinical practice, wherever it takes place, is grounded in an ethic of caring which essentially means caring for individuals in order to meet their health needs (Melia 1992).

Healthcare professionals cannot ignore the principle of justice since, according to Melia (1992), 'in everyday practice they [nurses and doctors] face competing claims for scarce resources and have to make decisions about how to proceed'. In trying to reconcile these problems, a utilitarian approach is attractive because of its ethical simplicity, but the approach belies the complexity of the demands made by individuals for health care and it fails to ensure justice for those most in need.

In the past the issue of how healthcare resources were to be allocated was primarily a clinical one, that is, it was left to doctors to determine whose needs for treatment took priority. Traditionally, access to health care has always been rationed but the process of rationing has been arbitrary and obscured.

In Oregon in the US, the problem of allocating resources at a macro level has been dealt with explicitly. The state's health commission, following extensive interviews with members of the population who were asked to rank in order of priority a list of 709 medical conditions, adopted a utilitarian approach to allocating its healthcare resources in order to maximise the 'common good' for society as a whole (Bowling 1992). The aim of the endeavour was 'not to seek specific opinions about health care, but rather to make explicit the value system the public use in reaching their decisions and formulating their opinions' (Bowling 1992). The Oregon proposals do not attempt to equalise access to health resources, but rather to determine which treatments will be available and which not, in order to ensure the most beneficial distribution of scarce resources. A balance was struck in favour of primary care services and those treatments which have a quality of life plus a cost benefit. Such an approach has its merits; in particular it makes public the covert rationing that has taken place, and does take place, in all healthcare systems (Warner 1991).

Issues relating to resource allocation and justice are probably ethically unsolvable, but what is important is that the means of determining who gets what and why is open to public as well as professional scrutiny. Health care is not simply about treating or preventing diseases or illness, it must also involve maintaining the rights and dignity of individuals. If as a professional body CHCNs are committed to patient welfare, then they must defend the demands made upon them through the principle of justice, and raise the level of debate about issues such as funding and provision of health care which affect everyday practice.

FAMILY-CENTRED CARE

One of the most distinctive features of the CHCN's role lies in the notion that the family is a distinct unit and is one of the focuses of care. The most prominent interpretation of family-centred care is that the CHCN has a commitment to the

well-being and safety of the family, as well as to individual clients, such as children, who live in it. It is this aspect of the CHCN's role that creates one the most serious ethical conflicts for her (Duncan 1992). The conflict encompasses:

- Children's rights
- The assessment of children's best interests
- The focus of care and the CHCN's role.

Children's rights

The Children Act 1989 and the United Nations Convention on the rights of children (1989a,b), emphasise the unique rights that children now hold. Some of these rights have direct significance for the CHCN's role. According to the UN, all children under 18 years of age have certain rights (Box 13.1, Beattie & O'Grady 1996).

It is clear that the the ability of children to make informed choices (autonomy) is to be respected wherever possible and taken into consideration when decisions about them are being made. 4 essential criteria were identified earlier as being prerequisites for the exercise of autonomy:

- Capacity (intelligence)
- Knowledge
- Rationality
- Resources.

The question arises, however, as to when children reach an age at which they are capable of autonomous choice. In the past the measure of a child's autonomy relied on the chronological age of the child (Beattie & O'Grady 1996), and this was supported by law in the form of the Family

---

Box 13.1 Children's rights

Children have the right to live with parents unless this is deemed incompatible with the child's best interests. Children have the right to express opinions and have them taken into account. Children have the right to freedom of thought. They have the right to expect freedom from neglect and abuse. They have the right to the highest possible level of health care. And they have the right to protection of their human rights under the law.

Law Reform Act (1969) in which children under 16 years were deemed incapable of making choices about their health. More recently, the Gillick ruling has set a legal precedent. Children under 16 years who seek contraception without parental consent and who are deemed to have sufficient knowledge and understanding, are allowed to have their right to self-determination respected (Gillick v Wisbech and West Norfolk AHA 1985).

The issue of developing and respecting children's autonomy is discussed at length by Alderson & Montgomery (1996).

In terms of the CHCN's role, the ethical issues raised by the idea of children's right to autonomy are difficult and uncertain. The law adds to the uncertainty as it does not always uphold a child's right to autonomy and each case has to be weighed according to individual circumstances and conditions. This is particularly so in cases involving children in potentially life-threatening situations.

What does the CHCN do if she feels a child's choice, for example to remain in an abusive family situation, is not in that child's best interests? This is balanced by the CHCN's recognition of the fact that compulsory interventions are only acceptable in extreme circumstances as they cause distress and suffering. There will always be circumstances in which the choice of the CHCN will conflict with a child's choice and in these circumstances the nurse's duty is to act in the best interests of the child (Children Act 1989).

Assessment of children's best interests

According to Duncan (1992), it is in the area of caring for vulnerable families, what she terms 'high risk parenting', that CHCNs face their greatest ethical challenge. The CHCN must be able to assess the degree of risk to children and when a family situation warrants professional and/or legal intervention. As Harris (1985) contends 'parenting bad enough to warrant intervention by the state is a less difficult concept than is the concept of good enough parenting'. In other words, how is the CHCN to know that the criteria against which she is to assess when

recommending intervention, for example for compulsorily removing a child from a potentially harmful situation, is morally as well as professionally desirable and in the best interests of that child?

The ethical dilemma for the CHCN centres on a conflict between the two fundamental ethical principles, beneficence versus the autonomy of the parent or parents. In other areas of community nursing, autonomy is considered to be an influential ethical principle; however, where children are at risk it might be the case that the CHCN has to recommend overriding the autonomy of parents or, indeed, the child, in order to promote the child's best interests.

The Children Act 1989 provides the CHCN with useful guidelines against which decisions concerning children's best interests can be assessed. The Act requires that several factors be taken into consideration when decisions are being made (Box 13.2, Beattie & O'Grady 1996).

The focus of care

The CHCN also faces conflict in determining where the focus of care lies; is it with the health of the child or the long-term health of the family (Duncan 1992)? By intervening in high risk situations, the CHCN has the potential to jeopardise the integrity and health of the family as well as her long-term relationship with that family. CHCNs have to work hard to build and maintain trusting relationships with vulnerable families who may be suspicious of their motives. According to Duncan

---

Box 13.2 Factors affecting decisions regarding children

- The wishes and feelings of the child, bearing in mind the child's understanding and maturity
- The effects of any proposed decision upon the child
- Any harm which the child has suffered or is at risk of
- The child's age, gender and social background
- The capability of the child's parents or significant others in meeting his needs
- The range of legal powers available

(1992), CHCNs feel 'that protective intervention for children contradicts their attempts to develop the skills and confidence of high risk parents'. Moreover, Duncan maintains that once intervention has been instigated, it remains highly probable that the child will be returned to the parent or parents with little evidence that the issues or situation that led to the intervention in the first place have improved. Duncan (1992) gives one poignant description of a CHCN's experience: 'Legally I had to report this high risk situation but it resulted in this family being unwilling to have further contact with me. They have received sporadic help from other agencies (when in crisis) but there has been no long-term help which I feel I could have provided'.

In this incident the consequences of intervening have been detrimental to the well-being of the family in the long term, and the one agency that could have offered ongoing support to this family is no longer able to monitor the situation and protect the long-term well-being of the child.

Quite clearly the dilemma here is not easily resolvable; however, it does seem important that CHCNs weigh up carefully the long-term repercussions of short-term interventions and that professional bodies as well as the law support nurses in making long-term, potentially hazardous decisions which may well result in vulnerable families and children having continous support, thus reducing the overall risk.

ETHICAL DECISION MAKING

The ethical issues raised by the concept of clients' rights in terms of the principles of respect for persons, autonomy, justice and beneficence force CHCNs to make moral choices and resolve moral conflicts. If these conflicts cannot be satisfactorily resolved, then the CHCN is left with feelings of anger, frustration and guilt (Duncan 1992).

In order for CHCNs to be able to cope with these emotions they need first to understand what it is they are experiencing and why, and second, to have strategies for dealing with the dilemmas that confront them on a daily basis.

This requires support within the workplace, sound knowledge and good decision making skills.

WHAT IS AN ETHICAL DILEMMA?

According to Thompson et al (1992), an ethical dilemma involves conflict between competing moral principles and values and making a difficult choice between apparently equally unacceptable outcomes. A dilemma asks the question 'what ought we to do?' What options are available and how can choices be defended in the light of the principles and values involved? It is important to note at this point that Thompson et al (1992) make a clear distinction between making moral choices and resolving moral dilemmas. They argue that not all moral choices are dilemmas since in many situations in health care, professionals know what ought to be done and the essential question relates to whether it will be done. In a dilemma, it is not clear which course of action is the most desirable. For example, when ethical dilemmas associated with the CHCN's health promotion role occur and the ethical principles of autonomy and beneficence come into conflict, there appears to be no course of action that would produce a satisfactory outcome in terms of upholding both of these ethical principles.

A model for ethical decision making
(Box 13.3)

The model suggested in Figure 13.1 and Box 13.3 utilises what is known as the 'principles approach' to ethical decision making. In this method, the application of ethical principles such as respect for persons, respect for autonomy, non-maleficence, beneficence, and justice, can act as a framework for clarifying the ethical dilemma (Curtin 1982, Edwards 1994).

The model offers practitioners help in making sense of dilemmas they experience, and draws heavily on the works of Aroskar (1980) and Curtin & Flaherty (1982). It follows the principles of the nursing process, its aim being to structure

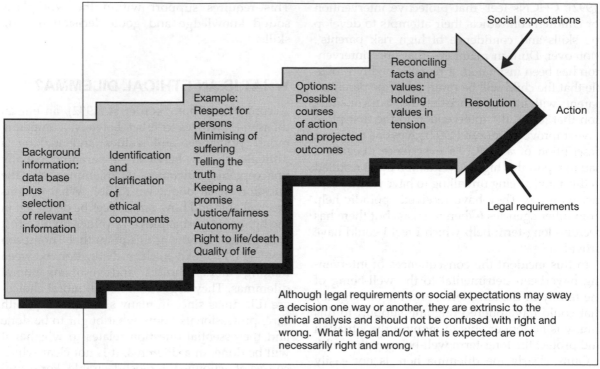

Figure 13.1 A model for ethical decision making. (Reproduced with kind permission from Elizabeth Pask.)

the ethical dilemma for clarification, decision making, and taking action (Aroskar 1980).

ETHICAL THEORY

Teleological or utilitarian theories

The term 'teleological' is derived from the Greek word telos meaning end or purpose, and teleological theory seeks to justify moral decisions in terms of the overall goal achieved. The goal being pursued is the personal happiness and fulfilment of the individual as well as that of the majority within human society. Happiness 'relates to the state of the whole person...and may persist even if the person is experiencing pain' (Thompson et al 1992). In other words, happiness is seen as a general state of being.

Over many years this approach has been redefined and reinterpreted, resulting in one of the most well known telelogical theories, namely the Utilitarian philosophy of John Stuart Mill. Mill's Utilitarianism, which is popular with modern Utilitarian thinkers, interprets happiness as a psychological state. It relates to feelings of pleasure and pain and emphasises three aspects:

- The consequences of one's actions. The approach looks at the right and wrong action in so far as it produces good and bad consequences
- The contribution of actions to human happiness and the prevention of suffering
- Acting for the greatest good for the greatest number.

In other words, the action which ought to be performed is that which produces the maximum beneficial outcome for society as a whole. According to Mill's Utilitarian thinking, there is ultimately only one moral aim – to act in order to contribute to the greatest happiness for the greatest number. According to Utilitarians such as Mill, acts are ethically correct if they either max-

Stage 1: clarification
At this stage, relevant information is gathered in order to ascertain:

- Who are the people involved in the situation?
- What are their histories in the situation?
- In what context is the dilemma occurring?
- What are the main ethical principles involved in the dilemma; is it, for example, a conflict between respect for persons and their rights and the allocation of healthcare resources?
- What is the intention of any action proposed?
- What are the likely consequences of any action taken?
- What other alternatives are available?

Stage 2: decision making
At this stage, consideration needs to be given to the following questions:

- Who should make the decision, for example, the nurse, patient, family or doctor? And why?
- For whom is the decision being made?
- What ethical principles are being used or negated in order to make the decision?

Stage 3: ethical theory
At this stage, consideration needs to be given to justifying the moral choices made for action. There are two fundamental approaches:

- Utilitarianism
- Deontology

imise pleasure or minimise suffering for everyone. According to Thompson et al (1992), 'The things which count as contributing to the greatest happiness for the greatest number are to be measured by the criterion of greatest benefit to all'. In a pure consequentialist approach, the end justifies the means if it produces more benefit than an alternative course of action; for example, it can be justified to override a competent person's right to autonomy if the consequences of doing so would lead to substantial benefits for the rest of society, in terms of either economic benefit or overall well-being. An example of this philosophy is the moral justification for public health interventions and measures such as seat belt legislation.

Modern philosophers distinguish between two types of Utilitarianism.

Act Utilitarianism. This determines the rightness or wrongness of an action depending on the consequences of the action, that is, how much happiness was produced and for how many people as a result of the decision made.

Rule Utilitarianism. In this approach, any action is measured not in terms of the results produced by a particular action, but by whether the action taken was based on moral rules and principles which, when followed, are likely to lead to the best consequences for all.

Strengths and limitations of Utilitarianism

The appeal of the approach is its simplicity for the CHC practitioner. A decision made from a Utilitarian stance will resolve the dilemma by examining the consequences and calculating the benefits that will result for the greatest number from any action taken. For example, the complex issue of justice and resource allocation would be solved simply by looking at the needs of the majority. However, the adoption of this approach alone within a health care context raises many issues, not least questions about fairness (as was seen in the section on resource allocation, p. 254). These issues include how one quantifies happiness or the common good, how the benefits of any action are calculated and who determines those benefits and for whom.

Utilitarianism fails to explain why the happiness of the majority is morally more desirable than that of the individual (Downie & Calman 1994). After all, if as members of a society and as healthcare practitioners, CHCNs wish to endorse the view that respects the rights of individuals, then surely this precludes a system of ethical decision making based on the maxim of the greatest good for the greatest number.

Utilitarian theory does possess some strengths in relation to resolving ethical dilemmas. Campbell (1984) offers a view of its merits, writing 'It [Utilitarianism] merits consideration because it acts as a good corrective to personal bias and idealistic decision making of principles'. In other words, its strength lies in its ability to be objective and rational and to move ethical decision making away from the subjectivity of the individual and his conscience. According to Thompson et al (1992), Teleological and Utilitarian theories emphasise three primary aspects of ethical experiences:

1. Goals are an important part of human existence.
2. These approaches help us to explore the practical implications of applying principles and to understand that the consequences of any action must be taken into account when making ethical decisions.
3. Any choice made should have a defined purpose or goal.

Deontological theories

Deontology is derived from the Greek word *deos* meaning duty. The most well known deontological philosopher is Immanuel Kant. Kant believed that as human beings, we are all capable of moral will. It is this moral will, determined by God and intrinsically part of man's rational nature, which allows universal moral laws and principles which must be obeyed to be adopted. Moreover, it is man's ability to be rational and to reason which sets him apart from other species.

Kant's (1972) moral theory centres around the idea that moral principles are to be regarded as a binding duty if they can:

- Be universal
- Be unconditional
- Be an imperative.

This means that if the principle of the sanctity of life is taken as a universal and God-given law, then according to Kant, killing a person would always be wrong because life is a good thing and therefore its preservation is an essential moral requirement. Thus, ending a life, whatever the circumstances and quality of that life, is always a bad thing to do.

The deontologist's principal concern lies with the duty and obligation individuals owe to each other. Duty requires that the moral agent acts according to universal, unconditional moral principles and laws and that it is the obligation of individuals to follow these at all times, irrespective of consequences and circumstances. This approach argues that it is not the consequences

of an act which make it right or wrong, but the moral intention of the agent to do good and act in accordance with binding moral principles even if the results are undesirable. In other words, the end does not justify the means as it does in utilitarian decision making.

Strengths and limitations of deontology

In relation to health care, the deontological approach has its limitations in that it asks fundamental questions about whether unconditional, imperative, universal moral principles can really be applied in all situations regardless of circumstance and utility. Thompson et al (1992) make this point when they suggest that the weakness of deontological thinking lies in the dichotomy it raises between the theory and its practical application. In the example cited earlier, the principle of sanctity of life was presented as an absolute moral principle which, from a deontological perspective, all CHCNs would have a duty to maintain. This can lead to conflict for the CHCN who may be faced with a terminally ill patient who does not want his life preserved and in fact wants to die. It is important to remember here that deontologists such as Kant also argue that to respect a person is to respect his rationality and hence his autonomy, and that this too is an absolute. Essentially, the CHCN is faced with a conflict between equally important ethical principles, namely the principle of sanctity of life and the principles of autonomy and respect for persons.

In these circumstances the nurse's code of conduct requires that she acts in a manner which promotes and safeguards the interests of individual clients (UKCC 1992). How then does the CHCN ascertain what her duty is in relation to deontological theory and the code of conduct? How does the nurse ascertain what is in the client's best interests? What happens if there is disagreement about where patients' best interests lie?

The strength of the theory for CHC practitioners lies in the deontologist's belief in human rationality and in unconditional human moral worth. This means that human beings are to be treated with respect and not used as a means to an end. It is this approach towards persons and their individual needs that best matches community nursing philosophy because it requires that moral decisions should not be made at the expense of individuals. In deontological terms, as each human being is important and has intrinsic worth, his individual needs and rights must be considered rather than ignored, as they would be by the utilitarian whose only concern is to benefit the greatest number.

Despite the apparent limitations of both utilitarianism and deontology, both theories can offer the CHC practitioner some rational grounds for the moral principles that govern her decision making in practice. After all, the practitioner's professional accountability demands that decisions, whether of a clinical or moral nature, are not made capriciously or arbitrarily, but rather must be explainable, reasonable and defendable.

Summary

This chapter has sought to raise some of the ethical issues that confront community health care nurses and to offer a model for clarifying the issues involved. The aim has been to aid them in their decision making. In order for community health care nurses to be able to fulfil their duties and responsibilities, much more attention must be paid to the issues that they experience every day. They need support and clarification on what is expected of them not only at a practice level, but at a strategic level as well.

REFERENCES

Alderson P, Montgomery J 1996 Health care choices: making decisions with children. IPPR, London

Aroskar M 1980 Anatomy of an ethical dilemma: the theory. American Journal of Nursing 80:658–663

Bandman E L, Bandman B 1978 Bioethics and human rights. A reader for health professionals. Little Brown, Boston

Beattie J, O'Grady 1996 Morals and ethics in children's nursing. In: McQuaid L, Husband S, Parker E (eds) Children's nursing. Churchill Livingstone, Edinburgh

Beauchamp D 1987 Lifestyle, public health and paternalism. In: Doxiadis S (ed) Ethical dilemmas in health promotion. John Wiley, Chichester

Beauchamp T L, Childress J F 1983 Principles of biomedical ethics, 2nd edn. Oxford University Press, New York

Beveridge W 1942 Social insurance and allied services. CMND 6404. HMSO, London

Bowling A 1992 Setting priorities in health: the Oregon experiment. Nursing Standard 6(37):29

Buchanan A 1984 The right to a decent minimum of health care. Philosophy and Public Affairs 13(1):55–78

Campbell A V 1984 Moral dilemmas in medicine. Churchill Livingstone, Edinburgh

Children Act 1989 HMSO, London

Cohen M (ed) 1961 The philosophy of John Stuart Mill. Modern Library, New York

Curtin L 1982 No rush to judgement. In: Curtin L, Flaherty M J (eds) Nursing ethics, theories and pragmatics. R J Brody, Bowie, Maryland

Curtin L, Flaherty M J (eds) 1982 Nursing ethics, theories and pragmatics. R J Brody, Bowie, Maryland

Department of Health 1989 Working for patients. CM555. HMSO, London

Department of Health 1991 The patients' charter. HMSO, London

Department of Health and Social Security 1985 Government response to the second report from the social services committee 1984–5 session: community care, Cmnd 9674. HMSO, London

Downie R S, Calman K C 1994 Healthy respect. Ethics in health care, 2nd edn. Oxford University Press, Oxford

Duncan S M 1992 Ethical challenge in community health nursing. Journal of Advanced Nursing 9(17):1035–1041

Edwards S 1994 Nursing ethics. Nurse Education Today 14:136–139

Family Law Reform Act 1969 HMSO, London

Fenner K M 1980 Ethics and the law in nursing. Van Nostrand and Reinhold, New York

Fried C 1982 Equality and rights in medical care. In: Beauchamp T L, Walters L (eds) Contemporary issues in bioethics, 2nd edn. Wadsworth, Belmont, California

Fry S T 1985 Individual versus aggregate good: ethical tensions in nursing practice. Journal of Nursing Studies 22(4):303–310

Gillick v Wisbech and West Norfolk Area Health Authority (revised) 1985 1 ALL E R 533 CP

Gillon R 1986 Philosophical medical ethics. Wiley, Chichester

Glover J 1990 Causing death and saving lives. Penguin, Harmondsworth

Gorovitz S 1976 Moral problems in medicine. Prentice Hall, London

Harris E E 1966 Respect for persons. In: de George R T (ed) Ethics and society. Macmillan, London

Harris J 1985 Child abuse and neglect: ethical issues. Journal of Medical Ethics 11:138–141

Hollis M 1991 Market equality and social freedom. In: Almond B, Hills D (eds) Applied philosophy, morals and metaphysics in contemporary debate. Routledge, London

Hunt G 1990 Patient choice and national health service review. Reprinted from Journal of Social Welfare no 4. Sweet and Maxwell, London

Jackson J 1992 Coming to ethical terms: 'ethics'. European Review 1(1):62–64

Jensen U J, Mooney G 1990 Changing values in medical and health care decision making. John Wiley, Chichester

Johnstone M J 1989 Bioethics. A nursing perspective. Saunders and Baillière Tindall, London

Jones C 1990 A fair share for all. Nursing Standard 5(9):49

Kant I 1972 The moral law (Paton H G trans). Hutchinson University Library, London

Kleining J 1983 Paternalism. Manchester University Press, Manchester

Loewy E H 1990 Commodities, needs and health care: a communal perspective. In: Jensen U J, Mooney G (eds) Changing values in medical and health care decision making. John Wiley, Chichester

McCormick R A 1981 How brave a new world? Dilemmas in bioethics. Doubleday, New York

Margolis H 1982 Selfishness, altruism and rationality. Cambridge University Press, Cambridge

Matthews H 1991 Can it be right to restrict freedom in order to promote health? Unpublished essay. Thames Valley University, London

Melia K M 1992 Everyday nursing ethics. Macmillan, London

Pellegrino E D 1984 Autonomy and coercion in disease prevention and health promotion. Theoretical Medicine 5:83–91

Rawls J 1971 A theory of justice. Oxford University Press, Oxford

Rayner M, Heughan A, Pearson G, Brunner E 1990 Why don't people living in Hackney take more exercise? Health Education Journal 49(2):64–68

Rowson R 1990 An introduction to ethics for nurses. Scutari Press, Harrow

Rumbold G 1993 Ethics in nursing practice, 2nd edn. Baillière Tindall and Saunders, London

Sade R M 1983 Medical care as a right: a refutation. In:

Gorovitz S, Macklin R, Jameton A L, O'Connor J M, Sherwin A (eds) Moral problems in medicine, 2nd edn. Prentice Hall, Englewood Cliffs, New Jersey

Schrock R A 1980 A question of honesty in nursing practice. Journal of Advanced Nursing 5:135–145

Seedhouse D 1992 Ethics: the heart of health care. John Wiley, Chichester

Seedhouse D 1995 Editorial: breaking the ethics barrier. Health Care Analysis 3:1–4

Thompson I E, Melia K M, Boyd K M 1992 Nursing ethics. Churchill Livingstone, London

Tschudin V 1996 Moral responsibility in nursing. Unpublished conference paper. Thames Valley University, London

United Kingdom Central Council for Nursing, Midwifery and Health Visiting 1992 Code of professional conduct for Midwifery Nurses, Midwives and Health Visitors. UKCC, London

United Nations 1978a The international bill of human rights. United Nations, New York

United Nations 1978b The international bill of human rights, article 25. United Nations, New York

United Nations 1989 Convention on the rights of children. United Nations, New York

Warner M 1991 Best for Britain? Health Service Journal 101(5266):19

World Health Organization 1978 Report on a primary health care conference. WHO, Alma Alta

World Health Organization 1994 A declaration on the promotion of patient rights in Europe. WHO Regional Office for Europe, Geneva

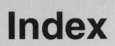

Index

Numbers in **bold** refer to tables